AF803447

The Impact of AIDS

The Impact of AIDS Psychological and Social Aspects of HIV Infection

Edited by

José Catalán
Charing Cross and Westminster Medical School, London, UK

Lorraine Sherr
Royal Free Hospital School of Medicine, London, UK

Barbara Hedge
University of London, UK

Routledge
Taylor & Francis Group
LONDON AND NEW YORK

First Published 1997
by Harwood Academic Publishers.
Reprinted 2004
by Routledge,
2 Park Square, Milton Park, Abingdon, Oxon OX14 4RN
711 Third Avenue, New York, NY 10017, USA

First issued in hardback 2017

Routledge is an imprint of the Taylor & Francis Group, an informa business

Copyright © 1997 OPA (Overseas Publishers Association) Amsterdam B.V.
Published in The Netherlands by Harwood Academic Publishers.

All rights reserved. No part of this book may be reprinted or reproduced or utilised in any form or by any electronic, mechanical, or other means, now known or hereafter invented, including photocopying and recording, or in any information storage or retrieval system, without permission in writing from the publishers.

Notice:
Product or corporate names may be trademarks or registered trademarks, and are used only for identification and explanation without intent to infringe.

British Library Cataloguing in Publication Data

The impact of AIDS: psychological and social aspects of
HIV infection
1. HIV infections - Psychological aspects 2. HIV infections
Social aspects
I. Catalán, José II. Sherr, Lorraine III. Hedge, Barbara
362.1'969792

ISBN 13: 978-1-138-41716-8 (hbk)
ISBN 13: 978-90-5702-041-4 (pbk)

Contents

Preface

The psychological and social implications of HIV infection became apparent from the start of the epidemic. Not only was HIV a condition with an unpredictable course, which often had fatal consequences and was therefore likely to lead to psychological distress and social disruption – in addition, the fact that in developed countries HIV infection affected individuals already stigmatised and in developing countries typically reached people facing adverse economic and social conditions, meant that this new syndrome was likely to have a substantial psychological and social impact beyond its purely medical and biological implications. Furthermore, the absence of effective treatments to treat the infection or prevent its transmission has meant that psychological and social interventions have provided the main method for prevention of the spread of HIV by focusing on behavioural change.

The psychological response to the HIV epidemic has evolved and grown through a number of phases over the last fifteen years. At first, behavioural change was seen as the main focus of action and much effort was spent on public education and in the dissemination of information. A very strong strand at the outset of the epidemic was the concern about the rights of individuals with HIV infection, and a good deal of effort was put into fighting discrimination and stigmatisation. Next came the realisation that behaviour change and its consequences were a much more complex process than anticipated, and this occurred in parallel with increased interest in counselling and support, both in relation to HIV testing and to the provision of support for individuals and families affected by HIV. New areas of interest have developed more recently –

first, concerns about the neuropsychological consequences of HIV infection, and second the issue of access to treatment, and in particular the involvement of people with HIV infection in the setting up of the agenda for treatment trials and access to sources of care. Finally, as the global nature of the epidemic has become clear and the epidemiological patterns of infection have begun to change, the role of socio-economic factors has become more prominent. While the emphasis of each one of these areas of concern has changed over the years, the relevance of each has not been in doubt.

From the start of the epidemic efforts have been made to bring together the medical, psychological and social dimensions of HIV, in some ways providing a model for other medical disorders and for psychosocial interventions. International AIDS conferences soon became a forum for integration of effort and communication between groups working in developed and developing countries. An example of such international co-operation has been provided by the experience of the International AIDS' Impact Conferences, which have focused on the interaction between psychological, social and biological factors in HIV infection.

This volume highlights major themes by including papers based on the AIDS' Impact Conferences, the first of which was held in Amsterdam in 1991, the second in Brighton, UK, 1994, and the third of which is scheduled for Melbourne in 1997.

The contents of this volume are structured in four thematic sections which emerged from the Brighton Conference: Prevention, Drugs, Gender Issues and Care and Treatment. Each section contains a selection of papers which illustrate the complexity of the subject and which review a particular topic or highlight a specific form of intervention which has important theoretical and practical implications.

The Prevention section is introduced by Manderson and colleagues who present a thorough review of research into the use of condoms in heterosexual sex, examining the methodological problems involved in the field, and then detailing the factors that contribute to or hinder condom use. Wanigaratne and co-workers complement Manderson's chapter with a practical review of group interventions to help gay men initiate and maintain safer sexual behaviour, illustrating the difficulties involved in carrying out and evaluating this kind of preventive work. Svenson, Johnsson and Hanson in Chapter 3 describe the process of developing peer education within a university campus to reduce the risk of transmission of HIV, while Gadd and Goss illustrate the process of HIV education in the workplace and the difficulties encountered in the work setting. The role of the media in providing information (or misinformation in many cases) and in shaping attitudes to HIV infection in those affected by it is examined by Cunningham and co-workers in the final chapter of the Prevention section through the discussion of ten years of AIDS images in the Puerto Rican press.

In the second section on Drugs three chapters focus on the way the HIV epidemic has spread amongst drug injectors. Stimson provides compelling and disturbing evidence about the spread of HIV infection in South-East Asia and highlights the social, economic and political factors involved. Friedman and colleagues working in New York provide detailed ethnographic observations concerning the factors and processes that contribute to risk behaviours and risk of HIV infection in drug injectors, as well as the identification of interventions likely to make a contribution to the prevention of spread in this group of individuals. Finally, Klee discusses the lifestyle of women who inject amphetamines and their risk behaviours in the rather different setting of northwest England.

The next section is devoted more specifically to Gender issues. Hankins focuses her discussion on the psychosocial and economic impact of HIV infection on women living in developing countries who may already be facing higher levels of adversity than their partners or than women in developed countries. The impact on caregivers in developed countries is reviewed by Reidy, and the consequences for children born to mothers with HIV infection by Goldie and co-workers, who carried out an empirical study involving twenty five parents and thirty six children who lived with one or both parents. Bailey gives a biological perspective of the risk of HIV infection in young women. Finally, Meadows and co-workers discuss the setting of an HIV counselling and testing service in an antenatal clinic in London, illustrating some of the difficulties and opportunities such a service can face.

The final section of the book presents current thinking on the Care and Treatment aspects of HIV disease. King, in a seminal paper, highlights the need to ensure that scientific progress and research developments in HIV can be accessed meaningfully by those who require them. Stein and co-workers working in Soweto give a detailed illustration of the work of nurse-counsellors in an urban area in South Africa, highlighting the need for training and continuing supervision. Lea illustrates the work of community nurses with families in two very different settings, Edinburgh in Scotland, and a rural community in British Columbia. Everall contributes an up-to-date review of the effects of HIV infection in the brain, reviewing both clinical syndromes such as HIV-associated dementia and the neuropathological consequences of the infection. Some of the psychiatric consequences of AIDS are examined in the next two papers. Beckett reviews some of the ethical dilemmas that can face not only psychiatrists but also other mental health professionals working in the field of HIV, particularly in relation to euthanasia and physician-assisted suicide. Finally, Ayuso-Mateos and co-workers provide empirical information on the prevalence of HIV infection among acute psychiatric admissions to a psychiatric unit in Madrid, highlighting the implications for the mental health services.

Although each chapter provides a self-contained perspective on a particular topic, it is important to consider what is their combined message. As became apparent in the closing talks in Brighton, 'the whole was more than the sum of the parts'. The complexities of prevention and care cannot be disentangled from the reality of social, political, economic and gender issues. It is necessary periodically to review the multi-faceted aspects of the impact of AIDS. We, the

Editors, hope that this sample of papers will afford the reader the opportunity to consider a number of bio-psycho-social issues posed by HIV and will contribute to the understanding of its impact on individuals and societies throughout the world.

José Catalán
Lorraine Sherr
Barbara Hedge

About the Editors

José Catalán, Reader in Psychiatry and honorary Consultant Psychiatrist at the Charing Cross & Westminster Medical School, University of London and Riverside Mental Health Trust has been involved in research into the mental health aspects of HIV infection for over ten years. He is also in charge of the psychiatric services for people with HIV infection at the Chelsea & Westminster Hospital which is the largest centre in the UK for the care of people with HIV infection.

Lorraine Sherr, Senior lecturer, Clinical Psychologist at the Royal Free Hospital School of Medicine. An editor of the international journal *AIDS Care and Psychology Health and Medicine,* she has travelled to Africa, Canada and the USA as a Churchill Fellow to conduct research into AIDS and HIV and participates in numerous national and international research and clinical initiatives.

Barbara Hedge, Consultant Clinical Psychologist at St Bartholomew's Hospital and honorary senior lecturer in psychology at St Bartholomew's and the Royal London School of Medicine and Dentistry, is responsible for the clinical psychology services for people with HIV disease at St Bartholomew's and the Royal London Hospitals. For the last ten years she has studied the psychosocial factors affecting the quality of life of individuals infected with HIV and their partners and has been involved in the running of workshops and counselling courses in Africa and Eastern Europe.

About the Editors

Notes on Contributors

Cliff Allwood is principal psychiatrist at Tara Hospital and acting head of the Department of Psychiatry at the University of the Witwatersrand, South Africa.

Jose L. Ayuso-Mateos, professor of Psychiatry, Clinical and Social Psychiatry Research Unit, Hospital Universitario Marqués de Valdecilla, Cantabria University, Spain.

Mike Bailey has worked as a consultant in the UK and in Africa and Asia for ODA, EC, UNDP, UNICEF, WHO and non-governmental organisations such as Save the Children and OXFAM. He is an honorary lecturer in the Centre for International Child Health at the Institute of Child Health, London, UK.

Alexandra Beckett is a graduate of the University of Michigan Medical School. She completed her residency training and a research fellowship in Psychiatry at Massachusetts General Hospital. She is an assistant professor of Psychiatry at Harvard Medical School. Since 1991, she has served as director of the HIV Psychiatry Service at Beth Israel Hospital in Boston, Massachusetts. She is also the principal investigator of a study on 'The Epidemiology of Suicidal Ideation in AIDS' funded by the American Suicide Foundation.

Andrew Billington is health adviser at Camden & Islington Community Health Service NHS Trust, London, UK.

Pierre Brouard is a senior HIV/AIDS counsellor and counselling trainer at the AIDS Training and Information Centre, South Africa.

Tracey Chester is the HIV specialist counsellor for the Chelsea & Westminster Health Care Trust Maternity Unit, UK.

Ernest L. Cunningham is professor of Medicine in the School of Medicine at the University of Puerto Rico.

Ineke Cunningham is professor of Sociology and director of the HIV/AIDS Research & Education Center at the University of Puerto Rico, Río Piedras campus.

Richard Curtis has over 10 years of experience in studying the ethnography of drug use. His research has included work on HIV epidemiology and HIV prevention as well as on social networks among drug injectors.

Dale J. DeMatteo has been involved in research for ten years at the Hospital for Sick Children in Toronto, Canada.

Ian P. Everall is MRC clinician scientist fellow and senior lecturer in Psychiatry at the Institute of Psychiatry, De Crespigny Park, London, UK.

Samuel R. Friedman is a senior research fellow at NDRI (National Development and Research Institutes Inc.), New York City, USA.

Karen Gadd is a lecturer in Health Studies at the University of Central Lancashire, UK.

Juan J. Picazo de la Garza, Chairman, Department of Microbiology, Hospital Universitario San Carlos, Madrid, Spain.

Robyn L. Salter Goldie works with families in the HIV program at the Hospital for Sick Children, Toronto, Canada and is currently principal investigator on a national study of Canadian families living with HIV based on these pilot study results.

Marjorie F. Goldstein is a principal investigator at NDRI, and is an epidemiologist and health educator. She received her MPH from Johns Hopkins University and her PhD from Columbia University. Her research interests include the behavioural aspects of HIV prevention, the role of social networks in risk behaviour, and the processes of obtaining drug treatment and HIV-related services.

David Goss is professor of Organisational Behaviour at the University of Portsmouth Business School, UK.

Catherine Hankins is a community medicine specialist in the Infectious Diseases Unit of the Montreal Regional Public Health Department, Canada and an associate professor in the Department of Epidemiology and Biostatistics of McGill University.

Bertil S. Hanson is head of the division of Social Medicine and Community Health Programmes at the Department of Community Medicine, Lund University, Sweden.

Don C. Des Jarlais is the director of research of the Chemical Dependency Institute at Beth Israel Medical Center, professor of Epidemiology and Social Medicine at Albert Einstein College of Medicine, and a senior research fellow at the NDRI. As a leader in the fields of AIDS research and intravenous drug use, his bibliography includes over 200 publications, and he has made 1000 presentations on AIDS and AIDS-related topics that include plenary addresses at the third and fourth International Conferences on AIDS. He has served on numerous advisory committees for the CDC, NIDA, the National Commission on AIDS, and the National Academy of Sciences. He is Vice Chair of the Committee of AIDS Research and the Behavioral, Social, and Statistical Sciences that was established by the National Research Council of the National Academy of Sciences.

Kent Johnsson has been the health promotion nurse at Lund University's Student Health Programmes at the Department of Community Medicine, Lund University, Sweden.

Benny Jose is a project director at the Institute for AIDS Research, National Development and Research Institutes Inc., New York City, USA.

Alan Karstaedt is head of the HIV/AIDS Clinic and the Infectious Diseases Unit at Baragwanath Hospital, South Africa.

Edward King is director of the gay men's HIV prevention organisations; Gay Men Fighting AIDS and Rubberstuffers.

Susan M. King is Paediatric Infectious Diseases consultant and assistant director of the HIV program at the Hospital for Sick Children in Toronto, Canada.

Hilary Klee is professor of Research Psychology at the Manchester Metropolitan University, UK and director of the Centre for Social Research on Health and Substance Abuse (SRHSA).

Carl A. Latkin is a social psychologist on the faculty of Johns Hopkins University School of Public Health. His primary interests include the social context of disease transmission and HIV/STD prevention using social network and social influence models.

Amandah Lea is currently a doctoral nursing student at the University of British Columbia in Vancouver, Canada. For more than a decade, she was a community health nurse for First Nation villages located in rural British Columbia.

Paul Lewis has been a midwife for over 14 years and is currently academic head of Midwifery and Women's Health at Bournemouth University, UK.

Lenore Manderson is professor of Tropical Health (Anthropology) at the Australian Centre for International & Tropical Health, University of Queensland, Australia.

Ismael Lastra Martínez, research fellow in the Clinical and Social Psychiatry Research Unit, Hospital Universitario Marqués de Valdecilla, Spain.

Jean Meadows is a research psychologist in the Psychological Medicine Unit of the Chelsea & Westminster Hospital, UK.

Alan Neaigus is principal investigator at National Development and Research Institutes Inc., in New York City, USA and co-investigator on the Social Factors and HIV Risk project and the HIV among Youth project.

Francisco Montañes Rada, resident, Department of Psychiatry, Hospital Universitario San Carlos, Madrid, Spain.

Kiruba Rajanayagam was assistant director of the Red Cross Blood Transfusion Services of Papua New Guinea, and in Australia was briefly attached to the Tropical Health Program, University of Queensland as a research assistant. She is currently a full-time general practitioner.

Mary Reidy is full professor at the Faculty of Nursing, University of Montreal, Canada. She is also scientific director of a nursing research team (AIDS: care and caregivers, funded by FRSQ). She has received considerable funding, and has extensively published and presented conferences regarding the psychosocial and the family/natural caregiving aspects of those living with AIDS.

Lynnette Rivera-Rodríguez and **Sigfrido Steidel-Figueroa** are law students and research assistants in the HIV/AIDS Research and Education Center at the University of Puerto Rico, Río Piedras campus.

Jo L. Sotheran is a senior project director at NDRI, where she currently directs a multi-method study of injection practices in a New York neighbourhood. Her research interests in relation to networks centre on injection groups and on domestic groups among injecting drug users.

Joanne Stein is a senior researcher in the National AIDS Research Programme of the Medical Research Council, South Africa.

Malcolm Steinberg is leader of the National AIDS Research Programme of the Medical Research Council, South Africa.

Gerry V. Stimson is professor of the Sociology of Health Behaviour and director of the Centre for Research on Drugs and Health Behaviour, Charing Cross & Westminster Medical School, London, UK.

Gary Svenson has worked full-time since 1989 with the biopsychological aspects of HIV infection at the Department of Infectious Diseases, University Hospital of Lund, Sweden.

Lee Chang Tye is a consultant specialising in the field of Health Promotion Evaluation, currently evaluating a workplace health promotion model at Griffith University, Australia.

Shamil Wanigaratne is consultant clinical psychologist & head of Clinical Psychology at Camden & Islington Substance Misuse Service, National Temperance Hospital, London, UK.

John Wenston was principal research associate at NDRI. Other HIV-related research he has carried out centres on utilization of HIV treatment, and on the effects of syringe exchange on risk reduction.

Malcolm Williams is principal social worker St Christopher's Hospice London, UK, working with change, loss and bereavement.

1

Condom Use in Heterosexual Sex: A Review of Research, 1985-1994.

LENORE MANDERSON, LEE CHANG TYE AND KIRUBA RAJANAYAGAM

INTRODUCTION

The condom has been and will remain the major technology to limit sexual transmission of HIV in the foreseeable future, and thus issues related to its acceptance and use are a priority. Since the isolation of HIV, the establishment of its primary modes of transmission, and the development of HIV/AIDS prevention programs, hundreds of studies have been undertaken on the male condom. These include cross-sectional KABP (knowledge, attitudes, behaviour and practices) studies of condom and/or other HIV prevention strategies, condom interventions and evaluations, and recently, ethnographic studies that document the social, cultural and interpersonal contexts of safer sex and condom use. This paper surveys articles published in biomedical and social science journals from 1985 to early 1994.[1] In reviewing this literature, we examine critically the research assumptions and construction of categories used, and draw attention to inconsistencies in findings and inferences.

[1] Since the review concentrates on publications in scientific journals, the review is necessarily partial. Over the period 1989-1993 alone, a restricted search of MEDLINE (condoms + HIV + heterosexual sex) identified 558 articles; SOCIOFILE lists a total of 204 articles to 4/1994; and PsycLIT includes 372 papers for the period January 1987 - March 1994. There is some overlap in citations, but even so the relevant literature is extensive and space is a major limitation of a comprehensive survey. We excluded much of the material informally published and distributed, and books and chapters in books are also largely excluded. Further, the literature relating to AIDS is generated at an exceptional pace compared with other areas of public health and medicine, and hence any review is inevitably out-of-date by the time of its completion.

Factors associated with the use of condoms do not apply universally across cultures or populations. A variety of issues influence acceptability, frequency and consistency of use among the study populations defined as 'at risk', although the conceptualisation and operational definitions of risk and the definition of the populations are themselves often problematic. Reasons for non-use of condoms by heterosexual youths, for example, are different from those of homosexual/bisexual adult men. Similarly, reasons for non-use across cultural and national boundaries (for instance, between Americans and Zaireans) are marked, although there is some interesting concordance too. Variations in sexual situations and contexts have a strong influence over condom use. Here, we largely limit our discussion to the male condom, heterosexual sex, and industrialised countries, although for comparative purposes we allude to other condom research. The studies on which we base this review reflect research predominantly conducted in the United States and Europe. There is far less published which addresses issues of HIV prevention in developing countries; this bias is not surprising given the concentration of researchers in the United States and the relatively early response by funding agencies to support research and behavioural interventions.[2] The papers which we describe below, their subject matter, methodological approaches, conceptual frameworks and research questions suggest that they are reasonably typical of the literature, although some of the work being conducted within the humanities (e.g. in anthropology and cultural studies) has a very different focus (e.g. Clatts & Mutchler, 1989; Bolton & Singer, 1992; Herdt & Lindenbaum, 1992).

POPULATION SELECTION

For research purposes, studies on condom use for AIDS prevention have defined target populations in line with epidemiological classifications of 'at risk' populations (Murray & Payne, 1989). These are not coincident with the target populations for contraceptive condom use, with the exception of young people, and there has been little reflection back on that earlier literature in terms of its possible lessons for HIV prevention. Although the selection of research populations of condom studies largely reflects the current burden of infection, the volume of research is not proportionate: within the US, for example, while men who have sex with men, commercial sex workers and recreational injecting drug users are disproportionately affected by the disease, 'heterosexuals' and 'youth' are the most common target populations for research, accounting for around half of all published studies. Blacks, Hispanics and other ethnic minorities have been the subject of relatively little research (around 10% of all studies) despite their disproportionate share of infection (Lesnick & Pace, 1990: 173).

[2] For a discussion of Australian government responses to the epidemic and to research funding, see Manderson (1994). The preponderance of publications from USA-based researchers reflects the research culture of different places, with relatively more or less emphasis on publishing, as well as the easier task of researchers with facility in English to successfully submit their work for publication.

Recruitment procedures vary considerably among the studies. Research conducted with 'at risk' populations often draws participants from groups that have been labelled and stigmatised, e.g. as prostitutes, homosexuals, alcoholics, or drug users (or 'abusers'), who are usually recruited in urban areas where the behaviour by which they are identified is presumed prevalent. Hence drug users tend to be recruited through clinics or street locations (e.g. Watters *et al.*, 1990), adolescents/youth through schools (Mathews *et al.*, 1990) or probation or remand homes (Wilson *et al.*, 1990), and commercial sex workers from 'red light districts' and similar geographic concentrations. The identification of locales and the recruitment of participants is frequently undertaken through relevant social networks such as community service agencies (health/medical clinics), social organisations, local media, and so on (Valdiserri *et al.*, 1989; Fullilove *et al.*, 1990) and volunteers are consequently individuals who have self-identified with the population group or its defining characteristics. By maintaining this focus, the literature tends to represent these groups as homogenous. The contradictions in research findings suggests that this is a fallacy, and that there are as many differences - across class, race, ethnicity, gender, age, and sexual orientation, for example - as there are commonalities.

Population selection, appropriateness of the research tool, and the context of data collection limit and at times bias findings. Many of the study populations have been recruited through opportunistic or convenience sampling, limiting generalisability. For example, a KABP study among Black and Hispanic students in the Bronx was conducted because of lack of information of perceptions and risk factors of transmission of this population, which has a high prevalence of HIV. The study population, however, was entirely opportunistic: students attending English language classes in one college, the majority with 'limited' proficiency in English, completed a self-administered questionnaire as a compulsory classroom assignment (Lesnick & Pace, 1990). Other examples of limitations on population selection (and method) might include the work of de Graaf *et al.* (1992), who recruited clients of prostitutes through newspapers and used 'snowballing' to recruit prostitutes direct from workplaces and through intermediaries and referrals - here the problem is not in terms of population recruitment per se, but in terms of its limitations when the research aim was to generate quantifiable data. Contrast this, for example, with the study of Fox *et al.* (1993), designed to test the effectiveness of an intervention (through discussion groups and the distribution of condoms) among commercial sex workers, where the use of opportunistic sampling was clearly appropriate.

Sample size in the studies surveyed varied enormously. It includes as few as two (where the notion of 'sample' is not appropriate) (Kane, 1990) to over 8000 (e.g. Campbell & Baldwin, 1991; Catania, Coates, Stall *et al.*, 1992). While sample size is not entirely predictive of method, generally studies with smaller samples used qualitative methods whilst larger studies used cross-sectional surveys with a simple, standardised instrument. Although generalizability and representativeness is a problem even with some of the very large studies, the low number of respondents in some of the 'qualitative' studies is a particular concern, since these are rarely based in ethnography and 'qualitative' often simply means the use of an open-ended semi-structured interview rather than a structured one, with few other differences in study methods or design.[3] Abramson's comments on the quality of sex research have some resonance here, at least in terms of methodological rigour (Abramson, 1990, 1992), although one might also question the gate-keeping functions of journal reviewers who allow such work to press.

As anticipated above with reference to the employment of epidemiologic categories, population definition tends to be problematic. Many studies fail to define it adequately, and variation within the literature makes comparison and the cumulative goals of research difficult (see also de Zalduondo, 1991: 228). Prior criticism of population definition and inclusion has focused on prostitution (de Zalduondo, 1991), and in this area most caution has been exercised to differentiate between commercial sex workers and others who trade sex, since these factors may influence condom use. Two papers illustrate this point: one from The Netherlands distinguishes brothel, window, street, home and escort prostitution and then searches for difference in condom use among women working in each of these industry sectors (de Graaf *et al.*, 1992); the other, describing female sex workers in Zaire, distinguishes between home-based, hotel-based and street-based prostitution and defines women as 'prostitutes' on the basis of self-reports of multiple sexual partners in exchange for money or goods (Nzila *et al.*, 1991). Other papers from both the social and medical sciences emphasise the heterogeneity of this population due to social class, geographic location and site of prostitution, frequency of partners, price of transaction, the permanent, transitory or opportunistic nature of commercial sex, and women's full-time, part-time or casual commitment to commercial sex work (e.g. Cortes *et al.*, 1989; d'Costa *et al.*, 1985; Kreiss *et al.*, 1986; Lyttleton, 1994; Schoepf, 1992; Simonsen *et al.*, 1990). This has not broken the general distinction between 'prostitutes' and 'wives', however, as if there were no overlap (although see Carovano, 1991; Osmond *et al.*, 1993).[4]

The use of other categories to define 'target populations' and 'risk groups' presents similar problems. This is particularly pertinent to the classification of sexuality (homosexual, heterosexual, bisexual) where distinctions between self-identity, community membership and affiliation, and sexual practice may be quite different (e.g. Dowsett *et al.*, 1992; Kippax *et al.*, 1994).[5] Shifts in operational definitions occur also in the quantification of multiple partnering, assumed to be

[3] These small studies are not unique to the medical literature. One study, published in a humanities journal, draws on two, one-hour 'focus groups', respectively involving four black women and three white women recruited 'informally' (directly or through friends); on this basis the author concludes that 'unequal relations of gender make it particularly difficult for women to initiate or negotiate safer sex practices, because of the negative consequences they incur from men when they do so' (Miles, 1993: 497).

[4] The HIV epidemic in Thailand, for example, is represented chronologically as an infection which moved progressively from foreign homosexual men, to local 'homosexuals', to IDUs, to 'prostitutes', to the general (male) population, to 'housewives', to unborn children, without greater reflexivity on the construction of heterosexual men as 'general', for example, or on the apparent discrete categories of (a non-reproductive) 'prostitute' and (reproductive) 'housewife' (cf. Lyttleton, 1994).

[5] The distinctions between self-identity, community affiliation and sexual desire, orientation and practice however was well made some time ago (e.g. Warren, 1974).

high risk for infection with HIV insofar as the greater the number of partners, the greater the possibility that one partner will be infected and the virus transmitted. Whilst Uitenbroek and McQueen (1992:588) concede that 'there is no generally agreed definition for level of sexual activity', they somewhat conservatively define a 'multi-partner' respondent as anyone who reported that they or their partner had had another partner in the past year, or who had had more than three partners in the past five years.[6] Yet we might expect major differences in background, personality and personal attributes, as well as risk of infection, between those at the narrow end of this scale and those who have had 100 or more partners in a twelve month period.

Youth is another indeterminate category. The inclusion of young people ('teenagers', 'adolescents', 'youth') is in part informed by mean age at infection, as estimated back from age at diagnosis, as well as on the risk of infection for early adolescent women due to physiological vulnerability.[7] But in addition, the focus on youth appears to be justified on the basis of their presumed vulnerability as a result of sexual naivety and/or inexperience influencing sexual negotiation, coincident with the desire for experimentation, numbers of partners and frequency of partner changes, and low perception of risk of infection (Norris & Ford, 1991; Diclemente, 1991; Rotheram-Borus *et al.*, 1991; Tyden *et al.*, 1991b). Both the population category and the association of youth and 'risk' are problematic however. Age boundaries vary. For example, Quirk *et al.* (1993) define women aged 14-25 as 'adolescent and young adult women', an age range arguably too wide to be useful in reflecting similarities of sexual experience and/or exposure to infection, or to capture the variety among individuals depending upon life circumstance (class, education, employment, sexual history, marital status, maternity history, and so on). Much of the work on young people also, as noted, is based on the supposition that their behaviour is intrinsically 'risky', and that therefore they are least likely to use condoms. This characterisation is neither accurate nor well-defined (Warwick *et al.*, 1988; Frankenberg, 1992: 83-86; Kane & Mason, 1992; Brough, 1995).

METHODOLOGIES

Most condom-use studies are quantitative and use standardised structured or semi-structured questionnaires to generate quantifiable data. Instruments may be self-administered, administered by an interviewer face-to-face or by telephone, conducted as a mail survey or through computer-assisted technology. The advantages of quantitative methods, although arguably supported as a consequence

[6] Walter et al. (1992) for example, contrast those who had had 2-4 versus those who had had one or no sexual partners over the past year, although these low numbers are partially explicable by the study in a school attending population. Norris and Ford (1991) differentiate 'lifetime sexual partners' (0, 1, 2-3, 4-6, and 7+) by 'well-known' and 'casual partners'; Campbell and Baldwin (1991) also differentiate by specifying lifetime number of partners (to 25+) and number of partners in the past three months.

[7] We are grateful to Heino Meyer-Bahlburg (pers.comm.) for this point. In addition, the large number of college-student studies may reflect student research projects; this would explain the over-representation of this population as subjects of HIV/AIDS research.

of the use of particular scientific paradigms (Manderson, 1994), should be to generate data of high external validity and generalisability. This is not the case in many of these studies that use non-random sampling procedures, although many are at least able to suggest who may be at risk, to estimate prevalences of safe/unsafe sexual behaviour among various at-risk populations, and to identify certain social and behavioural factors associated with non-use of condoms. This is not, of itself, a problem: there is value in defining the areas where transmission is most likely to occur, where interventions are problematic, and where condom use is variable. The major limitation of this work, in the end - particularly for the earliest KABP research - relates to the use of standardised protocols and the limitations of these to explore the complexity of individual attitudes, belief systems, and behaviour.[8]

The increasing number of ethnographic studies and other careful qualitative research has been most useful in identifying the cultural, social, economic and personal contexts of sex and condom use, and in explaining motivations and practice. Most studies represented as 'qualitative', however, have used focus groups, face-to-face or telephone interviews. Only a few have used participant observation techniques or included ethnographic (anthropological) research, these most often in developing countries (e.g. Farmer, 1990, 1992, 1994; Ingstad, 1990; Lyttleton, 1994; Parker, 1987, 1989a, 1989b; Schoepf, 1992, 1993; Seeley *et al.*, 1992, 1994; de Zalzuondo, 1991); this may be due to the relative recency of research on HIV in Africa coincident with the increasing interest in the potential of qualitative research methods in applied health research (Manderson & Aaby, 1992). However, the trend also reflects professional and geographic domains.

The evaluation of interventions has led to some change in method, since evaluation research aims to demonstrate effect on behaviour, rather than simply describing knowledge/attitude. In general, the few published evaluation studies draw on a wider variety of methods to allow for triangulation and validation. Worth's study of women's attitudes to condoms (1989), for example, derives from participant observation in two interventions with women who inject drugs, and this is supplemented by self-administered questionnaires, focus group discussions, and interviews. Similarly, an evaluation of an intervention in Honduras used self-reports of condom use supplemented by before-and-after KAP surveys, and diaries of sexual encounters and condom use kept during the 10 week intervention period (Fox *et al.*, 1993).

DOES FEAR OF INFECTION CHANGE BEHAVIOUR?

Early mass education directed towards reducing transmission of HIV used fear-oriented material. This approach was criticised as resulting in stigmatisation of people already infected with HIV while achieving little by way of behavioural change. While Rhodes and Wolitski (1990), based on a study of response to experimental posters, argue that fear-oriented campaigns are effective in promoting

[8] See also Fife-Schaw & Breakwell (1992) for their criticisms of methods used in UK studies of young people.

the adoption of preventive behaviours, others (e.g. Struckman *et al.*, 1990) have maintained that high fear compaigns do not affect behaviour more than other educational campaigns. Further, while condom use tends to increase following targeted health education campaigns (at least in some places and with some partners, e.g. Uitenbroek & McQueen, 1992; Wielandt, 1993), knowledge of the sexual transmission of HIV alone appears to have little influence on condom use (Ishii & Whitbeck, 1990).

The correlation appears to relate to general knowledge, perception of risk, and condom use (Carroll, 1991; Cromer & Brown, 1992; Diclemente, 1991; Jemmott, Jemmott, Spears *et al.* 1992; Martin *et al.*, 1990; Moatti *et al.*, 1991), although factors such as changes in perception of risk and boredom/disregard of health information or subject matter may reverse trends that favour prevention (Herlitz, 1992). Fear and anxiety of HIV, knowledge of and attitudes towards risk of infection, knowledge of people with HIV, and advocacy of behavioural change have affected behaviour, although with variation within and among populations (Moore & Barling, 1991; Witte, 1991; Hobart, 1992; McQueen & Uitenbroek, 1992, cf. Brown *et al.*, 1992; Zimet *et al.*, 1992). Moatti *et al.*(1991), for example, suggest among French heterosexuals with multiple partners a correlation between condom use and voluntary testing for HIV, average or greater fear of STDs, and knowledge of HIV status in personal relations, implying also that people assess 'risk' on the basis of their own experiences and behaviour. Hobart's study (1992) of young Canadians, however, illustrates that this is not always so: those acquainted with others who were seropositive, and thus presumed to be more aware of transmission and infection, were paradoxically those who rated sex with briefly known partners as least risky, and were least inclined to use condoms with passing acquaintances.

PARTNERSHIP PATTERNS AND CONDOM USE

Condom use varies as a result of partnership communication, negotiation skills, and inequalities and power that exist in relationships. The literature indicates that partner reluctance affects use, regardless of intent to use (Weinstock *et al.*, 1993), and that condoms are widely disliked because both men and women believe they interfere with the 'spontaneity' and pleasure of sexual relations (Chapman & Hodgson, 1988; Jemmott & Jemmott, 1991; Johnson, Gant *et al.*, 1992; Kenen & Armstrong, 1992; Sonnex *et al.*, 1989; Strader & Beaman, 1991; Weinstock *et al.*, 1993). Women seem more willing to use condoms than their partners and are more likely to use condoms always (Kenen & Armstrong, 1992; Sonnex *et al.*, 1989), and increased self-efficacy and positive experiences in using condoms in terms of sexual enjoyment, partners' support for condom use, and parents', peer and partner's attitudes to condoms, all relate to increased condom use intentions (Jemmott & Jemmott, 1991, 1992; Strader & Beaman, 1991). However, fewer women than men may have ever used condoms and women will not insist where there are other personal reasons which affect communication and/or behaviour, underlining the importance of interpersonal communication and negotiation skills to increase and sustain condom use. Sexual communication skills emerge as a key influence on condom use across all social strata (Catania, Coates, Stall *et al.*, 1992). These findings suggest the significance of relationships of power between partners (Worth, 1989). Condom use is most likely to occur in couples in relatively egalitarian relationships, hence the emphasis of various interventions to strengthen negotiation skills of women (also Miles, 1993).

Even so, interpersonal issues inhibit condom use in primary relationships regardless of use outside of these relationships. Sonnex *et al.* (1989) reported among young people presenting to genitourinary medicine clinics less use of condoms among non-regular partners than with regular partners (cf. Evans *et al.*, 1991). Other studies suggest condom use is most likely with new sexual partners (Abraham *et al.*, 1992), especially among young people, and condoms were considered to be more appropriate in extramarital than marital relationships, with use declining as the couple established stronger affectional ties (Moore & Barling, 1991), regardless of other HIV-related risk factors (Serraino & Franceschi, 1992). Commercial sex workers (like other women) are disinclined to use condoms with primary partners, feel at risk from clients rather than from husbands or boy friends, and use condoms more frequently with clients rather than with steady partners (Dorfman *et al.*, 1992; Hooykaas *et al.*, 1989; van den Hoek *et al.*, 1990).

The use of condoms with new partners, multiple and casual partners, and in commercial transactions points to the extent to which people assess the risk of infection on a series of subjective criteria, including partner history of 'high-risk' activities and other such criteria (appearance, general health, and so on). Such 'screening' activities range from interviewing the potential partner about past sexual history (Wiktor *et al.*, 1990; McKusick *et al.*, 1991; Basen-Enquist, 1992; Mays & Cochran 1993) to making judgements on the basis of appearance, 'cleanness' or 'niceness' (e.g. Chapman & Hodgson, 1988; Brough, 1995). In the process of deciding to use or not use a condom, there appears to be considerable stereotyping of who might be an 'AIDS carrier' (Maticka-Tyndale, 1991; Ku *et al.*, 1992; Bortolotti *et al.*, 1992; Wiktor *et al.*, 1990).

In short-term and casual relationships, communication appears to be less problematic and condom use less invested in symbolic value. Several studies point to higher condom use with casual and/or short-term partners, although not with multiple partners per se, and the absolute numbers involved, changing patterns of use, and frequency of use are variable (Calsyn *et al.*, 1992; Hart *et al.*, 1989; van Haastrecht & van den Hoek, 1991). The pattern is not true for all populations, however, and condom use with casual or multiple partners is not necessarily consistent nor regular (e.g. Hobart, 1992; Valdiserri *et al.*, 1989). For example, a study conducted by James *et al.* (1991) among heterosexuals with multiple sexual partners indicated that 79% did not perceive themselves as at risk of HIV infection and 64% only reported infrequent condom use with casual sexual partners; Catania *et al.*'s work (Catania, Coates, Stall *et al.*, 1992; Catania, Coates, Kegeles *et al.*, 1992) also indicates low condom use in heterosexual sex even with 'risky' sexual partners.

A range of social, cultural and psychological factors appear to complicate communication and condom acceptability, although the subtle interplay of these remains to be explored. For example, women of seropositive partners (Mayes *et al.*, 1992) were inconsistent in use of condoms where they found condoms to be an unpleasant and unwanted reminder of infection, felt obligated to maintain normality in terms of sexual relations, felt false reassurance as a result of their own negative results, or in other ways felt inhibited in communicating or fearful that their partner would feel rejected, and believed that established patterns of sexual behaviour would be difficult to change. These factors all overrode their understandings of the risks involved (Mayes *et al.*, 1992).

Other factors appear to influence if not determine condom use. Uitenbroek and McQueen's work in Scotland (1992) suggests higher condom use correlates with higher education; Potter and Anderson's survey data (1993: 204), however, indicates that women with more than high school education, as well as lower levels of education, were less likely to use condoms than women with high school education. Health education interventions also affect condom use in various ways: in Scotland, increasing use among less educated women, but decreasing condom use among less educated men (Uitenbroek and McQueen, 1992); in the US, among young people, increasing condom use and decreasing number of partners (Ku *et al.*, 1992).

Cultural differences in male/female relationships are inferred in studies that suggest ethnic differences in condom use. According to Weinstock *et al.* (1993), Black and Hispanic women were more likely than whites to report difficulty in getting their partners to use condoms, and Johnson, Hinkle *et al.* (1992) have reported that black males react aggressively when asked by partners about previous sexual contacts or when a partner refused sex without a condom. Others report contradictory results: Campbell and Baldwin (1991), on the basis of interviews with 7,619 women, found that condom use was greater for black than white women (see also Sonenstein *et al.*, 1989 for similar findings for never-married men). Situational factors are also implicated where drug and alcohol use is alleged negatively to influence condom use some or all of the time (Weinstock *et al.*, 1993), but again, the findings associating drug and alcohol use with low or erratic use of condoms are, in the end, equivocal.

DOES GENDER MAKE A DIFFERENCE?

Much of the research undertaken, particularly with men, has used survey methods and offers little insight into the motivations that affect condom use, other than dislike due to sensation loss and/or impediments to performance. By contrast, more research on interpersonal communication, affective aspects of sexual relationships, attributions of condom use, gender stereotypes and so on, has been conducted with women, and this has extended to soliciting women's views about men's attitudes: women don't think they can influence men to wear condoms because they think men are embarassed, concerned with sexual performance, feel they lack control (of women and/or coitus?), strip sex of 'spontaneity' and are connotative of 'unnatural' or 'undesirable sex' (Worth, 1989).

The foregoing discussion suggests some differences between men and women with respect to primary relationships and negotiating skills.[9] In this section we explore further the impact of gender, which in general emerges as a powerful factor influencing condom use in various cultural settings and contexts (Johnson, Gant *et al.*, 1992; Rickert & Gottlieb, 1992; Schoepf, 1992; Zimet *et al.*, 1992). Discussions on gender are largely concerned with interpersonal and relational dynamics, not with gender differences in perceptions of risk and susceptibility. Zimet *et al.* (1992) suggest that perceptions of susceptibility and anxiety in sexual situations may interact with gender to influence condom decision-making behaviour, and that perceptions of susceptibility alone may not be a strong enough influence to initiate condom usage.

Although men and women are influenced by common factors, including the willingness of their partner, the behaviour of their friends and family, and concern about contracting a sexually transmitted disease (Svenson *et al.*, 1992), men would appear to be more familiar with condoms and their prophylactic role (Leland & Barth, 1992). But in addition, self-efficacy has a strong effect on condom use and frequency (Richard & van der Pligt, 1991; Basen-Engquist & Parcel, 1992; O'Leary *et al.*, 1992; Wulfert & Wan, 1993), and in this respect as well as absence of effective negotiating skills women appear disadvantaged (Ehrhardt *et al.*, 1992). Further, although women appear to be more positive towards the use of condoms than men (Severn, 1990; Sonnex *et al.*, 1989; Kenen & Armstrong, 1992), condoms have negative connotations for both men and women, as already noted. These are not all culture-specific, but for many women they are associated with contraception and for some women, with 'genocide', they contradict various religious attitudes, and are assessed by woman against ideas of their own reproductive ability. Hence Worth's remark (1989) that condom use implies that there are options other than motherhood to define women's self-identity and self-esteem, and that the significance of an individual woman's desire to have a child may influence condom use. Condoms may also symbolise extra-relationship sexual activity, and so may be difficult to maintain or to introduce them into a long-term partnership unless they are used for contraception. Issues associated with both male and female fidelity and trust surface here. In addition condoms may be associated less specifically with 'irresponsibility' and 'cleanliness', and a woman may neither introduce nor continue use of condoms if she fears rejection by the partner, assuming in the first place her ability to discuss the question at all (Osmond *et al.*, 1993; Kane, 1990; Kippax *et al.*, 1990; Mays & Cochran, 1988; Shayne & Kaplan, 1991; Worth, 1989).

Osmond *et al.* (1993) conclude that women's lack of negotiating skills and low condom use in a primary partnership are related to gender stereotypes, gender stereotypes define romantic sex, and romantic sex is gendered and unsafe. They also point out, contrary to stereotypes implicit in research with poor women and commercial sex workers, that US white college women are least likely to use condoms (cf. Kippax *et al.*, 1990). Hence whilst condoms are more affordable for wealthier women, and health education messages concerning modes and risk of

[9] Although it also provides comment on the researchers' identification of questions of gender and on some stereotyping of sex differences in sexuality.

transmission of HIV might be better understood and therefore presumed to result in greater middle class use of condoms, in fact this group is most vulnerable to romancing sexual encounters and least prepared to take control of sexual behaviour. Further, 'women's gender attitudes explain very little of their behaviour with regard to using condoms' (Osmond *et al.*, 1993). It should also be noted that the literature concerned with the metaphoric significance of condom use and its associations deals almost exclusively with heterosexual partnerships, and largely with the women therein.

DOES SEX WORK REPRESENT A RISK?

Although there is some suggestion that men who pay for sex may be less likely to use condoms than other men, particularly when young (Sonenstein *et al.* 1989), the converse is not the case: female commercial sex workers use condoms with paying partners despite pressure for unprotected sex in both industrialised and developing countries (van den Hoek *et al.*, 1990; Swaddiwudhipong *et al.*, 1990; Neequaye *et al.*, 1991; McKeganey & Barnard, 1992; Spina *et al.*, 1992). In one Belgian study (Mak & Plum, 1991), for example, condoms were not used only in 10-20% of professional sex contacts, and the initiative to use condoms was usually taken by the woman. Although this is not universal (cf. van Deele, 1989; Rao *et al.*, 1991), the general consistency among sex workers highlights the problem of target interventions, since in this case the targeted behaviour is more likely among those least likely to be 'captured'.[10] Among female sex workers, condom use in commercial sex is influenced both by appreciation of the risk of HIV infection and in response to absence of or the short duration of other sexually transmitted diseases (e.g. Donovan *et al.*, 1991). There is less research on male sex workers, but it is worth noting that Peterson *et al.*'s study (1992) among gay and bisexual African-American men suggests that situational factors may override knowledge of risk factors of infection. Fox *et al.* (1993) also suggest that high-priced sex workers are most likely to insist on condom use, although their explanation of the reasons for this are purely speculative; others question the degree to which price and autonomy are associated (de Zalzuondo, 1991: 231). Fox *et al.* (1993) also suggest that clients who patronise higher-priced sex workers are more likely to use condoms, thus associating at least income and acceptability of condoms. However the predisposing and determining factors remain to be explored and may not be consistent cross-culturally.

Despite arguments that sex workers lack negotiating skills and may yield under client pressure not to use condoms, in general issues of interpersonal communication and subjective assessments (trust, imputed infidelity, closeness, etc.) are far more likely to affect condom use among main partners and this is true for all women. Condom use with private partners appears to be exceptional (Mak & Plum, 1991; Spina *et al.*, 1992; van den Hoek *et al.*, 1990). Sex workers feel at risk of HIV

[10] A similar issue arises with interventions in the gay community, where men who have sex with men and do not identify as gay are often overlooked or are inaccessible to community workers (Kippax et al., 1990, 1994).

infection from clients rather than from husbands or boy friends (Dorfman *et al.*, 1992),[11] and therefore are more likely to use condoms with clients than with main partners (Osmond *et al.*, 1993), and with main partners in relationships of relatively short duration (ibid.; Rotheram-Borus *et al.*, 1991).

In general the sex worker-client relationship emerges as one where women have more rather than fewer negotiating skills, and this fits with Carovano's argument relating condom use to women's dependence on male co-operation (Osmond *et al.*, 1993). The missing piece here is client behaviour, and there is little in the literature that examines heterosexual men's attitudes towards condoms in paid sex. With respect to commercial sex, researching clients has proven difficult since the population is diffuse, the tasks of sampling onerous, and men's privacy represented as sacrosanct. There appears also to be personal reluctance to explore too closely a population that in other ways is no different from the 'general population' of men (de Zalzuondo, 1991; Leonard, 1990).

DO DRUGS AND ALCOHOL CONSTITUTE A SITUATIONAL RISK?

The research on drug and alcohol use with regard to sexual practice, condom use and HIV is predicated on a series of hypotheses: first, that drugs and alcohol impair judgement such that individuals may 'forget' to use condoms or opt to take a risk, whereas if they were not influenced by drugs they would use a condom (Tyden *et al.*, 1991a); second, that drugs and alcohol encourage risk-taking; third, that people who misuse drugs and alcohol are already taking risks, hence are less interested in avoiding HIV infection or less able to perceive risk of infection; and fourth, that the need for money to purchase drugs, or the trade of sex for drugs, may be associated with low condom use. Whilst some of these premises may be questionable - such as the notion of people being 'risk-takers', for example - the research findings are considerably more consistent in this area than others. Condom use is less frequent among injecting and other recreational drug users, even though the proportion of the study population who consistently use condoms varies depending on the drug of choice and the context of its use (Bortolotti *et al.*, 1992; Kramer *et al.*, 1991; Schilling *et al.*, 1991). Amphetamine, benzodiazepine, and heroin injecting drug users, crack cocaine smoking, and heavy alcohol comsumption are all associated with extremely low reported condom use where either partner used drugs or alcohol (Harris *et al.*, 1990; Darke *et al.*, 1992; Edlin *et al.*, 1992; McEwan *et al.*, 1992; Weinstock *et al.*, 1993). There appears to be general agreement too that condom use is compromised where sex is exchanged for drugs (or for shelter, food or money) (Turner *et al.*, 1992; Calsyn *et al.*, 1992).

[11] More recent research among sex workers (e.g. abstracts of papers and posters presented at the IXth International Conference on AIDS, Berlin, 1993) highlights the contradictory nature of research in this area, whilst also pointing to the lack of comparability across cultures/nations. Hence whilst study results are contradictory, the evidence in Thailand is that higher income, higher education and better establishment correlate with lower rather than higher use of condoms (Bhassorn Limanondai et al. [Abstract no. WS-C08-1] and Noppavan Chongvatana [Abstract no WS-D10-5]).

The role of alcohol has been explored independently to that of illicit drugs, with differentiation made on the basis of levels of consumption and age of drinkers. The particular focus has been on alcohol use and HIV risk activities among adolescents and college students. A common finding is that heavier drinkers are more likely to have unsafe sex as defined by casual associations, non-use of condoms, and sex with someone known to have had many partners (McEwan *et al.*, 1992). In addition, men who frequently combine alcohol and sex are less likely than others to use condoms (Bagnall & Plant, 1990), and young age tends to be associated with low condom use. Young injecting drug users are also less likely to use condoms - hence the key variable associated with low condom use would appear to be age rather than substance use.

Other studies emphasise the lack of association between sexual risk taking and drug use (O'Mahony & Barry, 1992). Condom use is low where sex is exchanged for drugs (Turner *et al.*, 1992). However, regular sex work and alcohol or drug use are not necessarily associated with 'risky' behaviour, and data presented by Thomas *et al.* (1990) indicates that only amongst males who have anal sex with males, is alcohol consumption related to condom non-use. Indeed, the reverse would seem to be the case, for whilst among injecting drug users condom use is uncommon (15%), in prostitution - regardless of drug use - condom use tends to be high (Plant *et al.*, 1990; Thomas *et al.*, 1990; Wolk *et al.*, 1990).

This regular use of condoms may be true less for clients than sex workers, but again, depending on age (Sonenstein *et al.*, 1989), and in this context van den Hoek *et al.*(1992) point to the interpersonal and situational factors that may influence decisions to use or not use condoms, and the extent to which people at risk make decisions in the light of their own understandings of risk factors. Condom use among drug injectors is, in Stimson's assessment (1991), selective and less easy to change following interventions compared with other risk-reduction changes (i.e. reduction in needle sharing) (Harris *et al.*, 1990; Morrison, 1991). However, various intervention programs appear to have made some difference to reported condom use (Martin *et al.*, 1990; Watters *et al.*, 1990; Edlin *et al.*, 1992; Longshore *et al.*, 1993). In a large-scale AIDS prevention campaign targeting IDUs in Amsterdam, for example, limited change in sexual behaviour was said to occur: even so, use of condoms increased in frequency with casual partners (from 30-49%), the proportion of female IUDs working as sex workers decreased (from 56-41%), and IUDs who knew that they were HIV-infected used condoms more frequently with their steady partners and tended to report fewer casual partners than those who knew they were not infected (van den Hoek *et al.*, 1992).

DOES YOUNG AGE AFFECT CONDOM USE?

Until HIV, condom research was family planning territory, and within that context, the condom was preferred as a method of contraception neither by providers nor the target population, the former because of risk of failure, the latter because of negative attitudes associating condoms with 'promiscuity', infection (STDs), lack of trust, infidelity, and difficulties in negotiating use, impairment of sensation and sexual function. These remain impediments to condom use today. Recent studies on condom use provide further evidence of the lack of acceptability of the technology, which have implications for their prophylactic as well as their contraceptive use within established relationships (Davidson *et al.*, 1985). Studies concerned with contraception indicate that, depending on the population, condom use is non-existent or acceptability poor and a temporary measure only, primarily as first method of contraception among those of older age at first intercourse. Among some groups, too, condoms are used for STD prevention (Strader & Beaman 1991).

Condom use is predisposed by parental advice of their contraceptive use, prior history of sexual conduct, and 'sexual scripts' (Maticka-Tyndale, 1991; Jemmott & Jemmott, 1991). Factors negatively influencing condom use include use of alcohol, low educational aspirations, and partner continuity, the latter influenced in turn by negative connotations of condoms and suspicion of the contraceptive protection offered by condoms (Tyden *et al.*, 1991a; Kraft *et al.*, 1990).

The interest in students and other young people is predicated on risk of age at infection and on the probable especial risks for early adolescent women due to physiological vulnerability, as well as to suppositions about 'antisocial' behaviour, sex in adolescence and sexual experimentation, and limited negotiating skills. A study by Barnard and McKeganey (1990) supports the general assertion that many adolescents find issues relating to sex awkward, embarrassing and difficult to discuss (Wight, 1992). Such factors are hypothesised to impede negotiation of condom use (Kenen & Armstrong, 1992). In a study by Kasen *et al.* (1992), students expressed uncertainty of their ability to refuse sex with a desirable partner, under pressure, after drinking alcohol or using marijuana, and were reluctant to purchase condoms or use them consistently after drinking alcohol or using marijuana. They were also doubtful of their ability to question partners about past homosexual history. Intervention programmes with young people appear to have been successful in increasing awareness of the value of condoms for disease prevention. In one, condom use in young men almost doubled among school students as a result of AIDS education and at the end of the intervention some 96% knew that condoms could protect infection (Nielsen & Hansen, 1990; Anderson *et al.*, 1990). Rickert *et al.* (1989) also report that although 62% reported that fear of AIDS had influenced their contraceptive behaviour, only 17% purchased or used condoms specifically to prevent AIDS transmission, and condom use was not consistent (Oswald *et al.*, 1992; Pennbridge *et al.*, 1992; Hingson *et al.*, 1990; Anderson *et al.*, 1990). Further, positive attitudes towards condom use do not necessarily translate into 'safer sex' practices, and in the study by Vicenzi *et al.* (1992), whilst most students report avoiding high risk partners, only 3% were using condoms. Poor availability and accessibility of condoms are frequently cited as reasons for non-use (Ross, 1990; Richwald *et al.*, 1989). Finally, perceptions of risk had implications for current and intended condom use (Tyden *et al.*, 1991b; Friedland *et al.*, 1991).

CONCLUDING REMARKS:

WHAT FACTORS AFFECT INTENTION TO USE CONDOMS?

In the course of this paper, we have highlighted the problems in condom use as a means of preventing HIV, insofar as a range of situational, interpersonal and structural factors appear to influence their use. A key factor is the general dislike of condoms, by both men and women, because they are perceived to interfere with the spontaneity and pleasure of sexual relations, although women - and possibly younger women in particular (Campbell & Baldwin, 1991) - appear more willing than men to use them. Secondly, however, condom use is not detached from cultural context - hence ideas about fidelity, trust, commitment, infection, as well as pleasure and physical and emotional closeness affect use of condoms. Knowledge of the benefits of using condoms for prevention of disease, and knowledge of how and when to use condoms, are only two components in decision-making influencing their use, and these in turn are influenced by type of partner and the situational conditions of coitus. Sexual communication and the sexual enjoyment value of condoms correlate with condom use across gender and sexual orientation (Catania, Coates, Kegeles *et al.*, 1992).

Intention appears to be a strong predictor of condom use among young US adults (Basen-Engquist, 1992), and a series of studies have been conducted along these lines: that is, changes in intention predict changes in behaviour (Abraham *et al.*, 1992; Shulkin *et al.*, 1991; Boldero *et al.*, 1992) despite some evidence of behaviour falling short of intention (de Vroome & Paalman, 1990). Factors influencing intention vary according to population, however: a study of young people's behavioural beliefs about the effects of condoms on sexual enjoyment, normative beliefs regarding partners and mothers' approval, and belief in technical skills at using condoms were all associated with intention to use condoms (Jemmott, Jemmott & Hacker, 1992). Increased self-efficacy and more favourable outcome expectancies regarding the effects of condom on enjoyment and partners' support for condom use were significantly related to increased condom use intentions (Jemmott & Jemmott, 1992; Breakwell *et al.*, 1991), and a number of studies emphasise the importance of parental, peer and partner support for women (e.g. Maticka-Tyndale 1991). Gaps in knowledge may make the translation from knowledge to practice difficult (Macintyre & West, 1993). Whilst some of the recent research has focused on intention to use condoms, and the ability of individuals to link action to intentionality, there is also evidence that condom use is in turn dependent upon intention to have intercourse (Fullilove *et al.*, 1990). Intention to use condoms appears also to be influenced by medical history, which in turn affects perception of the possibility of HIV infection (Bruce & Moineau, 1991; Rao, 1991; Svenson *et al.*, 1992). The interest in self-efficacy, and the role of this psychological variable in enabling an individual to 'follow-through' intention with action, has generated a considerable amount of social psychological research recently, with Wulfert and Wan (1993) concluding that self-efficacy was a major factor (a 'central mediator', in their terms) influencing condom-use.

A sub-set of the population not discussed above are people who have been tested for HIV: here the research question has related to outcome of HIV testing procedures and counselling on behaviour. The results are interesting, since they are generally consistent across populations; they suggest that testing, counselling and knowledge of serostatus all result in behavioural change, at least in the short term, in both industrialized and developing country settings (Frazer *et al.*, 1988; Kamenga *et al.*, 1991; Maticka-Tyndale, 1991; Wenger *et al.*, 1991; Allen, Serufilira *et al.*, 1992; Allen, Tice *et al.*, 1992). However, there is a cautionary note: according to Mayes *et al.* (1992) (also Landis *et al.*, 1992), the effect of HIV testing and counselling may reverse behavioural change: a negative HIV test resulted in falsely reassuring people who infrequently used a condom, and a number of other researchers provide a more cautious note of the immediate and longer term effects of testing on perceptions of risk, risk reduction behaviour, and the prevalence of safe sex (Schechter *et al.*, 1988; Wiktor *et al.*, 1990; Bagnall & Plant, 1991; Landis *et al.*, 1992). The data suggest, even so, that whilst knowledge of AIDS per se may not influence condom use, knowledge of personal vulnerability or heightened risk does.

Research points to plenty of contradictions in findings. These are hardly surprising. They occur at least in part because of the nature of the research and its positing of research questions - the search for the independent variable that will provide the key to prevention. In this context, as we have noted, the heterogeneity of the study populations is minimised. Yet differences among students in a classroom are not insubstantial. Among other populations - sex workers, for instance, or 'Blacks' or 'Hispanics' - they are sufficiently great to raise real questions about the utility of their being treated as a single community for the purposes of research.

Yet in this overview of research, some consistency of the above patterns of condom use emerges. In particular, perceptions of susceptibility appear to influence condom use, that may over-ride other aesthetic, emotional and tactile reactions to condoms. As noted, however, these considerations are highest in new, casual, and short-term sexual partnerships and lowest in regular partnerships (Moore & Barling, 1991; Abraham *et al.*, 1992). Those with high perceptions of susceptibility, such as injecting drug users who are seropositive and aware of the risk of transmission to others, appear to be more diligent with condom use with steady partners and by decreasing casual sexual contacts (Schechter & Craib, 1988; van den Hoek *et al.*, 1992).

Finally, despite a body of research suggesting that those who engage in 'high risk' behaviour are least likely to change behaviour or use condoms (Cromer & Brown, 1992; Stewart & deForge, 1991; Forster & Furley, 1989), at least some 'high risk' groups are not 'risk takers', and are more consistent than other populations in condom use. This would suggest the merit in pursuing perception of risk as well as the context of condom use, specifically the ability of individuals to insist upon condom use where there may be partner resistance. Consistent condom use appears to be associated with high levels of social support from informal sources of help, positive interpersonal ties, and negotiation skills; as a consequence, skill training, rather than the transfer of health information alone, would appear to be most successful in encouraging condom use (Valdiserri et al., 1989) regardless of population, sub-group, gender, or risk category.

ACKNOWLEDGEMENTS

We are grateful to Dr. Heino F.L.Meyer-Bahlburg, HIV Center for Clinical and Behavioral Studies, New York State Psychiatric Institute, for his valuable criticisms of an earlier draft of this paper; we maintain full responsibility for its limitations.

REFERENCES

Abraham, C., Sheeran, P. Spears, R. & Abrams, D. (1992) Health beliefs and promotion of HIV-preventive intentions among teenagers: a Scottish perspective, *Health Psychology*, **11**, 363-370.

Abramson, P. (1990) Sexual science: Emerging discipline or oxymoron? *Journal of Sex Research*, **27**, 323-246.

Abramson, P. (1992) Adios: A farewell address, Journal of Sex Research, 29, 449-450.

Allen, S., Serufilira, A., Bogaerts, J., van der Perre, P. *et al.* (1992) Confidential HIV testing and condom promotion in Africa. Impact on HIV and gonorrhea rates, *Journal of the American Medical Association*, **268**, 3338-3343.

Allen, S., Tice, J., van der Perre, P. Serufilira, A. *et al.* (1992) Effect of serotesting with counselling on condom use and seroconversion among HIV discordant couples in Africa, *British Medical Journal*, **304**, 1605-1609.

Anderson, J.E., Kann, L., Holtzman, D., Arday, S. *et al.* (1990) HIV/AIDS knowledge and sexual behavior among high school students, *Family Planning Perspectives*, **22**, 252-255.

Bagnall, G. & Plant, M.A. (1990) Alcohol, drugs and AIDS related risks: results from a prospective study, *AIDS Care*, **2**, 309- 317.

Bagnall, G. & Plant, M.A. (1991) HIV/AIDS risks, alcohol and illicit drug use among young adults in areas of high and low rate of HIV infection, *AIDS Care*, **3**, 355-361.

Barnard, M. & McKeganey, N. (1990) Adolescents, sex and injecting drug use: risks for HIV infection, *AIDS Care*, **2**, 103-116.

Basen-Engquist, K. (1992) Psychological predictors of 'safer sex' behaviours in young adults, *AIDS Education and Prevention*, **4**, 120-134.

Basen-Engquist, K. & Parcel, G.S. (1992) Attitudes, norms, and self-efficacy: A model of adolescents' HIV-related sexual risk behavior, *Health Education Quarterly*, **19**, 263-277.

Boldero, J., Moore, S. & Rosenthal, D. (1992) Intention, context, and safe sex: Australian adolescents' responses to AIDS, *Journal of Applied Social Psychology*, **22**, 1374-1396.

Bolton, R. & Singer, M. (Eds) (1992) *Rethinking AIDS Prevention: Cultural Approaches* (Chur, Switzerland; Gordon and Breach)

Bortolotti, F., Stivanello, A., Noventa, F., Forza, G. *et al.* (1992) Sustained AIDS education campaign and behavioral changes in Italian drug abusers, *European Journal of Epidemiology*, **8**, 264-267.

Breakwell, G.M., Fife-Schaw, C.R. & Clayden, K. (1991) Risk-taking, control over partner choice and intended use of condoms by virgins, *Journal of Community and Applied Social Psychology*, **1**, 173-187.

Brough, M. (1995) 'At risk' youth: AIDS, masculinity and the politics of prevention. *Unpublished PhD dissertation*, Brisbane: The University of Queensland.

Brown, L.K., Diclemente, R. J. & Park, T. (1992) Predictors of condom use in sexually active adolescents, *Journal of Adolescent Health*, **13**, 651-657.

Bruce, K.E. & Moineau, S. (1991) A comparison of STD clinic patients and undergraduates: Implications for AIDS prevention, *Health Values*, **15**, 5-12.

Calsyn, D.A., Saxon, A.J. & Wells, E.A. (1992) Longitudinal sexual behavior changes in injecting drug users, *AIDS*, **6**, 1207-1211.

Campbell, A.A. & Baldwin, W. (1991) The response of American women to the threat of AIDS and other sexually transmitted diseases, *Journal of Acquired Immune Deficiency Syndromes*, **4**, 1133-1140.

Carovano, K. (1991). More than mothers and whores: redefining the AIDS prevention needs of women, *International Journal of Health Services*, **21**, 131-142.

Carroll, L. (1991) Gender, knowledge about AIDS, reported behavioral change and the sexual behavior of college students, *Journal of American College Health*, **40**, 5-12.

Catania, J.A., Coates, T.J., Stall, R., Turner, H. *et al.*, (1992) Prevalence of AIDS related risk factors and condom use in the United States, *Science*, **258**, 1101- 1106.

Catania, J.A., Coates, T.J., Kegeles, S., Fullilove, M.T., Peterson, J., Marin, B., Siegel, D. & Hulley, S. (1992) Condom use in multi-ethnic neighbourhoods of San Francisco: the population-based AMEN (AIDS in Multi-Ethnic Neighbourhoods) study, *American Journal of Public Health*, **82**, 284-287.

Clatts, M.C. & Mutchler, K.M. (1989) AIDS and the dangerous other: metaphors of sex and deviance in the representation of disease, *Medical Anthropology*, **10**, 105-114.

Chapman, S. & Hodgson, J. (1988) Showers in raincoats: attitudinal barriers to condom use in high-risk heterosexuals, *Community Health Studies*, **XII**, 97-105.

Cortes, E., Detels, R., Aboulafia, D., Xi Ling, L. et al. (1989) HIV-1, HIV-2, and HTLV-1 infection in high-risk groups in Brazil, *New England Journal of Medicine*, **320**, 953-958.

Cromer, B.A. & Brown, R.T. (1992) Update on pregnancy, condom use, and prevalence of selected sexually transmitted diseases in adolescents, *Current Opinion in Obstetrics and Gynecology*, **4**, 855-859.

Darke, S., Hall, W. & Wodak, A. (1992) Benzodiazepine use and HIV risk-taking among injecting drug users, *Drug and Alcohol Dependence*, **31**, 31-36.

D'costa, I.J., Plummer, F.A., Bowmer, I., Fransen, L. *et al.* (1985) Prostitutes are a major reservoir of sexually transmitted diseases in Nairobi, Kenya, *Sexually Transmitted Diseases*, **12**, 64-67.

Davidson,A., Kye Chon Ahn, Chandra, S., Diaz-Guerrero, R. *et al.* (1985) *The Acceptability of Male Fertility Regulating Methods: A Multinational Field Survey*. Final report to the Task Force on Psychosocial Research in Family Planning. Geneva: World Health Organization.

Diclemente, R.J. (1991) Predictors of HIV-preventive sexual behavior in a high-risk adolescent population: the influence of perceived peer norms and sexual communication on incarcerated adolescents' consistent use of condoms, *Journal of Adolescent Health*, **12**, 385-390.

De Graaf, R., Vanwesenbeeck, I., Van Zessen, G., Straver, C.J. *et al.* (1992) Condom use and sexual behaviour in heterosexual prostitution in The Netherlands, *AIDS*, **6**, 1223-1226.

Donovan, B., Bek, M.D., Pethebridge, A.M. & Nelson, M.J. (1991) Heterosexual gonorrhoea in central Sydney: implications for HIV control, *Medical Journal of Australia*, **154**, 175-180.

Dorfman, L.E., Derish, P.A. & Cohen, J.B. (1992) Hey girlfriend: an evaluation of AIDS prevention among women in the sex industry, *Health Education Quarterly*, **19**, 25-40.

Dowsett, G.W., Davis, M.D. & Connell, R.W. (1992). Working class homosexuality and HIV/AIDS prevention: some recent research from Sydney, Australia, *Psychology and Health*, **6**, 313-324

Edlin, B.R., Irwin, K.L., Ludwig, D.D., Mccoy, H.V. et al. (1992) High-risk sex behavior among young street-recruited crack cocaine smokers in three American cities: an interim report, *Journal of Psychoactive Drugs*, **24**, 363-371.

Ehrhardt, A.A., Yingling, S., Zawadzki, R. & Martinez-Ramirez, M. (1992) Prevention of heterosexual transmission of HIV: barriers for women, *Journal of Psychology and Human Sexuality*, **5**, 37-67.

Evans, B.A., Mccormack,S.M., Bond, A.R. & Macrae, K.D. (1991) Trends in sexual behavior and HIV testing among women presenting at a genitourinary medicine clinic during the advent of AIDS, *Genitourinary Medicine*, **67**, 194-198.

Farmer, P. (1990). Sending sickness: sorcery, politics, and changing concepts of AIDS in rural Haiti, Medical Anthropology Quarterly, **4**, 6-27.

Farmer, P. (1992). *AIDS and Accusation: Haiti and the Geography of Blame* Berkeley: University of California Press.

Farmer, P. (1994). AIDS-talk and the constitution of cultural models, *Social Science and Medicine*, **38**, 801-809.

Fife-Schaw, C.R. & Breakwell, G.M. (1992) Estimating sexual behaviour parameters in the light of AIDS: a review of recent UK studies of young people, *AIDS Care*, **4**, 187-201.

Forster, S.J. & Furley, K.E. (1989) 1988 public awareness survey on AIDS and condoms in Uganda, *AIDS*, **3**, 147-154.

Fox, L.J., Bailey, P.E., Clarke-Martinez, K.L., Coello, M. *et al.* (1993) Condom use among high-risk women in Honduras: Evaluation of an AIDS prevention program, *AIDS Education and Prevention*, **5**, 1-10.

Frankenberg, R. (1992). The other who is also the same: the relevance of epidemics in space and time for prevention of HIV infection, *International Journal of Health Services*, **22**, 73-88.

Frazer, I.H., Mccamish, M., Hay, I. & North, P. (1988) Influence of HIV antibody testing on sexual behaviour in a 'high risk' population from a 'low risk' city, *Medical Journal of Australia*, **149**, 365-368.

Friedland, R.H., Jankelowitz, S.K., De Beer, M., De Klerk, C. *et al.* (1991) Perception and knowledge about the acquired immunedeficiency syndrome among students in university residences, *South African Medical Journal*, **79**, 149-154.

Fullilove, R.E., Fullilove, M.T., Bowser, B.P. & Gross, S.A. (1990). Risk of sexually transmitted disease among black adolescent crack users in Oakland and San Francisco, California, *Journal of the American Medical Association*, **9**, 851-855.

Harris, R.E., Langrod, J., Hebert, J.R, Lowinson, J. et al. (1990) Changes in AIDS risk behavior among intravenous drug abusers in New York City, *New York State Journal of Medicine*, **90**, 123-126.

Hart, G.J., Carvell, A.L., Woodward, N., Johnson, A.M. *et al.* (1989) Evaluation of needle exchange in central London: behaviour change and anti-HIV status over 1 year, *AIDS*, **3**, 261-265.

Herdt, G. & Lindenbaum, S. (Eds) (1992) *The Time of AIDS. Social Analysis, Theory and Method*, Newbury Park: Sage.

Herlitz, C. (1992) Condom use due to the risk of AIDS. Trends in the general population of Sweden, *Scandinavian Journal of Social Medicine*, **20**, 102-109.

Hingson, A.W., Strunin, L., Berlin, B.M. & Heeren, T. (1990) Beliefs about AIDS, use of alcohol and drugs, and unprotected sex among Massachusetts adolescents, *American Journal of Public Health*, **80**, 295- 299.

Hobart, C. (1992) How they handle it: young Canadians, sex, and AIDS, *Youth and Society*, **23**, 411-433.

Hooykaas, C., Van der Pligt, J., Van Doornum, G.J., Van Der Linden, M.M. *et al.* (1989) Heterosexuals at risk for HIV: differences between private and commercial partners in sexual behaviour and condom use, *AIDS*, **3**, 525-532.

Ingstad, B. (1990) The cultural construction of AIDS and its consequences for prevention, Medical Anthropology Quarterly, **4**, 28-40.

Ishii, K.M. & Whitbeck, L.B. (1990) AIDS and perceived change in sexual practice: An analysis of a college student sample from California and Iowa, *Journal of Applied Social Psychology*, **20**, 1301-1321.

James, N.J., Gilies, P.A. & Bignall, C.J. (1991) AIDS related risk perception and sexual behavior among sexually transmitted disease attenders, *International Journal of STDs and AIDS*, **2**, 264-271.

Jemmott, L.S. & Jemmott, J.B. (1991) Applying the theory of reasoned action to AIDS risk behavior: condom use among black women, *Nursing Research*, **40**, 228-234.

Jemmott, L.S. & Jemmott, J.B. (1992) Increasing condom use intentions among sexually active black adolescent women, *Nursing Research*, **41**, 273-279.

Jemmott, J.B., Jemmott, L.S. & Hacker, C.T. (1992) Predicting intentions to use condoms among African-American adolescents: the theory of planned behavior as a model of HIV risk, *Ethnicity and Disease*, **2**, 371-380.

Jemmott, J.B., Jemmott, L.S., Spears, H., Hewitt, N. *et al.* (1992) Self-efficacy, hedonistic expectations, and condom use intentions among inner city black adolescent women: a social cognitive approach to AIDS risk behaviour, *Journal of Adolescent Health*, **13**, 512- 519.

Johnson, E.H., Gant, L.M., Hinkle, Y.A., Gilbert, D.C. *et al.* (1992) Do African-American men and women differ in their knowledge about AIDS, attitude about condoms, and sexual behavior, *Journal of the National Medical Association*, **84**, 49-64.

Johnson, E.H., Hinkle, Y.A., Gilbert, D.C. & Gant, L.M. (1992) Black males who always use condoms: their attitudes, knowledge about AIDS, and sexual behavior, *Journal of the National Medical Association*, **84**, 341-352.

Kamenga, M., Ryder, R.W., Jingu, M., Mbuyi, N. *et al.* (1991) Evidence of marked sexual behavior change associated withlow HIV-I seroconvertion in 149 married couple with discordant HIV-I serostatus, *AIDS*, **5**, 61-67.

Kane, S. (1990). AIDS, addiction and condom use: sources of sexual risk for heterosexual women, *Journal of Sex Research*, **27**, 427-44.

Kane, S. & Mason, T. (1992) 'IV Drug Users' and 'Sex Partners': The limits of epidemiological categories and the ethnography of risk, in: G. Herdt & S. Lindenbaum (Eds) *The Time of AIDS. Social Analysis, Theory and Method.* Newbury Park: Sage.

Kasen, S., Vaughan, R.D. & Walter, H.J. (1992) Self-efficacy for AIDS prevention behaviors among tenth grade students, *Health Education Quarterly*, **19**, 187-202.

Kenen, R.H. & Armstrong K. (1992) The why, when and whether of condom use among female and male drug users, *Journal of Community Health*, **17**, 303-317.

Kippax, S., Crawford, J., Waldby, C. & Benton, P. (1990) Women negotiating heterosexuality: implications for AIDS prevention, *Women's Studies International Forum*, **13**, 533-42.

Kippax, S., Crawford, J., Rodden, P. & Benton, K. (1994) *Report on Project Male-Call: National Telephone Survey of Men who have Sex with Men,* Canberra: Commonwealth Department of Human Services and Health.

Kraft, P., Rise, J. & Traeen, B. (1990) The HIV epidemic and changes in the use of contraception among Norwegian adolescents, *AIDS*, **4**, 673-678.

Kramer, T.H., Mosely, J.A., Rivera, A., Ottomanelli, G. et al. (1991) Condom knowledge, history of use, and attitude among chemically addicted population, *Journal of Substance Abuse Treatment*, **8**, 241-246.

Kreiss, J., Koech, D., Plummer, F., Holmes, K. *et al.* (1986) AIDS virus infection in Nairobi prostitutes, *New England Journal of Medicine*, **314**, 414-418.

Ku, L.C. Sonenstein, F.L. & Pleck, J.H. (1992) The association of AIDS education and sex education with sexual behavior and condom use among teenage men, *Family Planning Perspectives*, **24**, 100-106.

Landis, S.E., Earp, J.L. & Koch, G.G. (1992) Impact of HIV testing and counselling on subsequent sexual behaviour. *AIDS Education and Prevention*, 4, 61-70.

Leland, N.L. & Barth, R.P. (1992) Gender difference in knowledge, intentions, and behaviors concerning pregnancy and sexually transmitted disease prevention among adolescents, *Journal of Adolescent Health*, **13**, 589- 599.

Leonard, T. (1990) Male clients of female street prostitutes: unseen partners in sexual disease transmission, *Medical Anthropology Quarterly*, 4, 41-55.

Lesnick, H. & Pace, B. (1990) Knowledge of AIDS risk factors in South Bronx minority college students, *Journal of Acquired Immune Deficiency Syndromes*, **3**, 173-176.

Longshore, D., Anglin, M.D., Annon, K. & Hsieh, S. (1993) Trends in self reported HIV risk behavior: injection drug users in Los Angeles, *Journal of Acquired Immune Deficiency Syndromes*, **6**, 82-90.

Lyttleton, C. (1994) Knowledge and meaning: the AIDS education campaign in rural northeast Thailand, *Social Science and Medicine*, **38**, 135-146.

McEwan, R.T. McCallum, A., Bhopal, R.S. & Madhok, R. (1992) Sex and the risk of HIV infection: the role of alcohol, *British Journal of Addiction*, **87**, 577-584.

Macintyre, S. & West, P. (1993) What does the phrase 'safe sex' mean to you? Understanding among Glaswegian 18 year olds in 1990, *AIDS*, 7, 121-125.

McKeganey,N. & Barnard, M. (1992) Selling sex: female street prostitution and HIV risk behavior in Glasgow. *AIDS Care*, **4**, 395-407.

McKusick, L., Hoff, C.C., Stall, R. & Coates, T.J. (1991) Tailoring AIDS prevention: differences in behavioral strategies among heterosexual and gay bar patrons in San Francisco, *AIDS Education and Prevention*, **3**, 1-9.

McQueen, D.V & Uitenbroek, D.G. (1992) Condom use and concern about AIDS, *Health Education Research*, 7, 47-53.

Mak, R.P. & Plum, J.R. (1991) Do prostitutes need more health education regarding sexually transmitted diseases and the HIV infection? Experience in a Belgian city, *Social Science and Medicine*, **33**, 963-966.

Manderson, L. (1994) Drugs, sex and social science: social science research and health policy in Australia, *Social Science and Medicine*, **39**, 1275-1286.

Manderson, L. & Aaby, P. (1992) An epidemic in the field? Rapid assessment procedures and health research. *Social Science and Medicine*, **35**, 839-850.

Martin, G.S., Serpelloni, G., Galvan, U., Rizzetto, A. *et al.* (1990) Behavioral change in injecting drug users: evaluation of an HIV/AIDS education programme, *AIDS Care*, **2**, 275-279.

Mathews, C., Kuhn, L., Metcalf, C.A., Joubert, G. *et al.* (1990) Knowledge, attitude and beliefs about AIDS in township school students in Capetown, *South African Medical Journal*, **78**, 511-516.

Maticka-Tyndale, E. (1991) Sexual scripts and AIDS prevention: variations in adherence to safer-sex guidelines by heterosexual adolescents, *Journal of Sex Research*, **28**, 45-66.

Mayes, S.D., Elsesser, V., Schaefer, J.H., Handford, H.A. *et al.* (1992) Sexual practices and AIDS knowledge among women partners of HIV infected haemophiliacs, *Public Health Report*, **107**, 504- 514.

Mays, V.M. & Cochran, S.D. (1988) Issues in the perception of AIDS risk and risk reduction acivities by black and Hispanic/Latina women, *American Psychologist*, **41**, 949-957.

Mays, V.M. & Cochran, S.D. (1993) Ethnic and gender differences in beliefs about sex partner questioning to reduce HIV risk, *Journal of Adolescent Research*, **8**, 77-88.

Miles, L. (1993) Women, AIDS and power in heterosexual sex. A discourse analysis, *Women's Studies International Forum*, **16**, 497-511.

Moatti, J.P., Bajos, N., Durbec, J.-P., Menard, C. & Serrand, C. (1991) Determinants of condom use among French heterosexuals with multiple partners, *American Journal of Public Health*, **81**, 106- 109.

Moore S.M. & Barling N.R. (1991) Developmental status and AIDS attitudes in adolescence, *Journal of Genetic Psychology*, **152**, 5-16.

Morrison, V. (1991) The impact of HIV upon injecting drug users: A longitudinal study, *AIDS Care*, **3**, 193-201.

Murray, S.O. & Payne, K.W. (1989) The social classification of AIDS in American epidemiology, *Medical Anthropology*, **10**, 115-128.

Neequaye, A.R., Neequaye, J.E. & Biggar, R.J. (1991) Factors that could influence the spread of AIDS in Ghana, West Africa: knowledge of AIDS, sexual behavior, prostitution, and traditional medical practices, *Journal of Acquired Immune Deficiency Sydnromes*, **4**, 914-919.

Nielsen, M.B. & Hansen, K. (1990) Young mens' knowledge of AIDS. Development from June 1987 to January 1989, *Ugessir Laeger*, **152**, 235-237.

Norris, A.E. & Ford, K. (1991) AIDS risk behaviors of minority youth living in Detroit. *American Journal of Preventive Medicine*, **7**, 416-421.

Nzila, N., Laga, M., Thiam, M.A., Mayimona, K. *et al.* (1991). HIV and other sexually transmitted diseases among female prostitutes in Kinshasa, *AIDS*, **5**, 715-721.

O'Leary, A., Goodhart, F., Jemmott, L.S. & Boccher-Lattimore, D. (1992) Predictors of safer sex on the college campus: A social cognitive theory analysis, *Journal of American College Health*, **40**, 254-263.

O'Mahony, P. & Barry, M. (1992) HIV risk of transmission behavior amongst HIV-infected prisoners and its correlates, *British Journal of Addiction*, **87**, 1555- 1560.

Osmond, M.W., Wambach, K.G., Harrison, D.F., Byers, J., Levine, P., Imershein, A. & Quadagno, D.M. (1993) The multiple jeopardy of race, class and gender for AIDS risk among women, *Gender and Society*, **7**, 99-120.

Oswald, H., Pforr, P. & Dills, M. (1992) Sexuality and AIDS: attitude and behaviors of adolescents in east and west Berlin, *Journal of Adolescence*, **15**, 373-391.

Parker, R. (1987) Acquired immunodeficiency syndrome in urban Brazil, *Medical Anthropology Quarterly*, **1**, 155-175.

Parker, R. (1989a) Bodies and pleasures: On the construction of erotic meanings in contemporary Brazil, *Anthropology and Humanism Quarterly*, **14**, 58-64.

Parker, R. (1989b) *Bodies, Pleasures and Passions: Sexual culture in contemporary Brazil*, Boston: Beacon.

Pennbridge, J.N., Freese, T.E. & Mackenzie, R.G. (1992) High risk behaviors among male street youth in Hollywood, California, *AIDS Education and Prevention*, **4**, 24-33.

Peterson, J.L. Coates, T.J., Catania, J.A., Middleton, L. *et al.* (1992) High-risk sexual behavior and condom use among gay and bisexual African-American men, *American Journal of Public Health*, **82**, 1490-1494.

Potter, L.B. & Anderson, J.E. (1993) Patterns of condom use and sexual behaviour among never-married women, *Sexually Transmitted Diseases*, **20**, 201-208.

Plant, M.L. Plant, M.A. & Thomas, R.M. (1990) Alcohol, AIDS risk and commercial sex: some preliminary results from a Scottish study, *Drug and Alcohol Dependence*, **25**, 51-55.

Quirk, M.E., Godkin, M.A. & Schwenzfeier, E. (1993) Evaluation of two AIDS prevention interventions for inner-city adolescent and yung adult women, *American Journal of Preventive Medicine*, **9**, 21-26.

Rao, A.V., Swaminathan, R., Baskaran, S., Belinda, G. *et al.* (1991) Behaviour change in HIV infected subjects following health education, *Indian Journal of Medical Research*, **93**, 345-349.

Rhodes, E. & Wolitski, R.J. (1990) Perceived effectiveness of fear appeals in AIDS education: relationship to ethnicity age and group membership, *AIDS Education and Prevention*, **3**, 1-11.

Richard, R. & Van der Pligt, J. (1991) Factors affecting condom use among adolescents, *Journal of Community and Applied Social Psychology*, **1**, 105-116.

Rickert, V.I. & Gottlieb, A.A. (1992) Is AIDS education related to condom acqisition? *Clinical Paediatrics*, **31**, 205-210.

Rickert, V.I., Jay, M.S., Gottlieb, A. & Bridges, C. (1989) Adolescents and AIDS. Female's attitude and behaviours towards condom purchase and use, *Journal of Adolescent Health Care*, **10**, 313-316.

Richwald, G.A., Friedland, J.M. & Morisky, D.E. (1989) Condom sales at public universities in California: Implications for campus AIDS prevention, *American Journal of College Health*, **37**, 272-277.

Ross, M.W. (1990) Psychological determinants of increased condom use and safer sex in homosexual men: a longitudinal study, *International Journal of STDs and AIDS*, **1**, 98-101.

Rotheram-Borus, M.J., Koopman, C., Haignere, C. & Davies, M. (1991) Reducing HIV sexual risk behaviors among runaway adolescents, *Journal of the American Medical Association*, **266**, 1237-1241.

Schechter, M.T. & Craib, K.J. (1988) Patterns of sexual behaviour and condom use in a cohort of homosexual men, *American Journal of Public Health*, **78**, 1535-1539.

Schilling, R.F., El-Bassel, N., Schinke, S.P., Nichols, S. *et al.* (1991) Sexual behavior, attitude towards safe sex and gender among a cohort of 244 recovering IV drug users, *International Journal of Addiction*, **26**, 859-877.

Schoepf, B.G. (1992). Women at risk: Case studies from Zaire, in: G.Herdt & S.Lindenbaum (Eds.), *The Time of AIDS. Social Analysis, Theory and Method*, Newbury Park: Sage.

Schoepf, B.G. (1993) AIDS, sex and condoms: traditional healers and community-based AIDS prevention in Zaire, *Medical Anthropology*, **14**, 225-242.

Seeley, J.A., Kengeya-Kayondo, J.F., & Mulder, D.J. (1992) Community-based HIV/AIDS research - whither community participation? Unsolved problems in a research programme in rural Uganda, *Social Science and Medicine*, **34**, 1089-1096.

Seeley, J.A., Malamba, S.S., Nunn, A.J., Mulder, D.J. *et al.* (1994) Socioeconomic status, gender and risk of HIV-1 infection is a rural community in South West Uganda, *Medical Anthropology Quarterly*, **8**, 78-89.

Serraino, D. & Franceshi, S. (1992) Condom use and sexual habits of heterosexual intravenous drug users in northern Italy, European Journal of Epidemiology, **8**, 723-729.

Severn, J.J. (1990) College students and condoms: AIDS and attitudes, *College Student Journal*, **24**, 296-306.

Shayne, V.T. & Kaplan, B.J. (1991) Double victims: Poor women and AIDS, *Women & Health*, **17**, 21-37.

Shulkin, J.J., Mayer, J.A., Wessel, L.G., De Moor, C. *et al.* (1991) Effects of a peer led AIDS intervention with university students, *Journal of American College Health*, **40**, 75-79.

Simonsen, J.N., Plummer, F.A., Ngugi, E.N., Black, L. et al. (1990) HIV infection among lower socioeconomic strata prostitutes in Nairobi, *AIDS*, **4**, 139-144.

Sonenstein, F.L., Pleck, J.H. & Ku, L.C. (1989) Sexual activity, condom use and AIDS awareness among adolescent males, Family Planning Perspectives, **21**, 152-158.

Sonnex, C., Hart, G.J., Williams, P. & Adler, M.W. (1989) Condom use by heterosexuals attending a department of GUM: attitudes and behaviour in the light of HIV infection, *Genitourinary Medicine*, **65**, 248-251.

Spina, M., Serraino, D. & Tirelli, U. (1992) Condom use and high-risk sexual practices of female prostitutes in Italy, AIDS, **6**, 601-602.

Stewart, D.L. & Deforge, B.S. (1991) Attitude towards condom use and AIDS among patients from an urban family practice centre, *Journal of the National Medical Association*, **83**, 772-776.

Stimson, G.V. (1991) Risk reduction by drug users with regard to HIV infection, *International Review of Psychiatry*, **3**, 401-415.

Strader, M.K. & Beaman, M.L. (1991) Comparison of selected college students' and sexually transmitted disease clinic patients' knowledge, about AIDS, risk behaviours and beliefs about condom use, *Journal of Advanced Nursing*, **16**, 584-590.

Struckman-Johnson, C.J., Gilland, R.C., Struckman-Johnson, D.L. & North, T.C. (1990) The effect of fear of AIDS and gender on responses to fear-arousing condom advertisements. *Journal of Applied Social Psychology*, **20**, 1396-1410.

Svenson, L.W., Varnhagen, C.K., Godin, A.M. & Salmon, T.L. (1992) Rural high school students' knowledge, attitude and behaviors related to sexually transmitted diseases, *Canadian Journal of Public Health*, **83**, 260-263.

Swaddiwudhipong, W., Nguntra, P., Lerdlukanavonge, P., Chaovakiratipong, C. *et al.* (1990) A survey of knowledge about AIDS and sexual behavior in sexually active men in Mae Sot, Tak, Thailand, *Southeast Asian Journal of Tropical Medicine and Public Health*, **21**, 447-452.

Thomas, R.M., Plant, M.A. & Plant, M.L. (1990) AIDS risks and sex industry clients: result from a Scottish study, *Drug and Alcohol Dependence*, **26**, 265-269.

Turner, N.H., Black, S. & Taylor, D.J. (1992) HIV risks among minority drug users in a small city, *Ethnicity and Disease*, **2**, 246-251.

Tyden, T., Norden, L. & Ruusuvaara, L. (1991b) Swedish adolescents' knowlege of sexually transmitted diseases and their attitudes to the condoms, *Midwifery*, 7, 25-30.

Tyden, T., Bjorkelund, C. & Olsson, S.E. (1991a) Sexual behavior and sexually tranmitted diseases among Swedish university students, *Acta Obstetrica Gynecologica Scandinavia*, **70**, 219-224.

Uitenbroek, D.G. & Mcqueen, D.V. (1992) Changing patterns in reported sexual practices in the population: multiple partners and condom use, *AIDS*, **6**, 587-592.

Valdiserri, R.O., Arena, V.C., Proctor, D. & Bonati, F.A. (1989) The relationship between women's attitudes about condoms and their use: implications for condom promotion programs, *American Journal of Public Health*, **79**, 499-500.

Van Deele, M. (1989) AIDs Hotline Flanders: Results in 1988, *Archives Belgium*, **47**, 165-169.

Van den Hoek, J.A., Van Haastrecht, H.J. & Coutinho, R.A. (1990) Heterosexual behaviour of intravenous drug users in Amsterdam: implications for the AIDS epidemic, *AIDS*, **4**, 449-453.

Van den Hoek, J.A., Van Haastrecht, H.J. & Coutinho, R.A. (1992) Little change in sexual behaviour in injecting drug users in Amsterdam, *Journal of Acquired Immune Deficiency Sydnromes*, **5**, 518-522.

Van Haastrecht, H.J. & Van den Hoek, J.A. (1991) Evidence for a change in behavior among heterosexuals in Amsterdam under the influence of AIDS, *Genitourinary Medicine*, **67**, 199-206.

Vicenzi, A.E. & Thiel, R. (1992) AIDS education on the college campus: Roy's adoption model direct enquiry, *Public Health Nursing*, **9**, 270-276.

De Vroome, E.M. & Paalman, M.E. (1990) AIDS in the Netherlands: the effects of several years of campaigning, *International Journal of STD and AIDS*, **1**, 268-275.

Walter, H.J., Vaughan, R.D., Gladis, M.M., Ragin, D.F. *et al.* (1992) Factors associated with AIDS risk behaviors among high school students in an AIDS epicenter, *American Journal of Public Health*, **82**, 528-532.

Warren, C.A.B. (1974) *Identity and Community in the Gay World*, New York: Wiley Interscience.

Warwick, I., Aggleton, P. & Homans, H. (1988) Constructing commonsense - young people's beliefs about AIDS, *Sociology of Health and Illness*, **2**, 213-233.

Watters, J.K, Downing, M., Case, P., Lorvick, J. *et al.* (1990) AIDS prevention for intravenous drug users in the community: street-based education and risk behavior, *American Journal of Community Psychology*, **18**, 587- 596.

Weinstock, H.S., Lindan, C., Bolan, G., Kegeles, S.M. *et al.* (1993) Factors associated with condom use in a high-risk heterosexual population, *Sexually Transmitted Diseases*, **20**, 14-20.

Wenger N.S., Linn, L.S., Epstein, M. & Shapiro, M.F. (1991) Reduction of high-risk sexual behavior among heterosexuals undergoing HIV antibody testing: a randomised clinical trial, *American Journal of Public Health*, **81**, 1580-1585.

Wielandt, H.B. (1993) Have the AIDS campaigns changed the pattern of contraceptive usage among adolescents? *Acta Obstetrica Gynecologica Scandinavia*, 72, 111-115.

Wight, D. (1992) Impediments to safer heterosexual sex: a review of research with young people, *AIDS Care*, 4, 11-21.

Wiktor, S.Z., Biggar, R.J., Melbye, M., Ebbesen, P. *et al.* (1990) Effect of knowledge of human immunodefeciency virus infection status on sexual activity among homosexual men, *Journal of Acquired Immununodeficiency Syndromes*, **31**, 62-68.

Wilson, D., Sibanda, B., Mboyi, L., Mismanga, S. *et al.* (1990) A pilot study for an HIV prevention programme among commercial sex workers in Bulawayo, Zimbabwe, *Social Science and Medicine*, **31**, 609-618.

Witte, K. (1991) The role of threat and efficacy in AIDS prevention, *International Quarterly of Community Health Education*, **12**, 225-249.

Wulfert, E. & Wan, C.K. (1993) Condom use: a self-efficacy model, *Health Psychology*, **12**, 346-353.

Wolk, J. Wodak, A., Morlet, A., Guinan, J.J. *et al.* (1990) HIV related risk taking behavior, knowledge and serostatus of intravenous drug users in Sydney, *Medical Journal of Australia*, **152**, 453-458.

Worth, D. (1989) Sexual decision-making and AIDS: why condom promotion among vulnerable women is likely to fail, *Studies in Family Planning*, **20**, 297-307.

De Zalduondo, B.O. (1991). Prostitution viewed cross-culturally: toward recontextualizing sex work in AIDS intervention research, *Journal of Sex Research*, **28**, 223-248.

Zimet, G.D., Bunch, D.L., Anglin, T.M., Lazebnir, R. *et al.* (1992) Relationship of AIDS related attitudes to sexual behavior changes in adolescents, *Journal of Adolescent Health*, **13**, 493-498.

2

Initiating And Maintaining Safer Sex: Evaluation of Group Work with Gay Men.

SHAMIL WANIGARATNE, ANDREW BILLINGTON, AND MALCOLM WILLIAMS

INTRODUCTION

Changes in sexual practices by gay men to reduce risk of HIV and other infections were widely reported in the mid-1980s (Van de Laar *et al.*, 1990; Winkelstein *et al.*, 1987; Johnson & Gill, 1989). Whilst the vast majority had changed their practices a small but significant proportion were reported to experience difficulties in changing unsafe behaviours (McKusick *et al.*, 1990; Fox *et al.*, 1987; Martin, 1987).

Longitudinal studies such as the MACS study (Adib *et al.*, 1991) and the San Francisco Men's Health Study (Stall *et al.*, 1990) were reporting high levels of relapse from safer sex practices among those who changed their practices initially. Reported failure to maintain safer sex in the above two studies in a 2-3 year follow up period ranged from 50% to 62%. A number of factors associated with the failure to maintain safer sex have been identified. Associated demographic factors include: lower levels of education, poor economic status, belonging to an ethnic minority (St Lawrence *et al.*, 1990) and age, (younger gay men are reported to be more likely to engage in unprotected anal intercourse than older gay men) (Ekstrand & Coates, 1990; Kelly *et al.*, 1990, Evans *et al.*, 1993). Inter-personal factors and social factors include: having a regular partner, unsafe sex signalling love, trust and commitment (Stall *et al.*, 1990; Ekstrand *et al.*, 1992; Adib *et al.*, 1991; McKusick *et al.*, 1990; Hunt *et al.*, 1992); sexual negotiation skills, which include communication skills as well as assertiveness, (Adib *et al.* 1991; Gold *et al.*, 1991; Kelly *et al.*, 1991); social norms, risk behaviours being associated with perceptions that social norms do not favour safer sex (CDC, 1991; Hays *et al.*, 1992). High risk sexual behaviours and lapses into unsafe sex are associated with perceptions that safer sex is unacceptable within the peer group (Stall *et al.*, 1990; Kelly *et al.*, 1990). Intra-personal factors include: low self-esteem (Horn *et al.*, 1989), enjoyment of unprotected intercourse (Stall *et al.*, 1990; Hays *et al.*, 1992), depression (Gold & Skinner, 1992; Kelly *et al*,. 1991); suicidality (Cunningham *et al.*, 1992); lack of coping skills (Phillips *et al.*, 1990) and negative attitude to condom use (Valdiserri *et al.*, 1988). Other factors associated with failure to maintain safer sex include alcohol and drug use (Stall *et al.*, 1990; Gold & Skinner, 1992; McKusker *et al.*, 1990; McEwan *et al.*, 1992; Klee, 1992; Myers *et al.*, 1992).

The problems of initiation and maintenance of safer sex appear to take place within a backdrop of a high knowledge base regarding HIV infection and sexual behaviours (Gold *et al.*, 1991, 1992). Hence interventions to address these problems need to go beyond education and public campaigns. A number of innovative community level and group interventions have been developed in response to this need around the world. Some of these interventions and their relative effectiveness are reviewed by Thornton & Catalan (1993). This chapter describes a small group intervention developed in a clinical setting in London UK which is aimed at a target population of gay men who are experiencing difficulties in initiating and maintaining safer sex. It also deals with the problem of evaluating interventions of this nature and proposes an instrument based on self efficacy to facilitate evaluation. A comprehensive evaluative framework is also proposed.

Theoretical Background

The theoretical rationale for much of the HIV prevention work has centred around the health belief model (Becker, 1974), a model of behavioural decision making. The model presumes that the individual acts to maximise net benefits of their action for behaviours under their control. For health related decisions the individual is assumed to weigh up both health related and non health related consequences of their actions. The immediate short term benefits of certain behaviours may lead people to disregard their long term negative consequences. The health belief model identifies a number of factors that interact in health related behavioural decision making process. These include knowledge of health risks and health promoting behaviours, perception of oneself as being at risk and relating risks to one's action, perceived effectiveness of behaviour change and response efficacy, belief in the power of technological cures or preventions, sociodemographic variables, social network affiliations and group norms. Whilst it provides an adequate explanatory framework, the health belief model falls far short of a comprehensive predictive model in the area of HIV risk behaviour. Using the health belief model in conjunction with models developed in the area of addiction, e.g. Prochaska & DiClemente (1986) model of change and Marlatt & Gordon (1985) model of the relapse process, appears to hold more promise towards developing interventions to initiate and maintain safer sex. The Prochaska & DiClemente (1986) model of change describes changes in highly reinforcing behaviours such as smoking, drinking and sexual behaviours, taking place through a series of discreet stages. These stages, namely pre-contemplation, contemplation, preparation, active change and maintenance, take place in a cyclical process (Prochaska & DiClemente, 1986). Individuals at each stage of change can be assisted or supported by different interventions, e.g. Motivational Interviewing (Miller, 1983; Miller & Rollenic, 1991) for pre-contemplation through to active change and Relapse Prevention (Marlat & Gordon, 1985; Annis, 1986) for the maintenance stage. The Marlatt & Gordon (1985) cognitive behavioural model of the relapse process is a comprehensive model dealing with both specific and global aspects of maintenance of behaviour change and has considerable implications for interventions to prevent relapse from safer sex. It is acknowledged that the term relapse has negative connotations and that the use of it to describe failure to maintain safer sex has been criticised by the gay community as pathologising gay men's sexual practices (Hickson *et al.*, 1991). The term relapse in this area has been used as a metaphor and has undeniable medical links. On the other hand, the model itself deals with conscious and practical aspects of maintaining change and has empowerment as its central philosophy. It is not a passive disease model. Because of its comprehensive nature, the potential of this model in providing a framework for interventions in this area is immense.

The intervention described in this paper based on the above models and incorporating aspects of group psychology (Yallom, 1975) was titled and publicised as "Changing Personal Practice: a Group for Gay Men".

Aims of the Workshops

The aims of the workshop were to:

- prevent the spread of HIV infection among gay men by helping participants change their personal sexual practices to safer ones and enhance the probability of maintaining these changes
- give participants a greater sense of command over their sexual behaviours which would minimise the risk of HIV transmission
- develop and enhance participants' sexuality
- help participants make global changes in their lives (e.g. increase their self esteem and confidence)
- help participants develop a greater understanding of HIV infection and its transmission

Evaluation

Evaluation of group interventions of this nature is challenging. Behaviour change towards safer sex practices would be the most objective and desired outcome measurement. Retrospective reporting biases makes the use of behaviour change data questionable in its reliability. The diary keeping method although more reliable, may also act as an intervention in itself, thus making it unsuitable for the evaluation of the workshops. A desired measure of outcome would include quantitative as well as qualitative measures. Quantitative measures should be broad and have predictive utility as well as measure change. Qualitative aspects should take more of a single case type approach to evaluation. The experience of individuals attending the workshops and the long term effects of that, could have a greater importance than simple quantitative measures of change.

Measures of self-efficacy appear to meet the criteria of a quantitative measure of outcome that has predictive utility. In the field of addictive behaviours measures of self-efficacy have been shown to predict up to 75% of relapses (Annis, 1986). The construct of self-efficacy involves the perception of confidence in the ability of the individual to carry out specific behaviours under a specific set of circumstances. "Situational Confidence" constitutes a measure of this. Since there were no available validated instruments measuring self-efficacy in the area of the personal sexual practice of gay men, an instrument in the form of a Situational Confidence Questionnaire (SCQ) was developed as an evaluation measure of the intervention.

Evaluation of the workshops over a three year period has also yielded a framework for qualitative feedback from participants. The Overall Evaluation Questionnaire which was developed for participants' feedback of their experience of the workshops and facilitators, has built-in quantitative measures of expectations, perceptions of outcome, and behaviour change. A Follow-up Questionnaire was also developed by modifying the overall evaluation questionnaire.

The self-efficacy measure (SCQ), the Schedule for Initial Interviews, the Overall Evaluation Questionnaire and the Follow-up Questionnaire, in combination, are proposed as a comprehensive evaluation framework for both individual and group interventions aimed at initiation and maintenance of safer sex with gay men.

METHOD

Recruitment

The workshops were publicised by advertisements and articles in gay newspapers and by leaflets placed in genito-urinary medicine (GUM) clinics in London and in some gay bars. Referrals were also made by GUM physicians.

All referrals (self-referred and clinic referred) were assessed by one of the facilitators as described in the pre-group interview section below. Those meeting the following basic criteria were offered a place in the groups:

1. Wanting to change some aspect of their sexual behaviour that might directly or indirectly put them at risk of HIV infection or of infecting others.
2. Experiencing difficulty in sustaining changes.
3. With no psychological or emotional problems that would make participating in the workshop detrimental to the individual or the group.

Intervention

The main aspects of the intervention are outlined below. The following objectives were presented to the participants in a pre-group pack.

To clarify reasons for changing to and maintaining safer sex.

- To recognise the feelings of loss that may result from changing familiar and often highly pleasurable sexual practices.
- To discuss the risk factors involved in transmission and check, or expand, knowledge and understanding about HIV and other sexually transmitted diseases (STDs).
- To decide on sexual goals which relate to personal sexual needs.
- To identify the attitudes that could get in the way of achieving these goals.
- To discuss and practice ways of negotiating safer sex, including some exploration of the way in which thinking may affect behaviour.
- To look at self-esteem and lifestyle factors that can support any changes and develop ways of enhancing emotional sexual well being.
- To identify longer-term goals and some strategies to continue working with them.

The Pre-Group Interview

All participants, regardless of their mode of referral, were assessed by one of the facilitators for their suitability to participate in the workshop. This was carried out in the form of a structured interview, the format of which was adapted from an interview developed for similar group work in the area of addictions (Keaney *et al.*, 1994). The interview investigated people's direct or indirect risk of HIV infection or transmission and their experience of difficulties in making and sustaining changes. It considered their personal sexual goals, and their previous experience of counselling. Previous attendance of groups and specific anxieties about attending this group were noted. The interview also explored potential barriers to attending the group, such as a previous history of psychiatric or psychological problems. The content of the sessions, the ground rules and other guidelines were also discussed at the pre-group interview.

Those meeting the criteria for the intervention were offered a place on the six session workshop. The workshop covered the following topics:

Setting Personal Goals

- High Risks and Safer Sex
- Body Image and Anxiety Management
- All in the Mind: Safer Sex and Lifestyle Balance

- Safer Sex Negotiation and Lifestyle Balance
- Review and What Now?

Follow-up sessions were held at three month intervals to enable participants to meet and review their successes and failures.

Measures

During the three year history of the workshops a number of evaluation and outcome measures were piloted. This resulted in streamlining outcome measurement and the development of four instruments for the purpose of evaluating the workshops.

1) The Schedule for Initial Interviews and Self Completion Questionnaire.
2) The Situational Confidence Questionnaire.
3) The Overall Evaluation Questionnaire.
4) The Follow-up Evaluation Questionnaire.

Situational Confidence Questionnaire (SCQ)

Measures of self-efficacy are generally regarded as reliable predictors of specific behaviours under specific circumstances. A measure of self-efficacy was designed and developed for the workshops which lists common "High Risk Situations" in which participants are likely to find themselves. The questionnaire has 19 items covering 7 categories (scales) of High Risk Situations. The scales of the SCQ are: 1) Pick up situations, 2) Sex with regular partner, 3) Sex in open relationships, 4) Situations when alcohol and drugs are involved, 5) When sexually aroused, 6) Low mood and 7) Environmental "Hot Spots". There is also an overall confidence item. The participants are required to rate their confidence in each situation in a 0 - 100 scale. The instrument has a simple scoring procedure with ratings for scales with more than one item being averaged to obtain a scale score.

Reliability analysis for the SCQ scales yielded Cronbach alphas ranging from 0.69 to 0.87. Mean = 0.8. The items have high face validity; the content and construct validity of the measure was established by pilot work with participants of earlier groups. The SCQ was given to the participants at the first and last sessions and they were required to complete them anonymously. The questionnaires were also given again at follow-up groups.

Overall Evaluation Questionnaire (OEQ)

This questionnaire was designed and developed to obtain quantitative and qualitative information on participants' experiences of the workshops and subsequent behaviour change. The questionnaire has 22 items which cover areas ranging from expectations, helpful and unhelpful aspects of the group, satisfaction, and behavioural changes made during the workshops, to how group members experienced the facilitators. Participants were asked to fill out the questionnaire at the last session. They were requested to fill out the questionnaires anonymously using only unique identification numbers.

Follow-up Questionnaire (FQ)

This questionnaire was designed for the workshops and comprises mainly behaviour change questions from the Overall Evaluation Questionnaire. Participants were requested to fill out the questionnaire at the follow-up session anonymously and include only their unique identification number.

Design and Data Analysis

A repeated measures design was used for the analysis of quantitative data with each participant acting as his own control. Appropriate non parametric tests were used to analyse the data using SPSSX software run on a Personal Computer.

RESULTS

Participants

Over 120 gay men participated in the workshops over the three year period. The results reported here focused on the evaluation of workshops run over the past six months. 26 gay men participated in three workshops run since January 1995. Their average age was 35.2 years. 85% of those who attended the first group completed all sessions. Follow up data reported in this paper are from 9 participants as the majority of participants failed to attend follow-up sessions and postal follow-up evaluation was not instituted at the time of reporting.

Situational Confidence Questionnaire (SCQ)

A summary of results of participants' responses on each scale of the SCQ is presented in Table 2.1 Levels of confidence show an increase across all scales at post group data collection compared to pre-group levels. These differences reach statistical significance (Wilcoxon matched pairs sign test) on all scales with the exception of Alcohol/Drugs, and Sexually Aroused, Scales. The confidence levels show a slight increase at three month follow-up in comparison with the post group measures. These differences failed to reach statistical significance.

Table 2.1
Overall Situational Confidence Questionnaire (SCQ)

	N	Mean%	S.D.
1) Pick up Situation			
Pre	25	63.6	22.2
Post	22	76.4**	17.2
Follow-up	9	87.5	12.6
2) Regular Partner			
Pre	25	61.6	23.1
Post	22	77.7*	17.0
Follow-up	9	79.7	14.3
3) Open Relationship			
Pre	25	61.6	23.1
Post	22	72.6***	15.2
Follow-up	9	68.3	23.3
4) Alcohol/Drugs			
Pre	24	45.8	25.9
Post	21	61.9	25.9
Follow-up	9	67.0	16.3
5) Sexually Aroused			
Pre	26	56.1	34.0
Post	23	74.0	24.0
Follow-up	9	76.6	20.0
6) Feeling Low			
Pre	26	38.1	34.0
Post	23	61.3*	30.2
Follow-up	9	63.3	22.3
7) Hot Spot			
Pre	25	44.0	26.3
Post	22	65.2***	20.9
Follow-up	9	70.0	20.6
8) Total			
Pre	26	51.9	24.0
Post	23	68.7	19.8
Follow-up	9	82.2	12.0

Pre-post difference: *P<0.05 **P<0.01 ***P<0.001

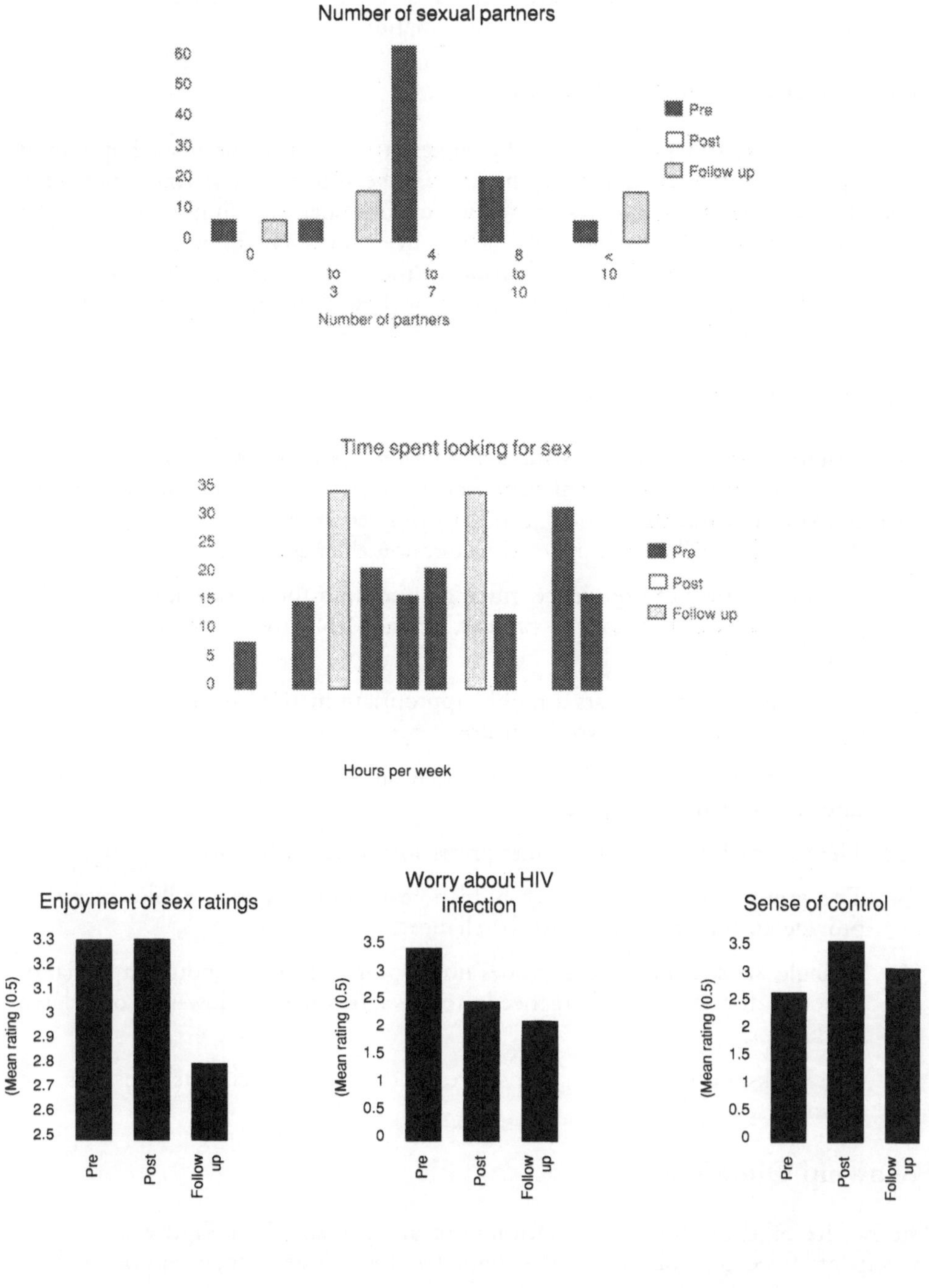

Fig. 2.1 Reported changes in participants at the end of the workshop and follow-up

Overall Evaluation Questionnaire

The overall evaluation questionnaire yielded quantitative responses of behaviour change as well as a wealth of qualitative information.

Behavioural and Other Changes

Figure 2.1 shows participants' reported changes at the end of the workshop and at follow-up. There are no significant changes in the number of partners per week reported at pre and post measures. In reports of time spent looking for sex, there is a trend towards shifting to less time. There were no changes in the ratings of enjoyment. Although there was a reduction in the mean worry about HIV and an increase in the mean sense of control, neither of these differences reached statistical significance.

Qualitative Feedback

The participants gave detailed feedback of their experiences of attending the workshops and of issues of current importance to gay men in the area of personal sexual practice. It is difficult to do justice to this feedback in the present context. The following is a distilled outline of the common themes.

1. Gay men appear to experience much guilt around their risk-taking behaviour and thus find it difficult to present, asking explicitly for help with unsafe sexual practices.
2. The group format appears a highly appropriate method of intervention as it can provide safety and avoid censure.
3. Gay men still require safer sex information and must feel able to relate it directly to their sexual practice.
4. The vast majority of participants prefer gay male facilitators.
5. The group process of making hidden fears and anxieties public seems to provide an important impetus for change.
6. A single, six session workshop does not appear to provide enough material or structure for change. There needs to be subsequent follow-ups or related workshops.
7. Any workshop must attempt to address individual participants' lifestyles and personal sexual strategies.

Follow-up Questionnaires

The results of the follow-up questionnaire are presented in Figure 2.1. Nine participants filled out follow-up questionnaires. Behaviour change reports at three months, compared with post group reports in the number of sexual partners does not show a significant increase. There was again a trend towards less hours per week spent looking for sex . However, there was a drop in the ratings of enjoyment of sex and of sense of control. Worry about HIV remained unchanged.

DISCUSSION

The method of evaluation described above provides a framework for predictive measures, behavioural and psychological change measures and qualitative feedback. The measurement process is brief and constitutes minimal intrusion into the intervention. Both quantitative and qualitative evaluation of the intervention show positive results. The self-efficacy measure (SCQ) shows a significant increase in situational confidence in most scales in pre - post comparisons and the levels of confidence appear to be maintained at three month follow-up. In terms of the theoretical model the intervention is based upon (Marlatt & Gordon, 1985), this points to global changes that should strengthen the probability of maintaining change. The behaviour change measures taken were those of the number of sexual partners per week and the time spent per week looking for sex. It is important to note that both these measures are not measures of unsafe sexual practice and hence cannot be correlated with the self-efficacy ratings. There were no significant changes in these areas compared to pre-group estimates. This is in sharp contrast to previous findings in these groups (Wanigaratne *et al.*, 1992) where significant changes were reported. The difference in findings may be a result of how the question was asked. In the previous study participants were asked to estimate the numbers the week before the group and report the numbers during the last week. The current study asked the participants to estimate their activities in terms of bands. Direct questions regarding penetrative sex and unsafe sexual practices have been incorporated into the Overall Evaluation Questionnaire and the follow-up questionnaire recently. The data from these questions should help establish the predictive validity of the SCQ. It is also acknowledged that the number of participants are relatively small and a larger data set is needed before broader generalisations are made.

The trends observed regarding the reduction in the worry about HIV and the increase in the sense of control are consistent with the positive, qualitative feedback received from participants. The validation received from the qualitative feedback appear to be crucial both in terms of the target population and the overall aims of the workshops.

Participants often approached the group with high expectations of what could be achieved in attending. Many aimed to make major changes in sexual behaviour and in other areas of their lives during or soon after the workshop. Some expressed these aims in general, sometimes vague terms, "I want to feel confident as a sexual person" or "I want to enjoy sex more". It became clear that many participants faced difficulties initially, in disclosing unsafe sexual practices and reframed or disguised these practices within these general statements. Gay men who have had or are having unsafe sex can often feel guilt and low self-esteem as a result. Ironically, much of this may stem from promotion of the condom as being the major if not only method of protecting oneself and others from HIV. Workers in the field of HIV prevention with gay men need to recognise ways of offering interventions which are sensitive to these feelings, which do not necessarily place emphasis on "admitting" to unprotected sex.

These difficulties were highlighted by comments made during the group sessions which often seem to be expressions of guilt associated with unsafe sex. Participants frequently described themselves as "bad" or "stupid" for not using condoms. Many stated that they had not talked about their risk-taking behaviour with others and had often not even voiced their concerns with their sexual partners with whom unsafe sex had occurred. Participants frequently expressed feelings of relief in being able to share their anxieties with their group members and to hear of similar behaviours – "knowing that other people do the same thing".

Most group members felt that one of the most positive aspects of the workshops was that the group was supportive and a good forum for sharing of anxieties without peer pressure or fear of censure. "Sharing with other gay men" and "talking about sex with strangers" was seen as helpful. Participants frequently stated how the feeling of safety in the group facilitated their ability to share experiences and thus gain from the group. This safety was felt to result from "group size" (never more than 12), from being "put at ease straight away and no pressure on us to talk made me open up better", from feeling "I had a lot in common (with other participants)", from "sympathetic facilitation" and from "the structure which enabled me to explore difficult/frightening areas".

Overall there was no one particular aspect of the group that any number of participants found unhelpful. Certain areas were identified as either more helpful than others or as requiring more time to be spent on them.

It appears that despite the wealth of material on HIV transmission and safer sex many gay men attending the group still felt either poorly informed or confused and stressed the importance of sessions which dealt with this. The clarity of the information given and the space for participants' personal anxieties to be addressed were noted as especially helpful. Participants were clear that information alone was not enough to facilitate change. Many identified low confidence and self-esteem as influencing their risk-taking behaviour. Some were either initially or subsequently able to go on and identify specific situations in which they wished for help such as "feeling more confident in negotiation" or "hoping to feel better about my body".

Some participants felt stress and anxiety influenced their sexual behaviour in that risk-taking behaviour frequently followed a stressful day or incident. Many requested more work around this topic.

All groups contained at least one or two participants who felt their risk-taking behaviour always followed drug or alcohol use. Many of these linked their drug/alcohol intake to a wish to improve confidence and to help them meet sexual partners but felt it led to "impaired judgement". However, some participants felt that although their drug/alcohol intake was high it played no part in risk-taking behaviour.

The "openness" and "friendliness" of the facilitators was identified as important by many group members as was their professionalism and awareness of boundaries. There was a definite preference for the workshop to be facilitated by gay men, a number of participants stressing they would not have attended if this had not been the case. Some members commented that they would not feel safe or relaxed enough to talk about their sexual behaviour if the facilitators had not been gay men.

The cognitive-behavioural group work format seems an extremely appropriate model of intervention since it can provide a safe an supportive area for making anxieties "public" firstly to oneself, then to other group members and finally to the whole group as appropriate. This appears to help reduce anxiety and promote an impetus for change. Clearly, the reasons for risk-taking are many and complex and relate to individual lifestyles. Most members thus inevitably felt that the groups were too short. Whilst, in effect, no group would have the resources to provide enough time and space to address all its members' needs this does highlight the need for further groups and workshops to address issues more relevant to particular participants. These would also be useful since participants often feel "dropped" at the end of a group and identify further input as important in confirming and maintaining change.

Any such workshop, although primarily focusing on sexual behaviour, must thus also address issues of lifestyle and personal sexual strategies. Furthermore, gay men attending recent groups have requested similar interventions to address risk-taking behaviour and sexual strategies within longer term relationships.

Taking account of the relatively small numbers of participants which these results are based on, the focused workshops do seem to be beneficial in promoting and maintaining safer sexual behaviours. This study shows clear evidence that the workshops were able to produce changes in an important predictor or relapse behaviour, 'Situational Confidence' in a sexual situation. The qualitative feedback confirms this finding and indicates the aspects of sessions which facilitated such changes. It appears that a focused workshop format with limited sessions can produce behaviour change constant with an increase in safer sexual behaviour. Whether individuals will be able to maintain the changes made for longer than three months still needs to be investigated.

ACKNOWLEDGEMENTS

Camden & Islington Health Promotion Service has made this work possible by funding it after its initial stage of development. We would particularly like to thank Ms Victoria George for her enthusiasm, interest and support. We would also like to thank all the doctors, nurses, psychologists and health advisers of University College and Middlesex Hospital GU Medicine Department for their support. We also acknowledge Ms Renee Aroney and Ms Julia Smith for their contribution during the initial stages of running these workshops.

Copies of questionnaires are available from the first author on request.

REFERENCES

Adib, S.M., Joseph, J.G., Ostrow, D.G., Sherman, A.J. (1991) Predictors of relapse in sexual practices among homosexual men. *AIDS Educ. Prevent,* **3**, 293-304

Annis, H. (1986) Relapse prevention model for treatment of alcoholics. In W.R. Miller & N. Heather (Eds) Treating addictive behaviours' process of change. New York: Plenum.

Becker, M. (Ed) (1974) The Health Belief Model. Thorofare, New Jersey, Slack.

Centers for Disease Control. (1991) Patterns of Sexual Behaviour change among homosexual/bisexual men - selected US sites. *MMWR,* **40**, 792-4

Cunningham, R., Stiffman, A.R., Earls, F., Dore, P. (1992) AIDS risk behaviour a new way of committing suicide? *Abstracts of the III International Conference on AIDS.*

Ekstrand, M.L., Coates, T.J. (1990) Maintenance of safer sexual behaviours and predictors of risky sex: the San Francisco Men's Health Study. *Am. J. Public Health,* **80**, 9732-8.

Ekstrand, M.L., Stall, T.D., Marlatt, G.A., Pollack, L.M., McKusick, L. (1992) Will the real relapsers please stand up. *Abstracts of VIII International Conference on AIDS.*

Evans, B.G., Catchpole, M.A., Heptonstall, J. *et al.* (1993) Sexually transmitted diseases and HIV-1 infection among homosexual men in England and Wales. *BMJ,* **306**, 426-8.

Faldiserri, R.O., Lyter, D., Leviton, L.C., et al. (1988) Variables influencing condom use in a cohort of gay and bisexual men. *Am J Public Health,* **78**, 801-5.

Fox, R., Ostrow, D., Valdisseri, R. *et al.* (1987) June 1-5th Changes in sexual activities among participants in the Multicentre AIDS Cohort Study. Paper presented at the III International Conference on AIDS, Washington DC.

Gold, R.S., Karmiloff-Smith, A., Skinner, M.J., Morton J. (1991) Situational factors and thought processes associated with unprotected intercourse in gay men. *Psychol Health,* **5**, 259-78.

Gold, R.S. & Skinner, M.J. (1992) Situational factors and thought processes associated with unprotected intercourse in young gay men. *AIDS,* **6**, 1021-30.

Hays, R.B. Kegeles, S.M., Coates, T.J. (1992) Changes in peer norms and sexual enjoyment predict changes in sexual risk-taking among young gay men. *Abstracts of VIII International Conference on AIDS.*

Hickson, F., Davies, P.M., Hunt, A.J. Weatherburn, P., McManus, TJ., Coxon, APM. (1991). Unsafe sexual behaviour among gay men; a critique of the relapse model. *Abstracts VII International Conference on AIDS.*

Horn, J. & Chetwynd, J. (1989) Changing sexual practices among homosexual men in response to AIDS: who has changed, who hasn't, why? Auckland: *New Zealand Department of Health.*

Hunt, A.J., Davies, P.M., McManus, T.J. *et al.* (1992) HIV Infection in a cohort of homosexual and bisexual men. *BMH,* **305**, 561-2.

Johnson, A.M. & Gill, O.N. (1989) Evidence for recent changes in sexual behaviour in homosexual men in England and Wales. Phil Trans R Soc Lond (Biol) **325**, 153-61.

Keaney, F., Wanigaratne, S., Pullin, J. (1994) The use of a structured assessment interview as an intervention to reduce dropout rates in outpatient relapse prevention groups for problem drinkers. *International Journal of Addictions* (in press).

Kelly, J.A., Lawrence, J.S., Brasfield, T.L. et al. (1990) Psychological factors that predict AIDS high risk versus AIDS precautionary behaviour. *J. Consult. Clin. Psychol.* **58**, 117-20.

Kelly, J.A. Kalishman, S.C., Kauth, M.R. *et al.* (1991) Situational factors associated with AIDS risk behaviour lapses and coping stragegies used by gay men who successfully avoid lapses. *Br. J. Public Health,* **81**, 1335-8.

Klee, H.A. (1992) New target for behavioural research - amphetamine misuse. *Br. J. Addict,* **87**, 439-46.

Marlatt, G.A. & Godon, J.R. (1985) Relapse Prevention: maintenance stragegies in the treatment of addictive behaviours. New York; Guildford.

Martin, J.L. (1987) The impact of Aids on gay male sexual behaviour patterns in New York City. *American Journal of Public Health,* 77, 578-581.

Miller, W.R. (1983) Motivational interviewing with problem drinkers. *Behavioural Psychotherapy,* **1**, 147-172.

Miller, W.R. & Rollnick, S. (1991) Motivational interviewing: Preparing people to change addictive behaviour. New York: Guildford.

McEwan, R.T., McCallam, A., Bhopal, R.S., Madhok, R. (1992) Sex and the risk of HIV infection; the role of alcohol. *British Journal of Addiction,* **87**, 577-84.

McKusick, L., Coates, T.J., Morin, S.F., Pollack, L., Hoff, C. (1990) Logitudinal predictors of reductions in unprotected and intercourse among gay men in San Francisco. *Am J Public Health,* **80**, 9978-83.

McKusker, J., Westenhouse, J., Stoddard, A.M., Zapka, J.G., Zorn, M.W., Mayer, K.H. (1990) Use of drugs and alcohol by homosexually active men in relation to sexual practices. *J. Acquir. Immune. Defic. Syndr.* **3**, 729-36.

Myers, T., Rowe, C.J., Tudiver, F.G., *et al.* (1992) HIV, substance use and related behaviour of gay and bisexual men; an examination of the talking sex project cohort. *Br. J. Addict.* **87**, 207-14.

Phillips, C., Folkman, S., Pollack, L., Chesney, M. (1990) Not stress. but how you cope with it, is related to sexual risk behaviour among gay men. *Abstracts of VI International Conference on AIDS.*

Prochaska, J.O. & DiClemente, C.C. (1986) Towards a comprehensive model of change. In W.R. Miller & N. Healther (Eds.) Treating addictive behaviours: process of change. New York: Plenum.

Stall, R., Ekstrand, Ml, Pollack, L., McKusick, L., Coates, T.J. (1990) Relapse from safer sex; the next challenge for AIDS prevention efforts. *J. Acquir. Immune. Defic. Syndr.,* **3**, 1181-7.

St. Lawrence, J. S., Brasfield, T.L., Kelly, J.A. (1990) Factors which predict relapse to unsafe sex by gay men. *Abstracts of the VI International Conference on AIDS.*

Thornton, S. & Catalan, L. (1993) Preventing the sexual spread of HIV infection - what have we learned? *International Journal of STD & AIDS,* **4**, 311-316.

Van de Laar, M.J.W. Pickering J., Van der Hoek, F.A.R., Van Grievsen, G.J.P., Coutinho, R.A., Van der Water, H.P.A. (1990). Declining gonorrhoea rates in the Netherlands, 1976-88; consequences for the AIDS epidemic. *Genitourin Med,* **66**, 148-55.

Wanigaratne, S., Wallace, W., Pullin, J., Keaney, F., Farmer, R., (1990) Relapse Prevention for Addictive Behaviours; a manual for therapists. Oxford : Blackwell.

Wanigaratne, S., Aroney, R., Williams, M., (1992). Initiating and maintaining safer sex; Description and evaluation of group work with gay men. *Abstracts, VIII International Conference on AIDS.*

Winkelstein, W., Samuel, M., Padian, N.S., Wiley, J.A., Land, W., Anderson, R.E. (1987) The San Francisco men's health study, III, Reduction in Human immunodeficiency virus transmission among homoseuxal-bisexual men. *Am J Publ Health,* **76**, 685-9.

Yalom, I.D. (1975) The theory and practice of group psychotherapy (2nd ed.) New York; Basic Books.

3

Utilising Peer Education and Target Group Empowerment to Induce Behaviour Change on a University Campus: "Projekt 6" at Lund University, Sweden

GARY SVENSON, KENT JOHNSON AND BERTIL S. HANSON

BACKGROUND

"Projekt 6" was initiated in 1991 by the Student Health Clinic, the Departments of Infectious Diseases and Dermatology, University Hospital of Lund, and the Malmöhus County Council. The goal at inception was to design a prevention model that would be adaptable to a target group's social norms and communication styles, capable of engaging both informational and social-normative influences, and able to induce a diffusional increase in safer sex practice from a minority of target group representatives to the target group majority. There was an interest in designing a prevention model that was adaptable to Lund University (33,000 students), as well as other cultures and subgroups.

A longitudinal research evaluation involving 3 anonymous and randomised yearly SAQ mail surveys, qualitative interviews (year 3) and clinical HIV-STD surveys was also instituted. The study is being conducted by Gary Svenson and Bertil S. Hanson via co-operation between the Dept's of Infectious Diseases and Community Health Sciences, University of Lund (Results from survey 1 and 2 presented in poster P016). It is funded separately by a grant from the Swedish Institute of Public Health.

THEORY

The biological influences on human sexual behaviour are conceivably minor in comparison to the influences of social and normative processes, which in turn affect not only communication styles, traditions and behaviour, but also identity. Sexual behaviour in its various manifestations involves communication, and for the individuals involved, some form of social or personal meaning (Ortner & Whitehead, 1981). Human sexuality is complex, and its various meanings are imbedded in a matrix of psycho social phenomena, including gender role, sexual identity, morals, religious beliefs and prestige. Within the traditional KABP model, the effect of social-normative influences on human sexual behaviour are often minimised or ignored. The designers of the model saw a need to expand this perspective. Additionally, the complexity of human sexuality and the variability of social-normative systems (and communication styles) was considered too great for a single top-down, expert-designed approach.

The productiveness of utilising directive blaming tactics, fear inducement and nagging was deemed from both personal field experience and current prevention research, to be questionable. Compliance can be outwardly induced (public self) using such techniques, but a permanent and internalised change in behaviour and attitudes (private self), that is adaptable to the long-term evolution of the HIV-pandemic, is debatable.

To design a prevention model adaptable to students at Lund University and other target groups' communication and social frames of reference, it was decided to incorporate peer education. To further augment target group adaptation as well as peer educator motivation, it was decided to allow the peer representatives to have over-reaching responsibility for the program approach, including strategies, planning, messages, materials, activities, goals, and even the 'culture' or 'spirit' of the program. Therefore target group empowerment was incorporated. E.M. Roger's (1983) theory on the diffusion of innovations was theoretically integrated and utilised in order to induce a slow diffusion of normative and behaviour change from a selected minority to the target group majority.

Roger's concept of "change agent" was adopted in order to define the role of the outside consulting expert. The outside expert often represents an agency or institution which desires to influence client behaviour in a certain direction. He or she is a peripheral figure to the group's norms and interpersonal communication channels and needs operative guidelines. Summarily, the concept of change agent implies that the expert is client-oriented rather than change agency-oriented; makes an active effort in contacting clients, has empathy for client norms, values and needs; does not impose his or her own norms and values on the client system; facilitates rather than directs; and has both competence credibility and trustworthiness in the eyes of the client. Such a role requires intense contact with clients during the early phases, but the goal is eventually to allow the client system to be self-sufficient.

APPLICATION

A step-by-step procedure was set up to make the model operational:

1. Locate the appropriate prevention experts (change agents).
2. Approach relevant student leaders and key individuals with the model.
3. Together with these leaders and key individuals
   - begin project planning
   - agree on the peer educator selection process, with the suggestion of using opinion leaders.
4. Assemble the peer educators and begin project development.
5. Train and educate the peer educators.
6. Begin application.

Project experts (change agents)

The first step was for the interested experts to agree on the model and its application. Funding was then formally applied for at the Swedish Institute of Public Health, and a grant of approx. 10,000 USD was received for the first year (May 1991 - April 1992). Continued funding was to be received from the Malmöhus County Council (May 1992 - May 1994).

Key individuals and leaders

The second step in the practical application of the model was to assemble student leaders or key individuals from the various college unions, clubs, pubs/discos, organisations and faculties. The reasoning behind this step is that group leaders and key individuals have formal influence and status within their group or organisation. They can be innovative if their group's norms are oriented to change, but if norms are opposed to change, these individuals will reflect it via resistance. Through gaining their confidence and co-operation they can be a valuable aid to peer educator selection as well as formally institutionalising a project. Institutional integration was considered important for long-term co-operation and project survival.

Student leader reluctance to an assembly concerning HIV and STD prevention was high, primarily due the boredom of the subject and dissatisfaction with previous nagging campaigns. However, once assembled and given the opportunity fully to define and design their own program, they became very involved. Guidelines and strategies were drawn up by way of focus group seminars and plenary discussions.

The most important conclusions by the student leaders at the meetings were:

1. Non-use of nagging, blaming and fear tactics. The project focus was to be on sex, sexuality, communication, and a generous use of humour.
2. The use of opinion leaders as peer educators was agreed upon. It was decided that these should be students who were socially active, popular, communicative and had an influential position in the group's interpersonal communication network (informal influence). These individuals were to be recruited on a voluntary basis by the individual student leaders.

Peer educators

The next step was to assemble and to begin actual planning with the newly recruited group of 40 opinion leaders. These individuals' attitudes toward prevention were fundamentally the same as those of the student leaders.

The group decided upon a 3-day weekend retreat, where the subjects of sex, sexuality, gender roles, communication, safer sex and peer education techniques were to be covered. Sexologists, approved by the students themselves, were eventually recruited. It was also requested that a HIV positive person their own age participated in the retreat.

Education on HIV/AIDS and STD, conducted by local medical specialists, was also requested and included. The retreat was to be followed up by small discussion/activity groups facilitated by project experts (change agents). The program was named 'Projekt 6', because in Swedish the number '6' and the word 'sex' have the same spelling and pronunciation.

The programme was to be divided into 2 components:

A. Local peer education activities on-site at the represented organisations.

B. University-wide media campaign arranged by groups of peer educators.

All materials were to be student designed, and project experts were to serve as facilitators and consultants. A central advisory committee (board) was created. It included student representatives and expert representatives from the Departments of Infectious Diseases and Dermatology, and the Student Health Clinic. The goal was to transfer the project completely over to the students after 2-3 years. The project was to be renewed on a yearly basis via the same procedure. The reason for this being:

1. To renew project ideas and goals via recruits from the majority in order to:
   - avoid minority polarisation.
   - keep the project in touch with trends.
   - allow majority feedback to the project.
   - keep up with student turnover.
2. To avoid student burnout/dropout.

The Association "Projekt 6"

The above procedure continued to be carried out in 1992 and 1993. In the Spring of 1994 the "Projekt 6 Association" was created and became certified as a non-profit student organisation. Control of the project had been completely transferred to the students. On the association board of directors sit 4 elected peer educators, the chairpersons of the university's 3 largest student unions, 1 representative from the student association of pubs/discos, and one representative each from the Departments of Infectious Diseases and Dermatology, and the Student Health Clinic.

RESULTING ACTIVITIES

Projekt 6 after 3 years has resulted in a wide range of student activities and is today integrated into the student community's social and political structures. Due to the large number of organisations involved (25), and because the students often operate independently, it is difficult to list them in their entirety. However, a brief description of the more interesting activities will follow.

Local peer education activities

The idea of the individual peer education activities is not only to have an effect on those witnessing the activities, but to induce a diffusion effect that will spread through the student communication network such as "ripples on a pond". The purpose is a horizontal student-to-student communication rather than a vertical authority-to-student communication.

- Plays and sketches dramatising typical communication problems concerning safer sex.
- Revues with distribution of "Projekt 6" condoms.
- Articles in student newspapers and newsletters on safer sex, "Projekt 6", sex, HIV, STD, gender roles, and so forth.
- 'Condom patrol' – students who "raid" pubs and discos and distribute condoms.
- Information to new members of local organisations concerning safer sex.
- Safer sex seminars.
- Discussion groups concerning sex, sexuality, safer sex, HIV, etc.
- Distribution of "Projekt 6" condoms at major events, dinners, seminars, festivals, concerts, etc.

- Distribution of "Projekt 6" brochures at a wide variety of occasions and events.
- Lectures within the various faculties and lecture circles on "Projekt 6", HIV, and safer sex.
- Co-operative efforts with local gay organisations and immigrant organisations at various events, for instance, during radio programmes and World AIDS Day.
- Displaying of project posters and brochures at strategic localities.
- Ongoing informal discussions, by the increasing number of peer educators, with other students.

University-wide media campaign

This campaign attempts to reach out to the student population as a whole, and is conducted by those peer educators who are interested in working with the various media. This media campaign has expanded at the peer educators' own pace, which is slower than if the involved experts had executed it themselves during working hours.

It has involved:

- **Poster series:** posters sensualizing and eroticising safer sex (7).
- **Brochure:** a student composed brochure covering HIV, the various STD and safer sex.
- **Weekly radio series** (2 hours) covering sex, sexuality, gender roles and safer sex.
- **Condom and safer sex radio jingles** daily on the student radio station.
- **Articles** in the major student newspaper as well as in the local press.
- "Projekt 6" T-shirts.
- "Projekt 6" condoms
  - distributed free at major events
  - sold at all student pubs/discos for 10-12 cents (retail price is 50-60 cents)
  - distributed free or given as change when ordering beer at student pubs/discos.
- Projekt 6 condoms available free of charge in the city of Lund's taxis.
- Information to new students at various colleges on registration day, including foreign students.

SUMMARY AND CONCLUSIONS

Three important basic questions need to be addressed:

1. is the model, as applied at Lund University, feasible and workable?
2. is the model, with its emphasis on communication and social norms, based on the correct prevention premises?
3. does the model in its application have any prevention impact on the target group?

Question 1

The model has after 3 years shown itself to be applicable within this target group. The student leaders' and peer educators' response has been enthusiastic, and this has led to a range of self-initiated activities. The main problems have occurred when the experts have drifted from the model and their role as "change agent", in order to expedite peer educator undertakings. However, the project was completely transferred into student control in April 1994, and the focus of power lies among them. A new balance will need to be found between the student organisation and the change agents. It is our experience that an open and trusting dialogue between project experts and target group representatives is essential at all stages.

The question of what motivates these students (and possibly other peer educator groups) to become involved naturally arises. The qualitative interviews (see introduction) are not yet concluded, but it appears from experience that the primary motivator is uncertainty. HIV and AIDS is not only a physical reality, but has metaphorically affected personal issues concerning sex, sexuality and sexual norms. There is a need to integrate a new situation (HIV) into an already existing belief system via a search for new information and meaning. Empowered to create and control their own prevention project allows a personal exploration of these issues, within the interpersonal context of a new peer group (project members).

As one involved opinion leader put it: "Having sex in the 1990s implies a risk for getting HIV, and people our age are adapting to this reality. Projekt 6 attempts to facilitate the process."

This particular target group has chosen sex, sexuality, gender roles and communication in their prevention focus. Condom use, in particular, is promoted by the group. It is, however, only one of several risk reduction behaviours discussed and practised.

Question 2

Two of the three planned SAQ mail surveys on undergraduate students between 19 and 28 years old have been completed. The response rate on the 1992 survey was 65.5% (n=442), and was 70.5% (n=492) on the 1993 survey. Contact with the project increased from 49% of students in 1992 to 70% in 1993. Perceived social norms negative to risk reduction behaviour and interpersonal communication barriers were found to be predictors of inconsistent condom use in both surveys. Level of HIV knowledge, degree of pleasure experienced using a condom, and high perceived risk were not predictive. Medium risk was predictive of inconsistent use in survey 1.

Using a model which attempts to adapt to this target group's communication and social frame of reference appears to be a good premise: the questionnaires revealed that only 1-2% of the student majority aware of the project had a negative opinion of it (both surveys), and 72% in 1992, and 76% in 1993, believed that the project's messages applied to them personally. Only 62% in 1992, and 64% in 1993, believed that national HIV-campaigns applied to them personally. It is also revealing that in the 1992 survey, 32% respective 39% believed that the health authorities and the mass media are not telling the whole truth about HIV.

Question 3

Students reached by the project had significantly higher condom use in both surveys, and logistic regression analysis (95% CI) found that contact with the project was a predictor of consistent condom use (OR=2.2, CI=1.3,3.6) in survey 2. In the one year interval between the surveys, consistent condom use with new partners among undergraduate students increased from 47% to 60% (P=.0001), perceived social norms negative to safer sex decreased 11.5% (P=.002) and low subjective knowledge (self-efficacy) decreased 7.5% (P<.05). The data could suggest that a minority of peer educators/opinion leaders can, under the conditions of this model, effect majority attitudes and behaviours. Such inferences concerning the project's impact, the durability of the student organisation, must wait until the conclusion of the entire study.

REFERENCES

Ortner, S.B. & Whitehead, H (1981). Sexual Meanings: the cultural construction of gender and sexuality. New York, N.Y: Cambridge University Press.

Rogers, E.M. (1983). Diffusion of Innovations. New York: Free Press.

Turner, J.C. (1991). Social Influence. Buckingham, UK: Open University Press.

4

HIV/AIDS Education in the Workplace: "It's not my responsibility..."

KAREN GADD AND DAVID GOSS

INTRODUCTION

The development of training and education relating to HIV and AIDS in the workplace remains an issue which many organisations are reluctant to tackle. This is surprising considering the fact that HIV/AIDS within the workplace has such far reaching consequences (including increased stress, fear and discrimination) for both the person living with HIV or AIDS, their colleagues and the organisation. Such consequences can be diverse, ranging from increased fear amongst the employees, which may lead to discrimination or stress related problems, to more serious incidents, such as refusal of fellow employees to work alongside an employee living with, or even suspected of living with, HIV or AIDS. (Tolley *et al* 1991; Slack *et al* 1992; Cone 1989).

Although the current economic climate is pushing AIDS education further down organisations' priority lists, waiting until an incident occurs can be much more expensive than implementing training. An examination of the literature however, reveals that some organisations have endeavoured to address this issue. (eg IDS 528, 1993). The strategies which have been adopted tend to fall into one of the following three categories: Information Giving which includes the provision of written information such as leaflets, Empowerment Strategies which enable individuals to identify the blocks to rational action, and Community Development Approaches which aim to enhance health by bringing about community change through collective action. (For more information concerning such strategies see Goss *et al.* 1994).

Implementing these strategies is potentially beneficial for organisations in terms of reducing the fear and misunderstanding which can ultimately affect productivity levels. However, confronting the issue of HIV/AIDS pro-actively in the workplace is often problematic. For example, many managers and personnel specialists dismiss AIDS as a non-issue for companies or as someone else's problem. They refuse to regard the issue as part of their responsibility.

The issue of responsibility inter-alia was addressed during the course of a large in-depth research programme conducted by the Centre for AIDS and Employment Research (CAER). The CAER research programme collected a comprehensive set of data relating to attitudes, values and definitions of HIV and AIDS as a workplace issue, both from a managerial and a workforce perspective. In total one hundred and six interviews were conducted in eleven organisations from a range of geographical locations and industrial sectors (Goss *et al* 1994).

Throughout this paper, the implications of the attitudes and responses which emerged from the research programme are appraised and their relevance to the debate concerning responsibility for information provision is considered.

AIDS TRAINING AND INFORMATION STRATEGIES

It is important to recognise that the widely perceived moral and threatening character associated with HIV/AIDS means that training and education can never be a simple matter. Clearly a precondition for any development in this area is the provision of good, reliable factual data about the virus. For instance: that becoming HIV positive is a result of behaviour not of social identity; that HIV can only be transmitted through blood to blood or sexual contact and not through ordinary workplace activity; that a person who is HIV positive can be perfectly healthy for many years and that someone with living with AIDS is not necessarily going to die immediately or be totally incapacitated. It is also necessary to address the attitudes, values and emotional responses of individuals because these can play an important role in determining the extent to which factual data is seen as credible (Goss and Adam-Smith 1993). For example, one chef who was interviewed by CAER was absolutely convinced that HIV could be transmitted upon money. He was willing to ask all his waitresses to wear rubber gloves. When it was pointed out that the information his judgements were based on was inaccurate, his response was: "It can't be wrong, I read it in The Sun!" Thus the attitudinal and behavioural dimension of training is likely to be important as more organisations develop formal policies relating to HIV and AIDS and expect employees to respond appropriately to them.

There are then a number of issues which education and training relating to HIV/AIDS must include: Medical Facts (factual information relating to individual risk); Legal Facts (factual information relating to conduct required by employment law in relation to HIV/AIDS); Organisational Information (relating to the nature and reasons for conduct required by the organisations policies/stance towards HIV/AIDS) and Individual Reasons (guidance relating to personal conduct, feelings, values and emotions). This means that managers will need to be aware of the basic medical facts connected with HIV/AIDS and with their legal responsibilities as representatives of the organisation towards employees with the virus. They will also need to understand the stance taken by the organisation and be able to act in accordance with this. Actually communicating such information is the key to effective education. Many of the organisations that have attempted to implement HIV/AIDS education have tended to use one or more of the three categories that were mentioned in the introduction:

Information Provision

This approach assumes that individuals will rationally avoid what they have been warned about, usually in the form of a leaflet drop. This is largely a 'do-it-yourself' approach which relies on top down communication from an 'expert' source. Many organisations have chosen this method because of the appeal of relatively low cost and broad coverage, however research has indicated that this approach alone is often insufficient to bring about clear and lasting behaviour change:

> "I think a lot more information should come down from the site to the shop floor people. Because you have to give people credit, they become more aware the more information that you give them.
>
> It might come down from a certain level through the management structure, but as it comes down, it is cascaded down through the structure. People get busier and busier and their jobs are more varied and it probably gets lost. I don't know but not enough information comes down" (shop floor worker).

Empowerment Strategies

These aim to reduce the incidence of illness and disease by enhancing people's ability to act rationally rather than on the basis of un-reflected emotions and feelings. The means of achieving this goal is via participatory learning, group work and self-exploration to help learners identify the choices they can make. These means also enable individuals to identify the extent to which emotions and attitudes may block an ability to act rationally and sensibly. However self empowerment strategies suffer from a number of deficiencies; most of them stem from their focus on the individual. For instance, someone who has been on an assertiveness course may feel more powerful at the end of it, but these feelings often disappear once the situation that led to the original feeling of powerlessness is encountered:

> "In the event of an accident, we would be required, like say a guy got his hand stuck in machinery, then it would be the job of the maintenance fitter to free him. If you see blood, it suddenly pops into your mind: 'God! HIV/AIDS!' and your job is to release the hand" (maintenance fitter).

As a result some health educators have favoured collective and community based approaches.

Community Development Approaches

These aim to enhance health by bringing about community change through collective action. The means of achieving this goal is via participatory learning and group work around shared experiences which lead to the identification of collective needs and planning to meet these. A particularly good example of this approach can be observed in a beauty products manufacturing company. The main feature of their HIV/AIDS awareness campaign was a series of awareness sessions, first for managers and then for all head office employees, staff were given the option of joining a single sex group if they wished. At the end of the sessions a questionnaire was circulated to enable those with questions to ask them.

In addition, the company bought in an interactive theatre company to run theatre workshops exploring the emotional issues raised by HIV and AIDS in the workplace. The actors performed a scenario, with one character revealing her HIV positive status and the other actors playing a colleague, a manager and the employee's husband; they frequently broke off to seek advice and comment from the audience. The manufacturing company was pleased with the response and is planning to repeat the sessions with the shop staff.

Implementation

Implementation of these strategies has been shown to be a worthwhile method of educating employees in the United States of America. For instance:

> Driving into the car park one morning, the Human Resources Director found employees milling around the back door of the company, refusing to enter the building. She knew that a long-time employee had called to say he would be returning to work that day after being hospitalised for Pneumocystis carinii pneumonia and wanted his co-workers to know his diagnosis. She put two and two together and came to the depressing conclusion that no-one wanted to work with a colleague who was living with AIDS.
>
> What happened next however surprised her. When the returning employee reached the car park, his co-workers wouldn't go inside until each person had offered him a hug, a card, flowers or some balloons. Astonished and laden with tokens of his co-workers goodwill and compassion, the employee began one of the best days of his working life! (Breuer 1992)

This is in stark contrast to how employees often react to the first case of HIV/AIDS in the workplace. When this happens there is often a stream of worried employees who are afraid of contact and visit personnel or occupational health departments posing hypothetical questions (Banas 1992). People are often afraid of what they don't comprehend and therefore are unhappy about working in the same environment as a person rumoured to be living with HIV/AIDS. However, having experienced thorough training, the employees should be aware that they are not at risk and their fear is likely to be greatly reduced.

In spite of the literature which proclaims the value of education, (Breuer 1992, IDS Study 528, Society of Occupational Medicine 1993), tackling the issue of HIV/AIDS in the workplace pro-actively is often problematic. For example, many managers and personnel specialists dismiss AIDS as a non-issue for companies or as someone else's problem. Alternatively they may not wish to have their name associated with such an emotive issue for fear that doing so will have a negative consequence for the business. The CAER research demonstrated that there was a widespread 'background concern' rooted in individuals inadequate understanding of HIV/AIDS and the exact nature of work related risk:

> "....I mean it flashes through your mind doesn't it? Um, there is always the thought at the back of your head, um, we have found that a lot of waiters or shall we say in inverted commas, "waitresses" are gay. You are always wary of that. Um, not so much chefs as far as I know in the trade again. It has only been recently the last few years I suppose that AIDS or HIV has come to life....... I'm in contact with raw meat and things like that so there is cross-contamination there..." (leisure centre chef).

This quote illustrates the still widely held, yet erroneous belief that HIV and AIDS is a 'gay disease', the respondent is also misinformed about the transmission routes of the virus: he is worried about cross contamination of blood when handling raw meat. This uncertainty means that many respondents, especially managers feel unprepared to deal effectively with issues attributable to HIV in workplace settings. For example:

> "Last year the local Health Education Council ran some training.... it made me very aware of how little I actually knew about the subject although I thought that I knew a fair amount.... I thought it was foolhardy to work on the assumption that it was never going to happen here, by the law of averages, I guess it's going to happen in most organisations at some point, and I am also perfectly aware of the fact that if we do get a member of staff with AIDS then the person they come to, to say, 'What do we do now?' is me. I thought I probably ought to be better aware than I am" (Personnel Manager).

However, an interesting paradox emerged in the course of the research; although many of the respondents felt unable to deal with the issue, HIV/AIDS was not considered to be of immediate and pressing relevance within the context of employment.

> "Nobody's ever talked about it specifically. Some years ago, when there was more of a scare we would talk about children in the schools and what was the potential likeliness of problems but none of us had any knowledge" (Administrative assistant).

For most managers, AIDS was not an issue that was high on their list of immediate priorities, and for most non-managers, it was not something that was at the forefront of their concerns regarding employment. Even among occupational health staff the subject of HIV and AIDS was something of a non-issue. HIV and AIDS education was something which was encompassed by the umbrella of health promotion. This is not encouraging for those who are keen to implement awareness training because in many organisations the umbrella remains closed. Health promotion is considered to be a 'nice-to-have', something that is more of a luxury, rather than a necessity. On many occasions during the interviews conducted, it emerged that although respondents regarded the provision of such information as both desirable and essential it was not a matter which was considered to be of great urgency. The extent to which this is prioritised is very much dependant upon the nature and significance of existing hazards to employees health in the workplace (eg. noise, chemicals, machinery). In particular, occupational health representatives from the 'heavy' industries were keen to explain that although they believed health promotion was an important aspect of occupational health, it was not on their priority list simply because the majority of their time was spent managing the day-to-day problems encountered in the work environment:

> "I think that the health promotion thing is obviously important..... Health promotion is probably, I'd have thought about a quarter of our work..... I think it is important that we devote time to it, and hopefully we will devote more time to it, but we have got other priorities" (CMO for a heavy industry).

Thus although the provision of education regarding health promotion issues is recognised as being of great importance, many managers and occupational health physicians must first deal with other issues considered to have greater priority.

RESPONSIBILITY

Managers, then, are faced with the challenge of reconciling an obligation to humanity, (ie. provision of education for their employees) and an obligation to organisation they belong to. It is clear that the majority of those likely to be affected by the virus are those who make up the bulk of the workforce at present (ie. those aged between 20 and 40 years). It is therefore important that HIV and AIDS be made a priority. Before long, most organisations will be affected by this issue, either because an employee is living with HIV or AIDS, or has a partner, member of the family or a friend who is living with HIV/AIDS.

Sooner, rather than later, it is likely that both the manager and the occupational physician will have to deal with an HIV or AIDS related matter concerning an employee, patient or colleague. Advance planning and preparation is more likely to lay the foundation for a reasoned, structured and appropriate approach when the time comes, rather than relying upon a reactive 'We'll tackle it when it arises' philosophy. Shaun Whelan (1992) put forward the important point that 'any exploration of HIV and AIDS is likely to raise issues which society on the whole finds difficult to face openly and objectively, (sexuality, death and disease) thus creating anxiety, fear and prejudice.....if handled sensitively education can go some way to alleviating such potentiality....the alternative is to manage the crisis...' The obligation to humanity and to the organisation need not therefore be mutually exclusive. Preparing for the likelihood of HIV/AIDS in the workplace fulfils both obligations to humanity and at the same time to the organisation. Education of the employees is likely to avert the crisis referred to by Whelan.

One way of encouraging employers to provide such training and information may be to emphasize the economic costs that the company may incur as a result of not implementing such educative strategies. Cameron (1993) cites Fox and Thomas:

> "Economists can predict the average costs for services for people living with AIDS. However these direct expenses pale in comparison with the loss to society of the potential economic productivity of relatively young people whose lives end prematurely. Add indirect costs generated by disruptions in social and economic activity caused by the fear of contagion and the resulting price tag is astronomical" (Fox and Thomas 1990).

The need for training has probably never been greater. It is shocking to discover just how much ignorance still exists. There are still many people who believe that, for instance, sharing of cups or toilets with people living with HIV/AIDS constitutes a major risk to their wellbeing, who also think that the virus can be transmitted by casual contact such as hand shaking, or by handling money. It appears that information is urgently needed in spite of all attempts to educate the general population. Perhaps a different emphasis is now required; rather than focusing upon transmission routes, an emphasis on how the virus cannot be transmitted would be more useful in dispelling the myths which abound. HIV/AIDS education within the workplace context offers many benefits which can be reaped by both employer and employee, for instance:

- Prevention of new infections among employees (and their families) by providing information about how HIV is and isn't transmitted.
- Preventing discrimination by fearful or misinformed employees by dispelling myths.
- Raising morale and alleviating fear and anxiety.

In order to be effective, health education must speak directly to the employees. The information must be relayed to them in a manner which facilitates understanding as to how HIV/AIDS relates to them as individuals. Not in a way which is so far removed from their everyday experience that it appears to have no significance to them.

The CAER research programme has provided support for the notion that obligations to humanity and the organisation are not in fact mutually exclusive, but are reconcilable. The question then, is not whose responsibility it is to provide such information, rather how such information can realistically be provided in both a time and cost-effective manner.

One way of achieving this is the use of the initiative developed by the Terrence Higgins Trust called Positive Management. This training package is the result of a research venture undertaken by the Terrence Higgins Trust and includes a video which raises many important HIV/AIDS related dilemmas managers are likely to encounter in the workplace. A training manual accompanies the video and gives full details on how to run interactive training options while the information pack contains briefing notes aimed to be an aid to policy makers. Use of this excellent training aid is cost effective and straightforward to implement, and is validated by the results of the CAER research.

To conclude, before managers dismiss AIDS as a non-issue for companies or as someone else's problem, they should recall Tedlow and Marram's (1991) point that 'For many adults, the workplace is the only place they receive this life saving information'. Instead of concluding that HIV/AIDS education is not a managerial or organisational responsibility, perhaps the likely responses of an uneducated and misinformed workforce should be contemplated. After all, even if no-one in the company today has been affected by HIV/AIDS, who knows what tomorrow may bring?

REFERENCES

Banas, G.E. (1992) Nothing Prepared me to manage AIDS, *Harvard Business Review, July-August*, pp. 26-33.

Breuer, N.L. (1992) AIDS issues haven't gone away, *Personnel Journal*, **71** (1), 47-49.

Cameron, M.E. (1993) Living with AIDS: Experiencing Ethical Problems, SAGE Publications, London.

Cone, L.A. (1989) AIDS and HIV in the workplace, *Mental and Physical Disability Law Reporter*, **13** (1) pp. 70-77.

Goss, D. and Adam-Smith, D. (1993) Empowerment or disempowerment? The limits and possibilities of workplace AIDS policy. Paper presented at The VII Social Aspects of AIDS Conference, South Bank University.

Goss, D., Gadd, K., Adam-Smith, D., and Meudell, K. (1994) "HIV/AIDS: The Implications for Training" Training Matters 1, 2.

IDS Study 528 (1993) AIDS returns to the agenda, April. Nov-Dec pp. 14-25

Slack, J.D. and Luna, A. (1992) AIDS related documents from 96 American cities and counties, Public Administration Review **52** (3) pp. 305-308.

Society of Occupational Medicine (1993) What employers should know about HIV AIDS, The Wellcome Foundation Ltd.

Tedlow, R.S and Marram, M.S. (1991) A case of AIDS, *Harvard Business Review*, **69** (6) 14-25.

Tolley, K., Maynard, A. and Robinson, D. (1991) HIV/AIDS and Social Care: Discussion paper 81, Centre for Health Economics, Institute for Health Studies.

Whelan, S. (1992) Managing a crisis: Employer policy on HIV and AIDS in North Nottinghamshire, North Nottinghamshire Health Authority.

5

Ten Years of AIDS Images in the Puerto Rican Press: 1983-1992

INEKE CUNNINGHAM,
LYNNETTE RIVERA-RODRÍGUEZ,
SIGFRIDO STEIDEL-FIGUEROA AND
ERNEST L. CUNNINGHAM

BACKGROUND

The impact of the AIDS epidemic on the Puerto Rican population has reached alarming proportions. From 1981 until mid-June, 1994, 13,517 persons have been diagnosed with AIDS in a population of some 3.2 million inhabitants (Department of Health, 1994). By 1991, AIDS was the fourth overall cause of mortality, and the first cause of death among men between 25 and 49 years of age and among women between 29 and 39 years of age (Department of Health, 1993). Since neither cure nor vaccine will be available in the near future, prevention is at present the only means toward minimizing the epidemic.

Prevention requires information about HIV and AIDS, the means of HIV transmission and methods of prevention, among others. Correct information must be given to the public if the HIV/AIDS epidemic is to be fought effectively. What we learn about a concept or a situation comes from observation, interpersonal communication, books, or the mass media. The mass media are certainly the most rapid and widespread means to disperse information to the public. However, they are not only a means of information dispersal. The media are also able to shape attitudes and focus attention. Thus, they are not only a major factor in determining what the public knows about important issues, but also what the public thinks about them.

No single component of the media includes all the information presented to the public, but the daily press leaves a printed record of all it has presented, so it can be studied in its entirety. Since we are interested in what information reaches people in Puerto Rico regarding HIV/AIDS, we have, therefore, been studying the Puerto Rican press.

Some theories of mass communication have conceived the mass media as the "transformers and interpreters" of reality in the gathering and transmission of information (Crane, 1992). They do not provide a neutral narration of the available information about what goes on in the world. An event becomes news not necessarily when it takes place, but when an editor decides that it is news (Klaidman, 1990). Reporters and editors select and structure information according to what they consider, from their own perspective, most important and "newsworthy". In this way, social reality is reconstructed by selectively including and ordering some information and excluding other, or giving alternate interpretations. Therefore, the information offered to the reader depends on the perceptions and ideology of the reporters, editors and owners of the newspapers, as well as on factors such as available space, what other stories are available at the moment, in which order they might be placed in the paper, and whether or not photographs or images are available to accompany the text. As cars and groceries, news is merchandise in a competitive market.

The language used in the reporting of events is part of their construction. It generally reflects the ideology of the management and the characteristics of the population which the newspaper wants to reach and, thus, it conditions how information is perceived and evaluated by the readers.

Visual images, whether they are illustrations, photographs, caricatures or graphs, not only attract attention to an article in particular, but also convey messages in themselves. They may help determine whether a reader reads a given article or not. Also, due to the haste with which society lives, readers frequently read the newspaper rapidly. Therefore, they sometimes note mostly the images, so these become a significant part of the message which the reader gets.

Like metaphors, visual images are also constructions. But the understanding of words may depend on the reading skills and the vocabulary of the reader, whereas it is relatively simple to perceive the message of an image, despite reading skills and level of education. Like words, though, images contain values and valuative implications, and are not simply photographs of reality.

The use of images in AIDS reporting has been studied in several contexts. Gilman (1988) has discussed how images of disease, including AIDS, have been used to construct definitions of diseases which will permit the general public to confirm to themselves that they are unlike those who are sick, and therefore do not have to fear the disease. Watney (1988) has shown how, earlier in the epidemic, images of AIDS enabled the British press to consider it as an exclusive problem for gay males, and therefore not a problem for heterosexuals. Another article illustrates how television can use images to neutralize the negative messages of homophobia and deterioration associated with AIDS (Gever, 1988).

The content and metaphors of AIDS reporting in the Puerto Rican press have also been studied. Cunningham (1989) analyzed all items relating to AIDS and HIV in daily newspapers from 1981 through 1987, with a particular interest in the local controversies at the time. She concluded that AIDS controversies had, for the most part, been viewed by the local press as party-level political bickering. A later study, covering the reportage through 1990, compared the content and metaphors with those used in the U.S. and concluded that whereas, like in the United States, earlier reporting had focused on risk groups and the danger their members posed to the population in general, more recent reporting tended to be more positive, emphasizing community efforts against the epidemic and the benefits of care (Cunningham & Cunningham, 1991). However, the visual images have not been studied, so in this article we will analyze those images which have been used to illustrate AIDS articles in the Puerto Rican press.

METHODS

All items in the five major daily newspapers of Puerto Rico which include the words AIDS or HIV or, prior to 1983, any reference to an immunologic disease related to homosexuals, have been reviewed and classified[1]. The accompanying illustrations to the items have also been classified and analyzed, and these visual images form the data for the present article. The analysis did not include photographs, nor any illustrations from advertisements.

A panel of 4 persons analyzed each image appearing in the newspapers through 1992 in terms of the themes it appeared to represent, and, separately, as to whether it conveyed a positive, negative or neutral impression. Both these classifications were made independently of the theme of the article illustrated by the image. In a few cases, it was not clear which of the accompanying articles mentioning the word "AIDS" was the one an image represented. Of the images examined, slightly more than 3% (35) were so imprecise that a classification by theme could not be carried out, but whether the impression was positive, neutral or negative was determined for all of them.

FINDINGS

A little over a 1000 (1,061) non-photographic illustrations or cartoons were analyzed. Figure 5.1 shows the distribution of these images by year. Prior to 1983, no illustrations were found for any of the newspaper items referring to what was to become AIDS. Very few images appeared before 1985. The greatest number appeared during the years 1987 (257) and 1988 (183). Marked increases in the

[1]The daily papers published during this time in Puerto Rico were El Mundo, El Nuevo Día, El Reportero, El Vocero and The San Juan Star. The latter is published in English, while the others are in Spanish. El Vocero and El Reportero are not published on Sundays. The San Juan Star was closed by a strike for several months during 1985, and El Mundo was not published for several weeks at the end of 1987. El Reportero ceased publication in 1987 and El Mundo, for the second time, in December, 1990.

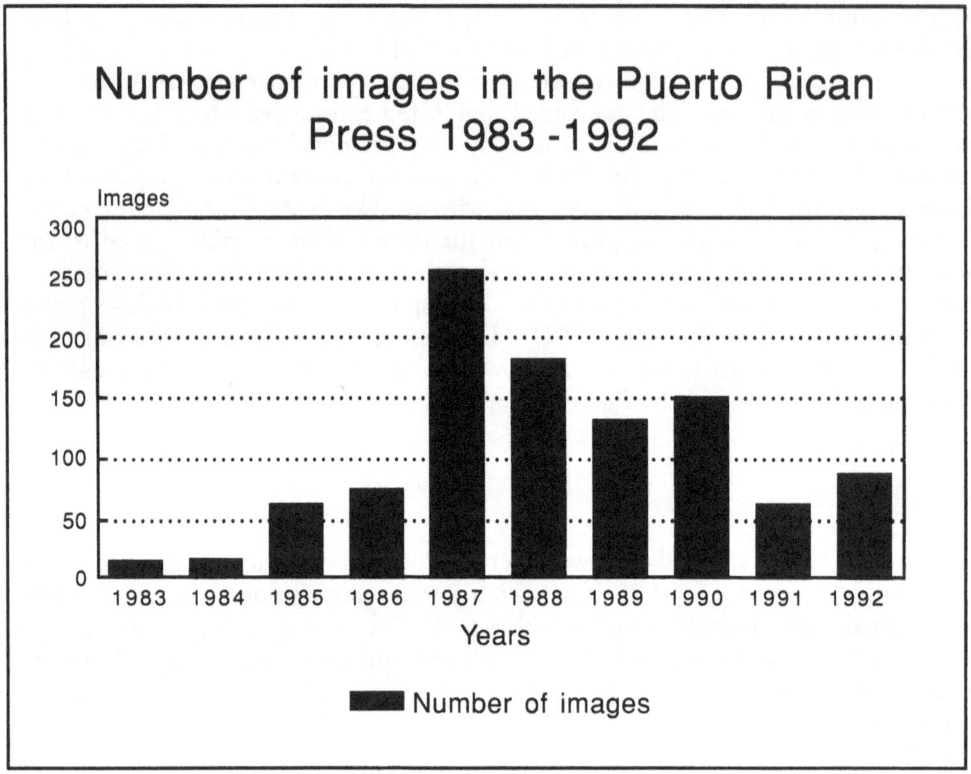

Fig. 5.1 Total number of visual images, both original and repeated, illustrating AIDS articles in the Puerto Rican Press by year, 1983 - 1992. No images appeared prior to 1983

number of AIDS articles in the Puerto Rican daily press in the years 1983, 1985, and 1987, resulted from specific occurrences in the AIDS epidemic[2], which corresponded to the years of increase in images. The number of AIDS articles decreased sharply as one of the newspapers ceased publication in December, 1990, and the Gulf War took over the press in January, 1991. Consequently, the number of images dropped as well.

The images are very diverse, differing in size, form and complexity. About half of these images (532) are original, the rest being repeats of images previously used. The great majority are repeated only once, but one image appears over 50 times, and 2 others appear over 20 times each. All told, 18 different images appear ten or more times.

[2]As Cunningham and Cunningham (1991) point out, the national press coverage of a medical article suggesting casual contact as a possible means of spread in May, 1983, the admission by Rock Hudson that he had AIDS in July, 1985, and a series of full page advertisements in the Puerto Rican press warning that it was unsafe to receive care from a health worker whose HIV status was unknown in September, 1987, were each related to a marked increase in press articles related to AIDS, with a maintenance of the new level for at least two years.

The most common theme, found in more than 43% of the images (460), is that of death. The percentage of images representing death, although higher among the few images of 1983 and 1984, change very little from year to year. This theme is usually identified by the presence of a skull or skeleton or, sometimes, the allegorical figure of death with a hooded cloak and scythe. However, not all images of death are this direct. Examples of other representations of death include candles burned to the candelabra, a vase with a wilted plant, and an empty baby carriage. In more than 70% of the images of death, the death figure or skeleton appears without any other figures, giving the simplified message that AIDS equals death. Five of the most frequently repeated images, including the one repeated more than 50 times, are of this nature. In the others, "death" is accompanied by a single figure, a couple, a group or a crowd.

The images of death frequently contain other themes as well. In one figure, for example, a couple is embracing inside a coffin, with the skeleton feet at the bottom making it clear that heterosexual sex equals death. In another, a couple is dancing on a cat's cradle woven by a death figure, suggesting that engaging in heterosexual sex is playing with death. Death is accompanied by symbols of sex, such as valentines, gender symbols or two persons, nearly 20% of the time (86 images), or of drugs, such as syringes or needles, nearly ten percent of the time (45 images). Other themes accompanying images of death occur, but are less common.

The next most frequent theme represented is sex or love. This is represented by couples (heterosexual or homosexual), gender symbols (at times intertwined), valentines, cupids, or some variation of these. Figure 5.2 shows cupid with a surgical

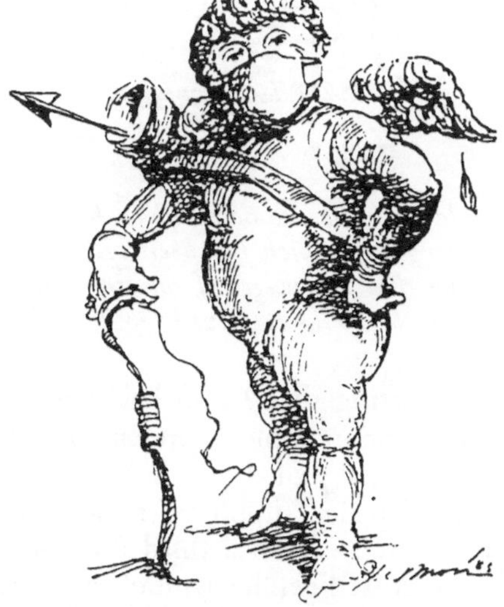

Fig. 5.2 Cupid, representing sex, wears a surgical mask, perhaps suggesting contamination through sex, and has a broken bow, indicating that casual sex has been to some degree crippled by AIDS. A feather dropping from his wing may indicate the slight deterioration of the concept of casual sex in the time of AIDS.
Published with permission of El Nuevo Dia, May 28, 1987.

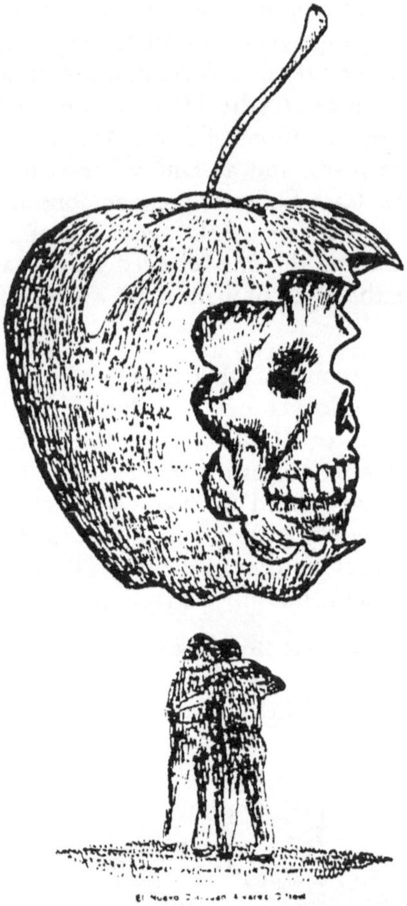

Fig. 5.3 A couple which could be either homosexual or heterosexual embraces underneath an apple, representing sin, which has been bitten, with the bite line forming the profile of a skull, indicating that the wages of the sin of sex is death. Published with permission of El Nuevo Dia, November 29, 1991.

mask and a broken bow, suggesting that AIDS has markedly limited casual love. Some images (the devil, a snake or an apple) represent sin and usually accompany a representation of sex, but occasionally of drugs or both, and sometimes death (see Figure 5.3). Despite the general belief, supported to some extent in the press, that AIDS is a homosexual disease, more than a third (77) of the images of sex refer specifically to heterosexual sex (mixed gender symbols or mixed couples), and only a quarter (52) to homosexual sex, always male (male couples or intertwined male gender symbols). Only 5% (10) refer to bisexual sex or multiple partners (a single gender symbol with both a cross and an arrow attached, several male symbols with only one female symbol). The rest are nonspecific. Although, like death, the percentage of all images representing sex does not change markedly from year to year, specific representations do change. Prior to 1985 there are no sex symbols of specific orientation, but from 1985 to 1990, the number of homosexual representations is approximately equal to the number of heterosexual representations. In 1991 and 1992 the number of heterosexual representations is significantly higher.

Although skulls or death figures are the most common representations of AIDS in these images, another representation is AIDS as a monster (see Figure 5.4). This takes such forms as a hairy monster consuming the island of Puerto Rico, octopus tentacles strangling the globe, or an iceberg with a dread visage labelled AIDS. Sometimes the letters are monstrous, such as the "A" of AIDS as a shark's head with many sharp teeth, or the "S" of SIDA (the Spanish acronym for AIDS) with teeth and a forked tongue. In one image, the monster is being chased by a globe wielding an axe. In this image, suggesting that the disease can be confronted and even overcome, AIDS is represented as a monster rather than a symbol of death. Generally the symbol of death dominates the illustration, no matter what other theme is included.

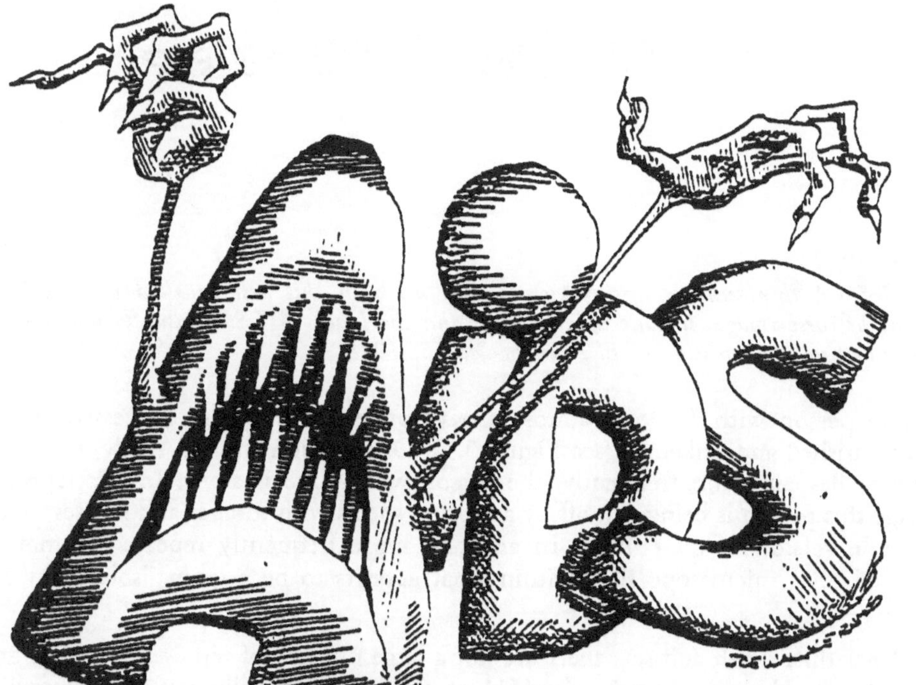

Fig. 5.4 AIDS as a monster, literally, with the first letter taking monstrous form. Published with permission of El Nuevo Dia, April 27, 1986.

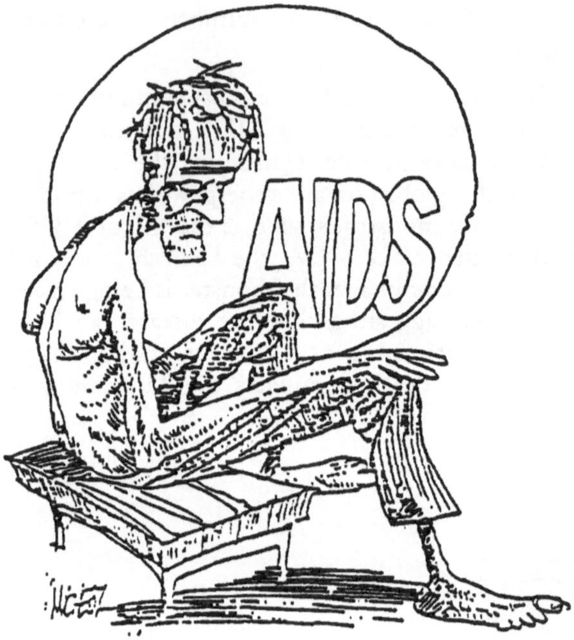

Fig. 5.5 A thin, unkempt, shirtless, shoeless man, in this case labelled with AIDS. Many of these images include a large disc, and the label "AIDS: is usually not present. Published with permission of El Mundo, May 5, 1988.

The person with AIDS is almost always presented as male, depressed, weak, malnourished and unkempt (see Figure 5.5). On occasions he (or, rarely, she) is in pain or despair. Most frequently, the person with AIDS is alone. In one repeated image this person is being run off by a mob in sheets with torches and crosses, in an extreme version of quarantine. In another, more frequently repeated, a man is trapped on a microscope slide within what appears to be a germ, isolated by his disease.

Other than death and sex, there are not a large number of representations of any one theme. However, nearly 5% (51) of the images are illustrations presenting graphs or tables of statistics, while over 3% (34) represent science or medicine. Nearly all of these are considered neutral in impact.

Many other themes are presented, but seldom, with fewer than 15 images each. Drug usage is represented, but usually accompanying death, sex, or both. Vertical transmission and transmission by blood are both represented, as are persons particularly affected by the disease, such as women and children, and the economic and political aspects of the epidemic. There are a few images of care and hope, the former usually consisting of one person showing concern for another, and the latter usually showing an individual or couple approaching a lighted area from the darkness, or looking up with a hopeful expression (see Figure 5.6).

Some of the images are complicated, appearing to contain many messages. For example, Figure 5.7 shows two different scenes at the same time. In the top part of

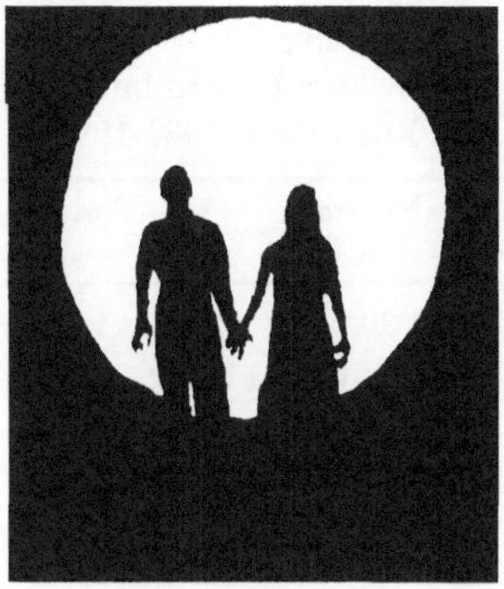

Fig. 5.6 A heterosexual couple, holding hands and walking towards a circle of light, is representative of the few messages of hope which have appeared.
Published with permission of El Nuevo Dia, May 1, 1988.

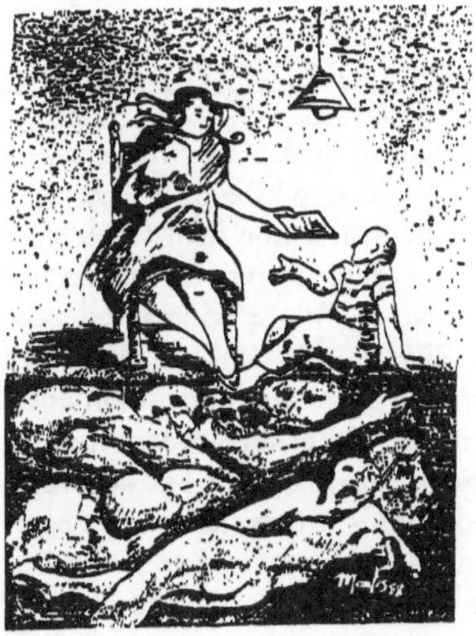

Fig. 5.7 A complicated image, described in the text. The word visible on the book cover is "SIDA", the Spanish acronym for AIDS.
Published with permission of El Nuevo Dia, June 28, 1987.

the scene, an adult woman without a mouth is holding out a book labelled "AIDS" to a child at her feet. There is a flow of information, even if it is diluted by the absence of the mouth, which may suggest that discussion of AIDS and sex is taboo. At the bottom of the picture is a field of cadavers, piled as in a mass grave, some of which are clearly women and children. Although giving information about AIDS to children is a positive message of prevention, the total figure is dominated by death. This illustration is used complete in some instances, while in some instances only the upper or the lower half is used. Therefore, essentially, the same image can give either a positive or negative impression.

Table 5.1
Positive, Negative and Neutral Images in the
Puerto Rican Press: 1983-1992

Year	Negative %	Neutral %	Positive %	Total %
1983	66.7	20.0	13.3	100 (N= 15)
1984	70.5	0.0	29.5	100 (N= 17)
1985	75.0	15.6	9.4	100 (N= 64)
1986	75.3	11.7	13.0	100 (N= 87)
1987	71.6	20.6	7.8	100 (N= 257)
1988	78.1	15.8	6.1	100 (N= 183)
1989	75.4	17.1	7.5	100 (N= 134)
1990	76.1	17.3	6.6	100 (N= 151)
1991	58.8	31.7	9.5	100 (N= 63)
1992	76.6	18.9	4.5	100 (N= 90)
TOTAL	73.2	18.9	7.9	100 (N= 1,061)

Table 5.1 shows the impressions given by the images. Nearly three quarters (73.2%) give a negative impression, while only 7.9 percent of the images are positive. The impression given by nearly one fifth (18.9%) is considered neutral. All images of death or isolation are determined to be negative. Of nineteen of 217 images representing sex, less than 10% are considered positive, while most of the rest are considered negative. Five of the positive sexual images represent safe sex. Other examples of positive images of sex include a man and a woman holding a rose between them. Gender symbols, whether intertwined or not, and cupids are examples of neutral sex images, and images of sex accompanied by death, a snake, drug paraphernalia or horned cupids are examples of negative images. Most of the drawings illustrating graphs and those representing science or medicine are neutral unless they include skulls or death figures, or suggest inordinate profit-making by groups of individuals such as pharmacists or physicians. All the messages of hope and care are considered positive.

In the course of the AIDS epidemic, the reasons for hope increase as more is learned about the condition, but positive images have not become more frequent.

Actually, the ratio of positive images to negative images is slightly higher in the earlier years of the epidemic than in the more recent ones. The actual percentage of positive or negative images has not changed much. Neither in the impressions given nor in the themes covered have the images used by the press in Puerto Rico in portraying AIDS changed much during the epidemic, although the epidemic itself has changed in several ways.

CONCLUSIONS

The press, in its important role in providing information to the public regarding HIV/AIDS, has two means at its disposal to portray the epidemic: metaphorical language and visual images. It uses each in different ways. While the language has taken AIDS from a "gay plague" dangerous to "risk groups" to a chronic disease which must be managed by those who have been infected, but which can be averted by avoiding certain risk behavior, the visual images continue to show that AIDS is death.

The language of the press demonstrates that, early on, AIDS was considered, basically, a disease of homosexuals, and it is only fairly recently that heterosexual spread of the disease has been covered as well. However, the images of homosexuality do not appear more frequently than those of heterosexuality at any time, and only in 1991 and 1992 are heterosexual images significantly more frequent than homosexual ones.

As the epidemic has evolved, increasingly we have more reasons to hope. HIV infection can be avoided through behavior modification. It is not rapidly and inevitably fatal. Some means of treatment have been shown to modify both the infection and its transmission. However this, again, is not reflected in the images. The small percentage of images which gives a positive impression has not increased over the years. Positive images appear from the beginning, but they have not increased in frequency when compared to the negative ones. Although the message one may receive from the metaphors and language of the press is that the disease is becoming more tolerable, and there is increasingly justification for, at least, faint hope, this message is not found in the images. In them, AIDS is still death, and what little hope is found is not more evident than it was earlier.

The press has considerable power to shape public opinion through its use of metaphors and visual images. Nevertheless, this power is accompanied by responsibility which the press cannot avoid. Through the use of non-judgmental language and images, the press can help to educate the public with regard to HIV infection and its prevention. Terms such as "risk groups", as well as illustrations representative of such concepts, should no longer be used, as they tend to categorize people and de-emphasize the importance of individual risk behavior. Homosexuality should be separated from HIV/AIDS, so that the gay population can confront HIV infection in the same way as everyone else in society. The representation of drugs in the images of AIDS should focus on the fact that it is the sharing of drug paraphernalia which constitutes risky behavior, and not the use of drugs themselves.

The continuing emphasis on AIDS equaling death should be modified to reflect the current state of knowledge about the disease, such as that more seropositive persons are living longer without developing AIDS, and the relationship between AIDS and death is changing as more treatments are becoming available, and the condition is becoming more manageable as a chronic disease. As a consequence, the articles and visual images should give greater emphasis to care and hope. Messages of safer sex practices should substitute the equation "sex = death", and sexuality should be treated with the same neutrality as other themes of interest. We exhort the press to take into consideration these recommendations so that they can better assume their significant role in HIV/AIDS education and prevention.

REFERENCES

Crane, D. (1992). The production of culture: media and the urban arts. Newbury Park, CA: Sage Publications. p. 14.

Cunningham, E. L. and Cunningham, I. (1991). La metaphora del SIDA en Puerto Rico: el reportaje de una epidemia. In I. Cunningham, C. Ramos-Bellido y R. Ortiz-Colón, Eds. El SIDA en Puerto Rico: acercamientos multidisciplinarios (pp. 85-105). Río Piedras: Universidad de Puerto Rico.

Cunningham, I. (1989). The public controversies of AIDS in Puerto Rico, Social Science & Medicine, **29**: 545-553.

Department of Health. (1993). Informe de estadísticas vitales, 1991. San Juan: Administración de Facilidades y Servicios de Salud, Oficina de Estudios de Salud.

Department of Health. (1994). Informe mensual de la Oficina Central para Asuntos del SIDA y Enfermedades Transmisibles Sexualmente. San Juan: OCASET, June 24, 1994.

Gever, M. (1988). Pictures of sickness: Stuart Marshall's bright eyes, in D. Crimp, Ed. AIDS: cultural analysis/cultural activism (pp. 109-126). Cambridge, MA: MIT Press.

Gilman, S.L. (1988). Disease and representation: Images of illness from madness to AIDS, pp. 245-272. Ithaca, NY: Cornell University.

Klaidman, S. (1990). How well the media report health risk. Daedalus, **119**: 119-132.

Watney, S. (1988). The spectacle of AIDS, in D. Crimp, Ed. AIDS: cultural analysis/cultural activism (pp. 71-86). Cambridge, MA. MIT Press.

6

Drug Injecting and the Spread of HIV Infection in South-East Asia

GERRY V. STIMSON

Drug injecting is now found in more than 120 countries, and HIV infection associated with drug injecting in over 80 of them (Stimson, 1996). The long established patterns of injecting which are found in developed countries - for example in Europe, North America and Australia - have now been joined by the spread of injecting in many developing countries. The recent spread of drug injecting has been noted in South America, in India, in many parts of Eastern Europe and in central Asia, and in some parts of Africa (Des Jarlais & Friedman, 1994; Wodak *et al.*, 1993a).

The diffusion of injecting has been particularly pronounced in drug producing and transport countries in south-east Asia, especially in the sub-region that embraces Thailand, Myanmar (formerly Burma), Yunnan in south-west China, and Manipur in north-east India (Figure 6.1). Production and transportation of drugs, the migration of drug users, and the rapid diffusion and adoption of injecting, has typically been followed by the extensive spread of HIV infection. Within just three years HIV infection among injectors in this sub-region reached record levels. HIV among injecting drug users occurred in Thailand by 1987, spread south to Malaysia by 1988, north to Myanmar and Yunnan in 1989, and to Manipur by 1990. Rates of HIV infection among drug injectors - peaking in some areas at over 80 per cent - are the highest that have been reported in the world. The epidemic is sustained at high levels due to the dynamic interaction between high risk syringe-sharing, the high prevalence rate which increases the odds of sharing injecting equipment with an HIV positive partner, the high infectivity of new cases of infection, and the extensive mobility and mixing between injectors in the region. The south-east Asian experience reflects missed prevention opportunities and a failure to address drug injection and HIV prevention as a sub-regional issue.

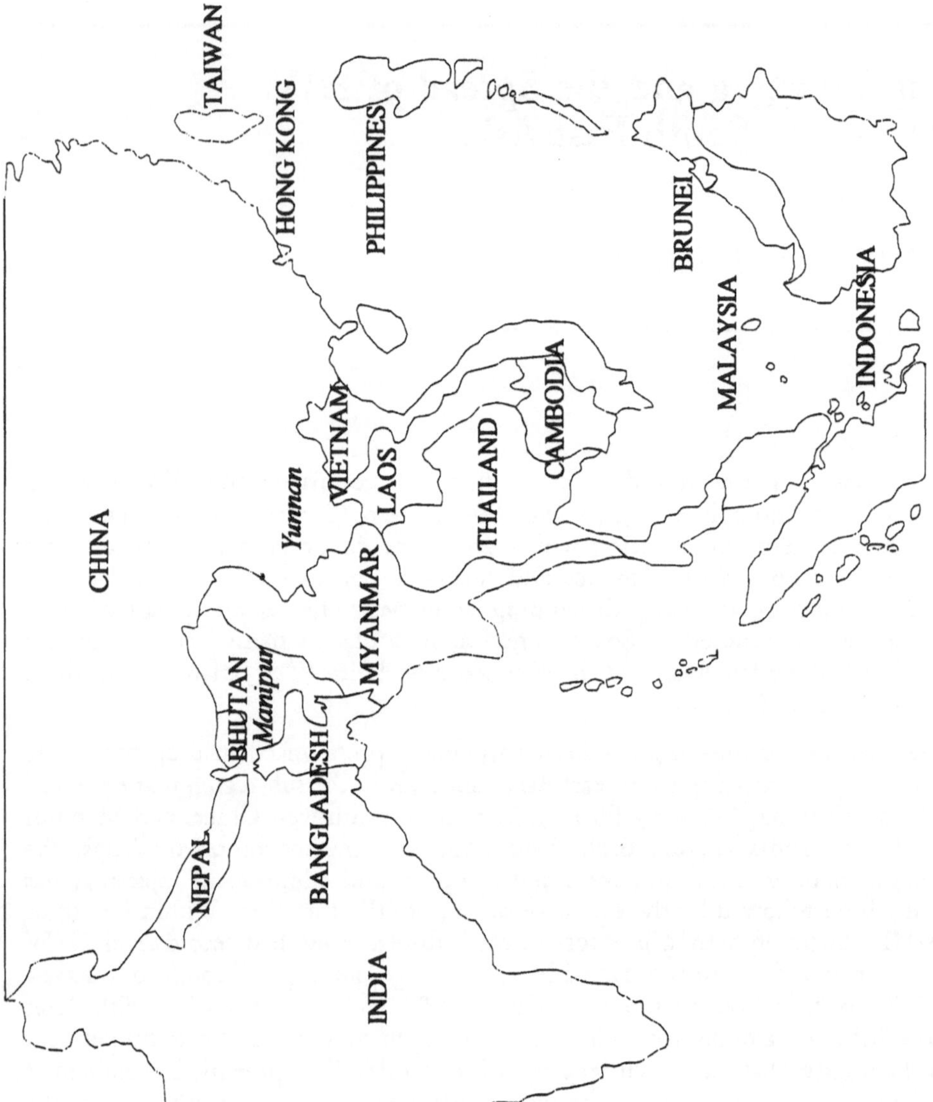

Fig. 6.1 South-East Asia

DIFFUSION OF DRUG INJECTING IN THE REGION

There has been a long-standing pattern of opium production and use in south-east Asia (Vichai Poshyachinda, 1994). The region includes the Golden Triangle which is the world's largest opium producing area and encompasses parts of Laos, Myanmar and Thailand (Cooper, 1989). Until the 1960s opium was produced for export for refining elsewhere (mainly in the Mediterranean basin) and local consumption was confined to opium. Heroin was unavailable locally unless imported (for example the first case of heroin addiction in Thailand involved heroin brought in from Hong Kong (Vichai Poshyachinda, 1988). The late 1960s onwards saw the expansion in this area of the refining of opium to heroin. The development of heroin refining, in refineries in or close to the growing areas, was influenced by the prospect of lower production costs, the growth of the world market, successful law enforcement against production in Mediterranean countries and later in Mexico, and local political conditions - control of opium and heroin being significant in local political control and in the financing of insurgent activity. In 1991 this area accounted for 70% of global opium production (Wodak *et al.*, 1993a). The refining and distribution of heroin - originally intended for export - in turn facilitated the local availability of heroin at (relatively) low prices: thus markets for heroin emerged.

Much of the heroin for world export went in transit through Bangkok but with enforcement and government activity against dissident groups in Myanmar, the cost of local 'taxes' on transport (ie. corruption) and the development of new transport networks, there was a shift in overland export routes through Shan State to Yunnan in China and on to Hong Kong. In the mid-1980s, an overland route north east of Myanmar through Manipur and north-east India also developed (Wodak *et al.*, 1993a; Wodak *et al.*, 1993b). More recently, the first major seizure of heroin at Ho Chi Minh City airport in Vietnam was reported, suggesting a new transit route.

Patterns of local drug consumption and modes of administration have been undergoing marked transformations here (Figure 6.2). The development of heroin injecting in Thailand was an early example of the diffusion of the practice of injecting. Local heroin use paralleled the trade in heroin for American servicepeople based in Vietnam, and the growth of world heroin markets. In a period of 20 years from the late 1950s, Thailand saw the gradual transition from opium smoking to heroin smoking, and then to heroin injection (Vichai Poshyachinda, 1988). A similar situation occurred in Malaysia and Singapore (Vichai Poshyachinda, 1992). Myanmar is the world's largest single source of heroin producing an estimated 200 tons a year and has major opium poppy growing and heroin refining areas, mainly in the eastern part of the country in Shan State. As in Thailand, the expansion of poppy growing and heroin refining occurred at the time of the United States' war in Vietnam. Myanmar itself became a major consumer of heroin from the mid 1970s onwards, and within a few years heroin injection began to take over from heroin smoking as the main problematic drug use. In Manipur as late as 1982, only 1% of known addicts preferred heroin (Pal *et al.*, 1990). Heroin smoking and then injecting became common in the mid-1980s. Manipur shares a long international

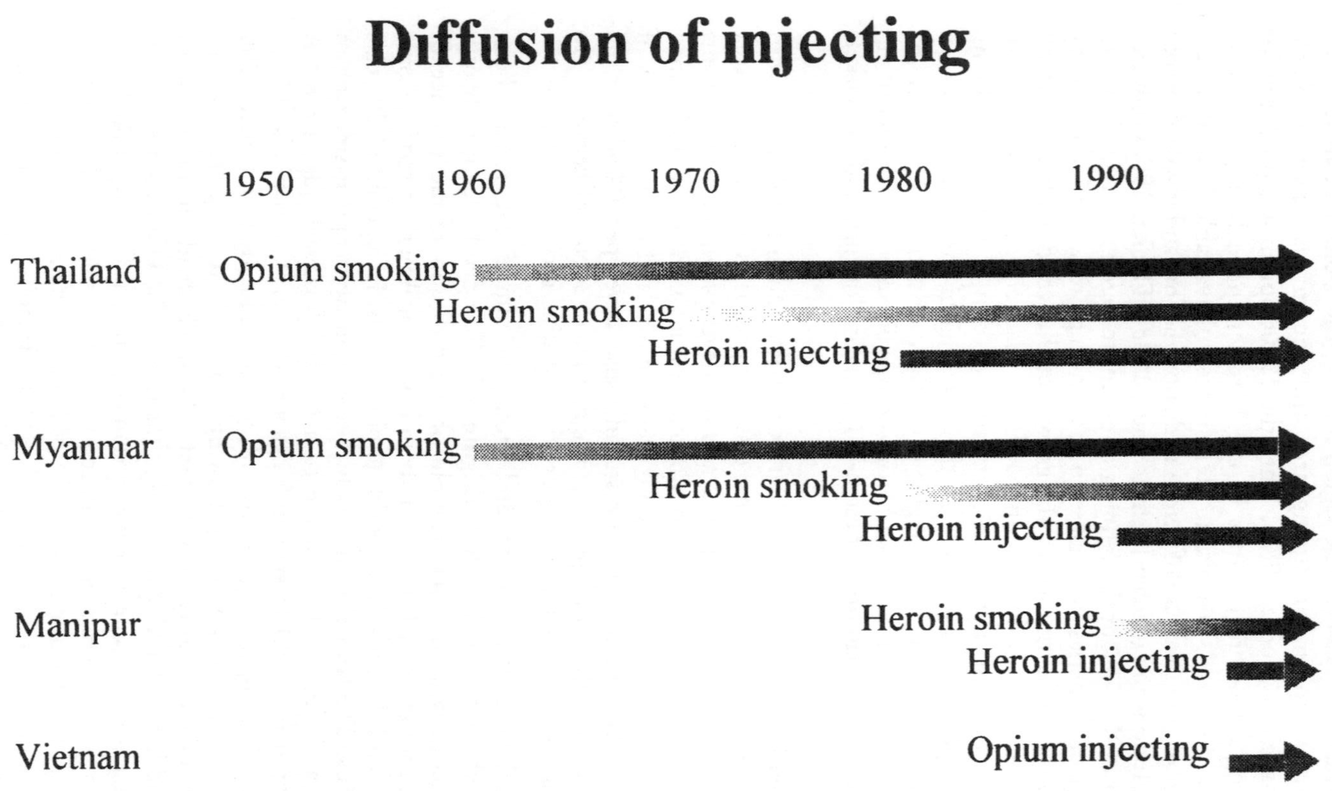

Fig. 6.2 Patterns of local drug consumption and modes of administration

border with Myanmar. The significance of drug distribution routes is exemplified in the fact that most of the heroin users are found along Highway 39. This is a heroin trans-shipment route starting at the Myanmar border and running through Manipur and north to Nagaland. In Vietnam, heroin injecting had not been reported since 1975, its use before then being linked with the occupation by US troops. The injecting of opium started in Vietnam in the 1990s. Heroin injection was reported in Hanoi and Ho Chi Minh City in 1993.

It is estimated that up to 95% of addicts in contact with treatment services in Myanmar and Thailand prefer to inject drugs (Vichai Poshyachinda, 1994). In Ruili in the border area of Yunnan and Myanmar the prevalence of injectors among treated addicts rose from 24% in 1990 to 36% by 1992 (Zheng *et al.*, 1994). In Vietnam, it appears that most opium users (97%) inject (Vichai Poshyachinda, 1994), boiling raw opium or the residue of smoked opium and injecting the liquid. Little is known about the situation in Laos or Cambodia. Opium use among rural communities is known in Laos but there are no reports of injecting (Vichai Poshyachinda, 1992).

The prevalence of drug injecting in the general population is unknown in these countries, as elsewhere. Estimates may be derived from surveys of special population groups and ad hoc studies. In Thailand, 2.3% of male conscripts to military service had a history of injecting illicit drugs at some time (Taweesak Nopkesorn *et al.*, 1993). A capture-recapture study estimated there to be 37,000 injectors in Bangkok (Mastro *et al.*, 1994). In Yangon (formerly known as Rangoon) in Myanmar in 1993, 1.4% of blood donors had a history of injecting drug use (Myo Thet Htoon *et al.*, 1992). Village and township surveys have found that up to 1.5% of the population are addicted, about half of whom are injectors. In Manipur social network studies in selected localities in urban areas with known population denominators suggest that the prevalence of injecting varies between one and two per cent. By 1990 it was estimated that there were approximately 15,000 injectors in Manipur, or 1.3% of the population (Pal *et al.*, 1990; Sarkar *et al.*, 1991; Sarkar *et al.*, 1994). High rates are reported in some villages in Thailand - 7% of the population in a fishing village were reported to be addicts (though the proportion injecting was not known (Wiebel, 1992)). The area continues to see new recruits to injecting, suggested by the short length of injecting reported in various samples: in Yangon in Myanmar 40% of patients had been injecting drugs for six months or less; in Manipur most are under 25 years old (Naik *et al.*, 1991; Sarkar *et al.*, 1991) in Malaysia most have been injecting drugs for less than 5 years (Singh and Crofts, 1993).

RAPID DIFFUSION OF HIV TO HIGH PREVALENCE LEVELS

These parts of south-east Asia have seen the most rapid diffusion of HIV infection among injecting drug users found anywhere in the world (Figure 6.3). Many areas reached a prevalence of 40% or more within approximately 12 months. In Bangkok HIV rates among drug injectors of zero or one per cent were found in various surveys from 1985 through to 1987 (Weniger *et al.*, 1991). HIV rates climbed

Prevalence rate reaching 40 per cent or more in approx 12-months

	1987	1988	1989	1990
Bangkok	1%	40%		
Chiang Rai		1%	61%	
Myanmar		0%	73-96%	
Yunnan (Ruili)			13%	58%
Manipur			9%	60%

Fig. 6.3 Rapid diffusion of HIV infection among injecting drug users

rapidly from the beginning of 1988 to reach between 32 and 43% by August and September of 1988. Extremely high sero-conversion rates were found in Bangkok: 20% of drug injectors who were negative in February 1988 had sero-converted by September of that year, giving an incidence of 3% per month, and a further 35% sero-converted between September 1988 and April 1989, giving an incidence of 5% per month. In Chiang Rai in northern Thailand, prevalence was 1% in 1988 and rose to 61% in 1989. Ad hoc surveys revealed similar high rates even among drug injectors in remote hill-tribe areas (Weniger *et al.*, 1991). In south-west China, in the town of Ruili, 13% of injecting drug users were positive at the end of 1989, and this increased to 58% by 1990 (Zheng *et al.*, 1994). In Manipur, the first sero-positive drug injector was not detected until October 1989; within 3 months 9% were positive, and in the next 3 months, the prevalence rate had increased to 56% - giving a rise from 0 to 56% within six months (Sarkar *et al.*, 1994; Naik *et al.*, 1991). In Myanmar, despite extensive HIV testing among various population groups, no HIV positive drug injectors were found in the years up to 1988. High levels of HIV infection were discovered among drug injectors from 1989 onwards in geographically distant parts of the country, with rates ranging from 73 to 96% (Department of Health Union of Myanmar, 1993a).

The high levels of HIV infection found in south-east Asia are unprecedented (Figure 6.4). Several towns have experienced prevalence rates among drug injectors of above 60%, and in one case of 96%. Extremely high rates have been found in Ruili in Yunnan – at 82% in 1992 (Zheng *et al.*, 1994), in Chiang Rai in northern Thailand at 61% in 1989 (Vichai Poshyachinda 1992), and in north-east

India in Manipur at 73% in 1992 (Sarkar *et al.*, 1994). In Myanmar rates of above 60% have been reported from most testing sites, for example 74% in the south in Yangon, 96% in Bhamo, 84% in Mandalay in central Myanmar, and 91% in Myitkyina in the north. Since the sentinel surveillance programme was introduced there in 1992 national rates for injectors have averaged between 60 and 75% (Department of Health Union of Myanmar, 1993a; Department of Health Union of Myanmar, 1993b).

Yunnan, China	Ruili	1992	82%
Myanmar	Myitkyina	1988	95%
	Bhamo	1988	96%
	Mandalay	1990	72%
Thailand	Chiang Rai	1989	61%
N.E. India	Manipur	1992	73%

Fig. 6.4 Towns experiencing extremely high prevalence rates among injecting drug users

The extremely high prevalence of HIV infection among injecting drug users shows no signs of decreasing. The prevalence over time in Manipur has continued at between 60 and 70% (Sarkar *et al.*, 1994), at around 75% across sites included in the sentinel surveillance programme in Myanmar (Department of Health Union of Myanmar, 1993a; Department of Health Union of Myanmar, 1993b), and in Thailand at between about 30% in Bangkok (Weniger *et al.*, 1991) and between 20% and 50% elsewhere.

There is evidence from Myanmar that many drug injectors become infected soon after commencing to inject, a pattern rarely found elsewhere. In Yangon in 1992, 41% of those who had injected for six months or less were already HIV positive. In the north of the country, among injectors of whom 91% were HIV positive, 48% had used drugs for 6 months or less (Ba Thaung, 1993).

HIGH RISK INJECTING PRACTICES AND THE SPREAD OF HIV INFECTION

The rapid and extensive spread of HIV infection among drug injectors in some parts of this region is linked to high risk injecting practices. In many places drugs are injected with home-made equipment rather than with hypodermic syringes. This includes blow-tubes – a length of polythene tube with a needle attached, reported from Yunnan (Kittelsen, 1991) and Myanmar, and with a variety of other improvised implements including needles which are attached to medical drip sets, to eye-droppers or to ink-droppers (Sarkar *et al.*, 1994). In Mandalay in Myanmar in 1989, 52% of injectors used self-made equipment (Sarkar *et al.*, 1994). In Manipur, only 3% used a regular syringe (Pal *et al.*, 1990). In Thai prisons, methods included the use of tubes from ballpoint pens.

Also significant for the spread of HIV infection is the use of professional injectors at drug injecting shops, and the injection of drugs at public gathering sites. Throughout Myanmar, drug injectors report using professional injectors, at locations where there would commonly be only one set of injecting equipment. Addicts pay to be injected and large numbers use each place during the day. Initiation into injecting commonly takes place in such settings. Injectors in Hanoi buy their drugs from shooting galleries, where the dealer supplies the syringes and the drug solution is drawn up from a common pot. The use of professional injectors has not been reported in Manipur, but needle-sharing is common, with 83% regularly sharing with between 3 and 5 people in a group of the same sex and of a similar age (Sarkar *et al.*, 1991). In Thailand, needle-sharing was common as was the use of equipment provided at or left nearby drug sellers' houses for use by multiple clients (Wright *et al.*, 1994) and syringe cleaning was rare (Suphak Vanichseni and Sakuntanaga, 1990). In many places sharing is often with multiple partners on one occasion, or over time (Singh and Crofts, 1993; Sarkar *et al.*, 1994). Bleach, which could be used to disinfect syringes, is often unavailable as a domestic product, or is not used.

DYNAMIC FEATURES SUSTAINING THE EPIDEMIC

HIV prevalence is sustained at high prevalence rates, with new sero-conversions, by the dynamic relation between several features of the epidemic (Figure 6.5). *Firstly,* there is continuation in most countries of high risk syringe-sharing behaviours with multiple-sharing partners, with consequent opportunities for transmission. *Secondly,* the high prevalence rate means that there are high odds that, when equipment is shared, the sharers will include those who are HIV-positive. *Thirdly,* there are many new cases of infection who will be at a highly infectious stage of HIV disease and who may more readily transmit it to others.

A *fourth* feature may also be especially important for the further spread of HIV in the south-east Asian context, both for understanding the past spread of infection and the significance for future spread: this is the mobility and mixing of injectors in

Epidemic sustained at high prevalence rates

High risk syringe sharing behaviours
+
High prevalence rate
+
New cases of infection
+
Mobility and mixing

Fig. 6.5 Dynamic relation between several features of the epidemic

the region. The mobility of drug users searching for drugs, treatment, or in the normal course of their employment or search for work, has been noted elsewhere. In most of these countries there is evidence that drug injectors travel extensively both internally and to other countries. In northern Malaysia, three quarters of drug injectors had travelled to Thailand in the previous 5 years and half had shared syringes whilst there (Singh & Crofts, 1993); nearly as many had travelled to other states in Malaysia, both injecting and having sex when they travelled. In Myanmar there is considerable mobility from villages and towns connected with trade and the search for employment.

A significant additional feature of the Myanmar HIV epidemic is the existence of *epidemic focal* areas. These are the jade and gem mining areas which attract large numbers of the population. It is estimated that the population of just one of these rural mining areas is upwards of half a million. Many drug injectors visit such places – as also do young women engaged in casual sex work. In some village tracts up to 10% of the population – mainly younger people – may be absent at a time working in such areas. Extremely high risk injecting and sexual behaviours have been reported.

SEXUAL TRANSMISSION FROM MALE INJECTORS TO FEMALE PARTNERS

Almost all drug injectors in this region are male. Most are sexually active with spouses, some with casual partners, and some with female commercial sex workers

(Vichai Poshyachinda, 1992; Sarkar *et al.*, 1994; Weniger *et al.*, 1991). Condom use is rare, both among drug injectors and in the general population (Singh and Crofts, 1993). In one group of injectors studied in northern Myanmar over 80% had never heard of condoms (Ba Thaung, 1993). In Manipur only between 3 and 5% reported even the occasional use of condoms (Department of Health Union of Myanmar, 1993a) and 10 to 16% had sex with commercial sex workers. Condom use was low in Bangkok, but rates of use are now higher with 12% of injectors in Bangkok in 1990 reporting condom use with a primary partner – but even this was lower than a comparison group of injectors in New York (Weniger *et al.*, 1991; Suphak Vanichseni *et al.*, 1993).

There is evidence of early and rapid sexual transmission to spouses. In Ruili in Yunnan, 10% of wives of drug injectors tested were HIV positive and, based on the duration of infection among drug injectors, it was estimated that the heterosexual transmission rate was 6.4% per annum per person (Zheng *et al.*, 1994). Similarly in Manipur, within one year of HIV spread among drug injectors, 6% of wives who were tested were HIV positive (Department of Health Union of Myanmar, 1993a). This was self-selected group – but even so, by the same time 2% of antenatal mothers who were tested were HIV positive.

PROFILE OF EPIDEMIC SPREAD IN SOUTH-EAST ASIA

We see in south-east Asia a distinctive profile of epidemic spread. Injecting drug users are a major vector for the regional spread of HIV infection: they are widespread, form a large pool of infection, are mobile, sexually active, and have unprotected sexual intercourse. In many countries they are the largest and earliest group with HIV infection. In Manipur for example drug injectors made up 95% of the 899 known HIV-positives by 1990 (Pal *et al.*, 1990). In Yunnan in 1991, 88% of the known HIV-positives were injecting drug users, and in Vietnam 94% of the 926 known HIV-positives were drug injectors (in 1993) (Anon). In this region, drug injectors and others engaged in high risk behaviours appeared to kickstart the epidemic (Weniger *et al.*, 1991).

The second important conclusion that may be drawn from the data is the importance of epicentres to sub-regional spread (Stimson, 1994). Figure 6.6, attempts to reconstruct the pattern of epidemic diffusion. Although it is possible that there were varied sources of the epidemic in the region, and that it might have commenced simultaneously in several sites, there is considerable evidence to suggest the pattern of diffusion shown here. This is based on the chronology of the epidemic, the geography of spread, and known travel and migration patterns. Figure 6.6 shows the approximate date of first cases, and then the approximate date of epidemic take off, defined as an increase in prevalence to 30%. The first cases were found in Bangkok in 1987 followed by a rapid take off in early 1988. A few months later, the same pattern was repeated in the south of Thailand near the Malaysian border and a few months later in northern Malaysia. Going further south, two years later the first cases of HIV infection among drug injectors in Singapore were

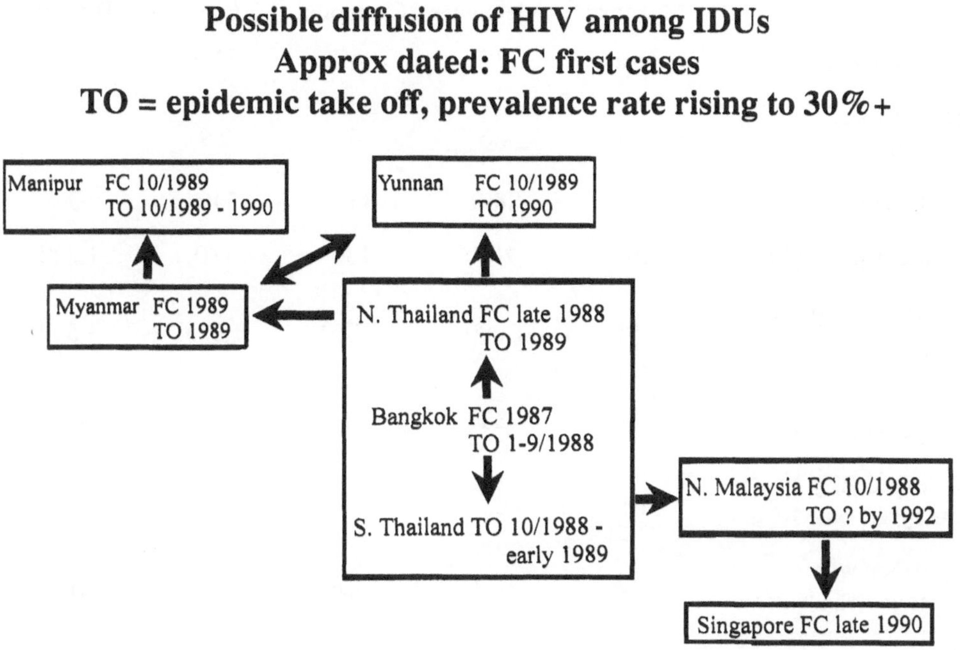

Fig. 6.6 Approximate dates of first cases and epidemic take off

identified in 1990. North from Bangkok, HIV infection among injecting drug users was identified in northern Thailand about 8 months later than Bangkok. HIV infection was not identified in Myanmar until 1989 but, when it was discovered, it was already present at high epidemic levels throughout geographically disparate parts of the country. As in Myanmar, the first cases in Yunnan were picked up in 1989. Manipur, which is on a direct heroin trading link from Myanmar, had its first cases in 1989 and take off in 1990. Going to the east of the region, there are no data for Cambodia and Laos. There is little information available for Vietnam, but the first case of HIV infection was found in December 1990 (National AIDS Committee of Vietnam, 1994).

SOCIAL, ECONOMIC AND POLITICAL FACTORS AND HIV PREVENTION

Social, economic and political features of these countries raise enormous problems for HIV prevention. Within south-east Asia there is a wide diversity of characteristics between and within countries ranging from the rapid economic growth seen in Singapore, Malaysia and Thailand to some of the world's poorest countries (Thailand, Indochina and Burma Handbook, 1992).

Many of the impoverished countries have populations living in poor social conditions, and lack the infrastructure on which prevention campaigns in much of the developed world have been based. They have 75% or more of the population

	Myanmar	Vietnam	Cambodia	Laos	Thailand
Rural Population	75%	78%	88%	81%	77%
Mean years of schooling	2.5	4.6	2	2.9	3.8
Adult literacy rate	81%	88%	35%	54%	93%
Income: $ per capita	200	200	130	180	1,220
$ purchasing power parity	595	1,000	1,000	1,025	3,569
Communications - TVs per 1000 pop.	2	38	8	5	109
Life expectancy at birth (years)	61	63	50	50	66.1
Population with access to clean water	32%	46%	na	29%	81%

Fig. 6.7 Impoverished countries having populations living in poor social conditions

living in rural areas and depending on agriculture for their livelihood (Figure 6.7). Educational levels are low. They are ethnically diverse, with many different population and language groups. In Myanmar for example there are 135 nationalities recognised by the government and over two hundred languages and dialects. Yunnan has 24 ethnic groups and Manipur has 33. Such countries have low per capita income. They also have poor communications systems - including undeveloped mass media and poor access to the media. In many countries most people do not have a clean water supply. There are major health problems apart from HIV including tuberculosis, diarrhoea and dysentery, and malaria, with life expectancy at birth much lower than in developed countries, and an absence of adequate local resources to respond efficiently.

Communication and transport are difficult due to geography, climate and poor infrastructure. Dry season journey times are slow, but are improving in some places with road development. Many parts of these countries are only accessible on foot. Despite this, there is considerable population mobility connected with trade and employment. There are few natural borders and a long-standing tradition of cross-border movement for trade and visiting relatives.

There have been huge population dislocations connected with the political history of this region over the last 60 years, including the impact of the Second World War, independence and nationalist struggles, and the wars in Vietnam and Cambodia. In Myanmar, parts of the country have been under the control of nationalist and insurgent groups and opium war lords, each of which has controlled the opium and heroin trade or has benefited from it, as have others. Separatist and autonomist aspirations have been intertwined with the control of heroin production and distribution.

The area has also been subject to extensive (and changing) United Nations interventions to control the production of heroin. A conflict may occur between drug control and HIV prevention, for example, by prioritising funding to activities aimed at reducing production of drugs (supply reduction), rather than to activities which reduce demand for or the harmful consequences of drug use. Unintentional effects of successful law enforcement include the shift of drug distribution routes to new areas, subsequently exposing new populations to drug use.

PREVENTION LESSONS AND OPPORTUNITIES

South-east Asia provides a case study of the failure of both drug prevention and of HIV prevention. A number of lessons may be learned which are applicable for the region and for many developing countries.

Firstly, what has happened in south-east Asia illustrates that drug producer and transit countries in turn become drug consumer countries. The regional experience points to the rapidity with which new drug use patterns may emerge. *Secondly,* local drug problems are often overlooked. Activity in these countries by national governments and international organisations has often focused more on reducing production than on reducing local demand. Some international donor countries restrict their bilateral and UN drug control funding to activities that may have an impact on the supply of drugs to the donor country, and neglect drug problems within the producer and transit countries. National governments, aware of what appeals to funders, often ignore (and sometimes conceal) domestic consumption problems in favour of projects that target production: this usually means enforcement and economic development projects.

Thirdly, with hindsight it would have been possible to predict the spread of HIV infection in this region: this might have encouraged the introduction of prevention activities while there was a window of opportunity. Among the errors made include: (a) the neglect of the role of drug injectors in the early stages of HIV epidemic spread. Their role was underestimated both by national governments and the World Health Organization: it may have been assumed that drug injectors were marginal members of society and could thus be ignored. (b) A further error was the difficulty of persuading governments to act on early signs. Some governments and leaders think that their countries are different from others - they fall into the trap of the "national immunity myth". They assume that their politics, national identity, religion, or culture provide some protective factor - and therefore believe that their country is immune from the spread of HIV infection. (c) Next there was the absence of sub-regional cooperation in the prevention of drug injecting and of HIV infection. The spread of HIV infection in one country has rapid implications for epidemic development in adjacent countries. This suggests that the focus for assessment and for planning of prevention should to be sub-regional rather than just the nation state.

Fourthly, much of the success of the region's efforts to limit the spread of HIV infection will depend on the success of public health prevention measures related to injecting. This task is difficult because many areas have entered that dynamic relationship between high HIV prevalence, high risk behaviours, and new cases of infection. Once HIV infection is present at high levels, it is hard to break the cycle of further transmission that in turn sustains the epidemic. Greater changes in risk behaviour are required than in countries with lower prevalence. However, the reduction of risk in high prevalence areas in south-east Asia has already been shown among Bangkok injectors (Des Jarlais *et al.*, 1994). The focus for prevention has to be broad and to target various groups, of which current injectors are only one. HIV prevention has to find ways of discouraging the transition to injection, and to avoid measures that might encourage its spread. Thus far, there is little experience with this. Innovative prevention projects will need to be developed that try to prevent the diffusion of injecting into new areas and groups. HIV prevention will also need to encourage risk reduction in neophyte injectors. The problem here is that injectors in some of these countries are becoming HIV positive early in their injecting careers, often before they contact prevention and treatment services. Ways to reach these people will need to be developed. HIV prevention will also have to target sexual transmission from HIV positive injectors to their sexual partners.

Fifthly, the south-east Asian epidemic experience points to the desirability of early prevention to encourage changes in risk behaviours before prevalence takes off, a possibility that still exists for some countries and towns in the region, and for countries that are only just facing the spread of injecting. In contrast to the experience in south-east Asia, countries which have sustained low and stable prevalence rates have often introduced risk reduction before epidemic take-off, and this risk reduction has proved sufficient, in combination with low prevalence and few new infectious cases, to sustain low and stable prevalence (Des Jarlais and Friedman, 1994; Stimson, 1995; Bloor *et al.*, 1994).

The patterns of diffusion of injecting and of HIV infection observed in this region has implications for many countries that are facing new drug use patterns. This includes other parts of south-east Asia. Social changes are occurring linked to political developments, improvement in transportation, new trade links, and to urbanisation and modernisation; these factors make certain population groups vulnerable. Trade, cultural and migration links between the epidemic epicentre and neighbouring areas suggest that south India, Cambodia, Laos, and Bangladesh may be susceptible to both drug injecting and HIV infection.

Other regions also face these problems, including Central and Eastern Europe, Central Asian republics, south-west Asia, West Africa, and South America. For example, Nigeria has long been a drug transit country for cocaine from South America and heroin from south-east Asia, en route to Europe and North America. Nigeria now has its own indigenous problems with the consumption of heroin and cocaine. Columbia is the largest exporter of cocaine for world markets. Within

Columbia, cocaine products are smoked, and its "national immunity myth" is that the population is culturally resistant to injection. Recently the country has seen the introduction of opium poppies and heroin refining, and there are now reports of the injection of heroin and other drugs.

The experience in south-east Asia shows that producer and transit countries create their own local demand for drugs. Knowledge of drug production, drug trading routes, drug use practices, current and potential diffusion of injecting, migration, and distribution of HIV infection, could be used to predict areas which are vulnerable to the diffusion of drug injecting and associated HIV infection.

ACKNOWLEDGEMENTS

Some of the material in this chapter appeared in a shorter version in a letter published in the journal AIDS (Stimson, 1994). The Centre for Research on Drugs and Health Behaviour is core-funded by North Thames Health Authority.

REFERENCES

Ba Thaung. (1993) Community Drug Control Programme, Union of Myanmar. (UnPub)

Bloor, M., Frischer, M., Taylor, A., Covell, R., Goldberg, D., Green, S., McKeganey, N., and Platt, S. (1994) Tideline and turn? Possible reasons for the continuing low HIV prevalence among Glasgow's injecting drug users. *Sociological Review*, **42**, 738-757.

Cooper, M.H. (1989) The Business of Drugs. Congressional Quarterly Inc, Washington.

Department of Health Union of Myanmar. (1993a) Annual Report of the AIDS Control Programme, Myanmar 1992.

Department of Health Union of Myanmar. (1993b) AIDS Prevention and Control Programme, Sentinel Surveillance Data, March.

Des Jarlais, D.C., Friedman, S.R. (1994) AIDS and the use of injected drugs. *Scientific American*, February, 56-62.

Des Jarlais, D.C., Kachit Choopanya, Suphak Vanichseni, Kanokporn Plangsringarn, Wandee Sonchai, Carballo, M., Friedmann, P., and Friedman, S.R. (1994) AIDS risk reduction and reduced HIV seroconversion among injection drug users in Bangkok. *American Journal of Public Health*, **84**, 452-455.

Kittelsen, J. (1991) Personal communication.

Mastro, T., Kityaporn, D., Weniger, B.G., Vanichseni, S., Vati Laosunthorn, Thongchai Ureklash, Chintra Ureklash, Kachit Choopanya, Khanchit Limpakamjanaret (1994) Estimating the number of HIV infected drug users in Bamgkok: a capture-recapture method. *American Journal of Public Health*, **84**, 1094-1097.

Myo Thet Htoon, Khin San Tint, Khin Ohmar San, Hla Htut Lwin and Min Thwe. (1992) A study on blood donors at Central National Blood bank with regard to their behaviours relating to HIV transmission. (UnPub)

Naik, T.N., Sarkar, S., Singh, H.L., Bhunia, S.C., Singh, Y.I., Singh, P. and Pal, S.C. (1991) Intravenous drug users - a new high-risk group for HIV infection in India. *AIDS*, **5**, 117-118.

National AIDS Committee of Vietnam (1994) Medium Term Plan for Prevention and Control of HIV/AIDS in Vietnam 1994-1995 and 1996-2000. Ministry of Health.

Pal, S.C., Sarkar, S., Naik, T.N., Singh, P.K., Tushi Ao, S.I., Lal, S. and Tripathy, S.P. (1990) Explosive epidemic of HIV infection in north eastern states of India, Manipur and Nagaland. *CARC Calling*, **3**, 2-6.

Sarkar, S., Mookherjee, P. and Roy, A. (1991) Descriptive epidemiology of intravenous heroin users - A new risk group for transmission of HIV in India. *Journal of Infection*, **23**, 201-207.

Sarkar, S., Das, N., Panda, S., Naik, T.K., Sarkar, K., Singh, B.C., Ralte, J.M., Aier, S.M. and Tripathy, S.P. (1994) Rapid spread of HIV among injecting drug users in north-eastern states of India. *Bulletin on Narcotics*, **XLV**, 91-105.

Singh, S. and Crofts, N. (1993) HIV infection among injecting drug users in north-east Malaysia. *AIDS Care*, **5**, 273-281.

Stimson, G.V. (1994) Reconstruction of sub-regional diffusion of HIV infection among injecting drug users in South-East Asia: implications for early intervention. *Letter to AIDS*, **8**, 1630-32.

Stimson, G.V. (1995) AIDS and drug injecting in the United Kingdom, 1987 to 1993: the policy response and the prevention of the epidemic. *Social Science and Medicine*, **41**, 5: 699-716.

Stimson, G.V. and Kachit Choopanya (1996) Global perspectives on drug injecting. In G.V. Stimson, D.C. des Jarlais and A. Ball (Eds.) Drug injecting and HIV infection: Global Dimensions and Local Responses (Forthcoming).

Suphak Vanichseni, des Jarlais, D.C., Kachit Choopanya, Friedmann, P., Wenston, J., Sonchai, W., Sotheran, J.L., Raktham, S., Carballo, M., and Friedman, S.R. (1993) Condom use with primary partners among injecting drug users in Bangkok, Thailand and New York City, United States. *AIDS*, 7, 887-891.

Suphak Vanichseni and Sakuntanaga, P. (1990) Results of three sero-prevalence surveys in IVDU in Bangkok. VI International Conference on AIDS, Abstract FC105.

Taweesak Nopkesorn, Mastro, T.D., Suebpong Sangkharomya, Sweat, M., Pricha Singharaj, Kanchit Limpankarnjanaret, Gayle, H.D., and Weniger, B.G. (1993) HIV-1 infection in young men in northern Thailand. *AIDS*, 7, 1233-1239.

Thailand, Indochina and Burma Handbook (1992). Trade and Travel Publications, Bath.

Vichai Poshyachinda. (1988) Future Outlook of Drug Dependence in Thailand. Institute of Health Research, Chulalongkorn University, Bangkok.

Vichai Poshyachinda. (1992) Drugs and AIDS in Southeast-Asia. *Forensic Science International*, **62**, 15-28

Vichai Poshyachinda. (1994) Drug injecting and HIV infection among the population of drug abusers in Asia. *Bulletin on Narcotics*, **XLV**, 77-90.

Weniger, B.G., Khanchit Limpakarnjanaret, Kumnuan Ungclusak, Sombat Thanprasertsuk, Kachit Choopanya, Suphak Vanichseni, Thongchai Ureklabh, Prasert Thongchareon and Chantapong Wasi. (1991) The epidemiology of HIV infection and AIDS in Thailand. *AIDS*, **5**, S71-S85.

Wiebel, W. (1992) Report on substance abuse in southern Thailand. (UnPub)

Wodak, A., Fisher, R. and Crofts, N. (1993a) An evolving public health crisis: HIV infection among injecting drugs users in developing countries. In N. Heather, A. Wodak, E. Nadelmann, P.O'Hare (eds), Psychoactive Drugs and Harm Reduction: From Faith to Science, Whurr Publishers, London.

Wodak, A., Crofts, N., and Fisher, R. (1993b) HIV infection among injecting drug users in Asia: an evolving public health crisis. *AIDS Care*, **5**, 313-320.

Wright, N.H., Suphak Vanichseni, Pasakorn Akarasewi, Chantapong Wasi and Kachit Choopanya. (1994) Was the 1988 HIV epidemic among Bangkok's injecting drug users a common source outbreak? *AIDS*, **8**, 529-532.

Zheng, X., Tian, C., Choi, K.H., Zhang, J., Cheng, H., Yang, X., Li, D., Lin. J., Qu, S., Sun, X., Hall, T., Mandel, J., and Hearst, N. (1994) Injecting drug use and HIV infection in south west China, *AIDS*, **8**, 1141-1147.

7

Network and Sociohistorical Approaches to the HIV Epidemic among Drug Injectors

SAMUEL R. FRIEDMAN, ALAN NEAIGUS, BENNY JOSE, RICHARD CURTIS, MARJORIE GOLDSTEIN, JO L. SOTHERAN, JOHN WENSTON, CARL A. LATKIN AND DON C. DES JARLAIS

INTRODUCTION

Most epidemiology, prevention efforts, and policies concerning HIV among drug injectors have thus far been based on the psychological assumptions of methodological individualism. That is, we have tended to focus on the individual, and to see his or her probability of becoming infected with HIV as simply a function of his or her own individual behaviors. These behaviors, in turn, have been seen as being an outcome primarily of his or her personality and knowledge as they direct him or her to react to opportunities or threats. Given these assumptions, then, we have tended also to see AIDS prevention in individualistic terms: as providing information to individuals so they can make better-informed choices, or as providing counseling, therapy, skills training, or other assistance so that individuals can make their personalities more appropriate to avoiding AIDS risk behaviors. In addition, some prevention efforts have distributed risk-reduction supplies – such as condoms or syringes – to individuals for their own use and, in some projects, to be passed on to other individuals.

Somewhat more sophisticated models have recognized that people who know each other have impacts on each other's behaviors. Such social influence can amount to a veto power on high-risk behaviors (or on lower-risk forms of these same behaviors) in circumstances where people might otherwise engage in risk behaviors together. Thus, one partner might refuse to have sex without a condom, or refuse to share injection equipment, or refuse to share drugs through syringe-mediated drug sharing ("backloading" – a behaviour which was first identified by Grund *et al.* (1991) and then was found to be related to seropositivity among drug injectors in New York by Jose *et al.*, [1993].) Our ethnographic observations in New York indicate that some drug injectors, at least, have developed such an awareness that they will refuse ever to share drugs again with anyone who has engaged in backloading–that is, again, using a potentially-infected syringe as a receptacle in which to mix or measure drug solutions for sharing drugs. In general, then, these more sophisticated social-influence models have been embodied in prevention projects that aim either at (1) conducting outreach directed to the friendship groups of IDUs or (2) holding group education and counseling sessions in which efforts are made to have the attendees become a reference group which exerts pressure for safer behavior on participants.

In this paper, we present evidence that the probability of being HIV-infected, the probability of engaging in risk behaviors, the probability that risk behaviors will lead to infection, and HIV prevention approaches can all be viewed usefully as depending on larger-scale social and historical forces, structures, and/or processes. First, we review previous work on how large-scale sociohistorical forces affect HIV spread. Then, we present evidence from recent research focusing on a much smaller scale (though still on a scale larger than the individual) – namely, the social network.

Large-Scale Sociohistorical Factors Have an Impact on the HIV Epidemic:

The HIV epidemic is deeply shaped by historical, geographic, and social dynamics. We will discuss this cluster of factors in terms of three concepts: (1) racial/ethnic subordination; (2) production and market dynamics; and (3) the geographic movement of people.

Racial/ethnic subordination and HIV among drug injectors:

HIV seroprevalence is greater in some racially/ethnically subordinated groups in the United States than it is among whites. AIDS case surveillance data reported through December, 1993 (CDC, preliminary data) find that–whereas 12% of the United States population is African-American and 9% is Latino–the corresponding percentages among men with AIDS are 28% African-American and 16% Latino; and among women with AIDS, 54% are African-American and 20% are Latina. As can be seen from Figure 7.1 and 7.2, African-Americans and Latinos are more likely to have been diagnosed with AIDS due to each of a wide range of risk behaviors than would be expected from their proportions in the population.

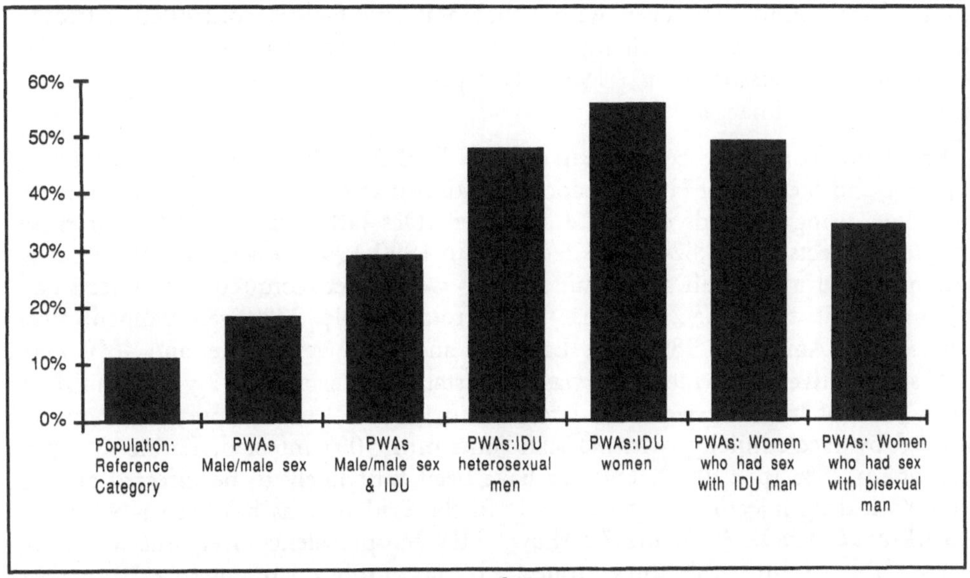

Fig. 7.1 African-Americans as Proportion of Category

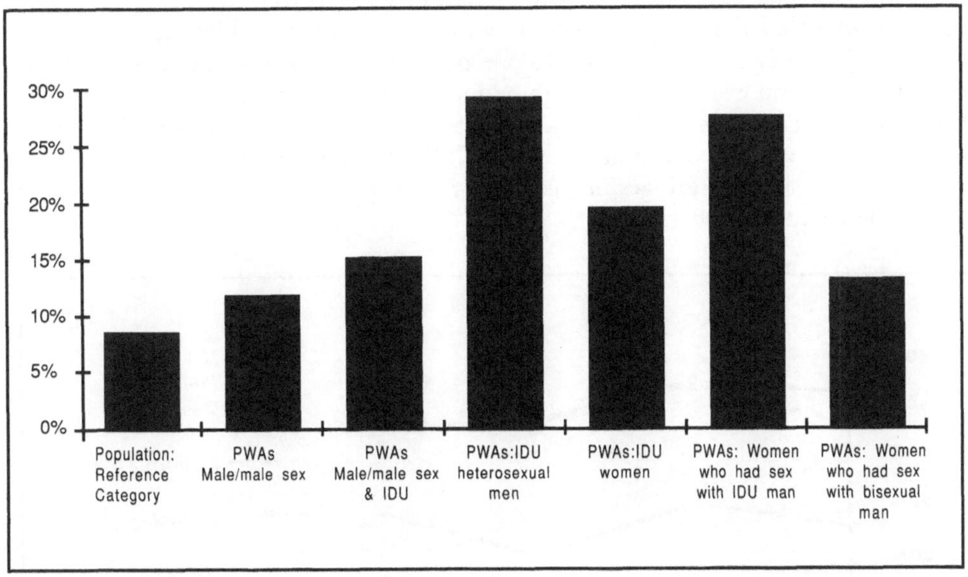

Fig. 7.2 Latinos as Proportion of Category

HIV seroprevalence data are available by race/ethnicity among injecting drug users (IDUs) for many areas in the United States. In many of these areas – but not all (Williams & Johnson, 1993) – African-Americans and those Latinos of Puerto Rican origin or descent are more likely to be seropositive than whites (Chitwood *et al.*, 1993; Friedman *et al.*, 1987, 1990, 1993a; Hahn *et al.*, 1989; Koblin *et al.*, 1990; LaBrie *et al.*, 1993; Marmor *et al.*, 1987; Nwanyanwu *et al.*, 1993). A number of studies have found that, even with behavioral risk factors controlled, African-American and/or Latino drug injectors are more likely than whites to be HIV seropositive (Chaisson *et al.,* 1989; D'Aquila *et al.,* 1989; Jose, 1993 or to seroconvert (Friedman *et al.,* 1993c).

The New York City component of the WHO's Multi-Site Study of Drug Injecting and the Risk of HIV Infection has studied seroprevalence by race/ethnicity over time, using methods elsewhere described (Des Jarlais *et al.,* 1994). For these analyses, subjects were 1,824 IDUs recruited in 1990-1993, of whom 929 were new entrants to a drug detoxification unit and 895 were street-recruited. All subjects had injected within the prior 2 months. Of the total sample, 23% were women; 39% were African-American, 38% were Latino/a, and 23% were white; and 46% were HIV seropositive. Their mean age was 36.5 (standard deviation 7.2 years) and their mean years of injection was 17.1 (standard deviation 9.1). Seroprevalence overall differed by race/ethnicity, with African-Americans 50% infected, Latino/as 52%, and whites 28% ($p < .001$). (Whites have been least likely to be infected among New York drug injectors since very early in the epidemic, as has been reported in Novick *et al.*, 1989). As Figure 7.3 shows, HIV seroprevalence over time was more or less stable within racial/ethnic groups, with no significant trends ($p \leq .10$) within racial/ethnic subgroups. White subjects interviewed in each year had lower seroprevalence than Latino/a or African-American subjects ($p < .05$). Interview data were available that described the people with whom subjects injected on the last occasion when they injected drugs. No one of a different race ethnicity was present at the last injection event at 84% of these most recent injection events for African-American subjects, 85% for Latino/a subjects, and 81% for white subjects. Thus, there are relatively few occasions in which HIV can be transmitted across racial/ethnic lines by sharing syringes or needles, or by engaging in backloading or other syringe-mediated drug sharing.

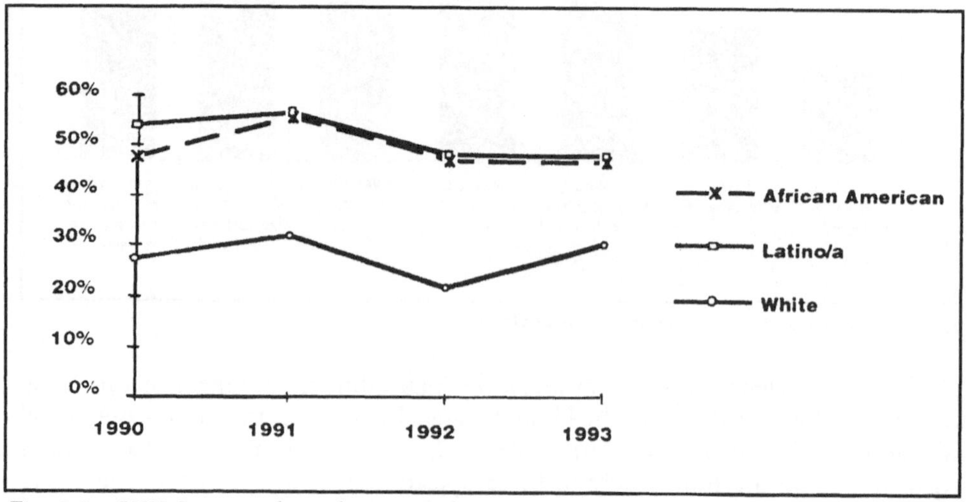

Fig. 7.3 HIV Seroprevalence by Race/Ethnicity over Time among New York City Drug Injectors

This implies that, historically, the probability that an African American or a Latino/a who shares syringes or backloads will do so with an infected person is greater than for whites. Thus, the racial/ethnic segregation that pervades American society has probably been a major force in maintaining HIV differences in seroprevalence by race/ethnicity in spite of the fact that in many cities, including New York, African American and/or Latino/a drug injectors may have engaged in more risk reduction, and may be engaging in less of a number of risk behaviors, than white drug injectors (Friedman *et al.,* 1990; Friedman *et al.,* 1993a).

Production and Market Dynamics in the Drug Industry

In recent decades, there has been a worldwide trend in many industries for production to become globalized. The production of semi-final and final products is no longer restricted to the developed countries; increasingly, it is conducted in low-wage areas and in areas where raw materials are extracted or grown. This pattern has also affected the growing and manufacture of the primary injected drugs, heroin and cocaine. Whereas the production of injectable forms of opiates and coca products used to be conducted in industrialized countries, now it occurs in the areas where poppies and coca grow (Des Jarlais *et al.,* 1992b; Lima *et al.,* 1992; Stimson 1993). This means that the final products are smaller in bulk and in mass, and are thus easier to hide from drug enforcement agencies and from competitors. It also means that injectable heroin and cocaine are now produced in southeast Asia and in Latin America (among other regions), and that they are often used as part payment of labor, and/or sold in local markets, throughout the distribution process. As a consequence, drug injection has spread in Asia and Latin America. There are now tens of thousands of drug injectors in Thailand, Vietnam, Myanmar, Malaysia, India, Brazil, and Argentina (Des Jarlais *et al.,* 1992b; Lima *et al.,* 1992; Mesquita 1991; Stimson 1993).

In each of these countries, unfortunately, large percentages of the drug injectors have become infected with HIV. Thus, seroprevalence rates among drug injector samples have been found to be as high as 75% in Myanmar, 50% in Manipur in northeast India, 40% in Bangkok, 34% in Rio de Janeiro, and 60% in Santos (Sao Paulo State in Brazil.) (Annual Report of the AIDS Prevention and Control Programme, Myanmar, 1992; WHO Collaborative Study Group, 1993; Sarkar *et al.,* 1993). Other life-threatening infections, such as hepatitis C, are also widespread among drug injectors in many of these countries (Waller & Holmes, 1993; Carvalho *et al.,* 1994).

Geographic Movement of People

HIV spreads from one geographic location to another when people move between locations. This can happen through many kinds of movement. Some of it is migration (whether for entire lives or for more limited periods). To some extent, also, HIV is transmitted along the transportation routes through which goods flow in commerce (as was discussed above for the drug industry). In addition, people can spread HIV through vacation travel or visits to family members who live elsewhere.

Hunt (1989) has shown that patterns of medium- and long-term labor migration have helped spread HIV throughout East Africa. Men and women have moved to cities for economic opportunity, and have become infected there through sexual transmission. When they later returned home, either as visitors to spouses or other members who had not come with them, or as return migrants, they took the virus with them, and this led to further sexual spread.

In the United States, AIDS case data demonstrate a pattern of diffusion over time from the large coastal cities to smaller, inland cities and to the countryside. One salient pattern of this spread has been diffusion along the main commercial highways (Gould, 1993).

Among gay and bisexual men, studies of the early AIDS cases showed a pattern of diffusion that could be traced among defined persons in different parts of the country (Auerbach *et al.,* 1984; Darrow, 1991.) It was possible to determine who traveled where and when, and when they had engaged in sexual activity with other people who also were diagnosed with AIDS.

Sociohistorical and Social Network Factors

This brief review has covered only some of the sociohistorical factors that have shaped the epidemic. It has not dealt with questions of prevention policy and politics, nor with questions of class or gender, nor with changes in land-use patterns that lead to sizable population movements within urban areas, nor with the large-scale structuring of risk behavior, risk reduction, and of barriers to risk reduction. On the other hand, it has indicated that structures of racial/ethnic subordination, patterns of production and distribution of drugs, and patterns of personal movement have had impacts on the epidemic.

These sociohistorical processes and structures clearly involve large-scale parts of the social economy. In addition, however, they have impacts that can be traced in terms of much smaller-scale patterns of social interaction. That is, these large-scale forces affect the epidemic through shaping person-to-person sexual and syringe-mediated interactions among persons. That is, these large-scale processes affect the social networks and thence the risk networks through which HIV and other blood-borne and sexually-transmitted pathogens get disseminated. The next section of the paper discusses recent findings about the networks of drug injectors and how these are related to the HIV epidemic.

SOCIAL NETWORKS AND RISK NETWORKS

Social networks and risk networks are smaller social structures that also affect both drug injectors' behavior and the probability that high-risk behavior will lead to becoming infected. Social networks are relationships that can influence ideas, norms, and behaviors. Risk networks are behaviors and material transfers (for example, of "anonymous" syringes in shooting galleries) that can transmit HIV from person to person to person. Social and risk networks often overlap. Recent evidence indicates that both kinds of networks have major consequences for HIV epidemiology and behavior.

First, we will present data from the Social Factors and HIV Risk (SFHR) project, which was conducted in the Bushwick neighborhood of Brooklyn, New York.

Social Factors and HIV Risk: Subjects and Data:

767 subjects were interviewed (with informed consent) from July 1991 to January 1993 in the Bushwick community of Brooklyn. They were tested for HIV antibody (double ELISA with Western blot confirmation) and hepatitis B core antibody. To enter the study, subjects had to have injected drugs within the prior year; those currently in drug abuse treatment were allowed to participate. Subjects were recruited through ethnographically-directed outreach in areas with heavy drug use or through chain-referral by other subjects.

Questionnaire:

A face-to-face interview gathered data on subjects' sociodemographic and biographical background; drug and sexual risk behaviors; medical history; health beliefs; social roles in the drug scene; peer norms; and networks.

Network Information:

Subjects were asked to provide information about up to 10 persons with whom they had injected drugs, had sex, or otherwise interacted in a non-casual way during the prior 30 days. They also provided information regarding how long they had known each network member, the nature of their relationship, the network member's risk behavior, and their risk behaviors together.

Network concepts and data:

Network data and concepts are relatively new. For reasons of clarity, we will briefly present a few terms and their relationships to the data that were collected and to the databases and variables to be used in the analysis.

Figure 7.4 presents a sociometric network among research subjects. Note here that only the 491 drug injectors who have been linked to at least one other subject are part of this sociometric network. For purposes of these analyses, furthermore, we have restricted the data to be analyzed here to 404 drug injectors who were also HIV

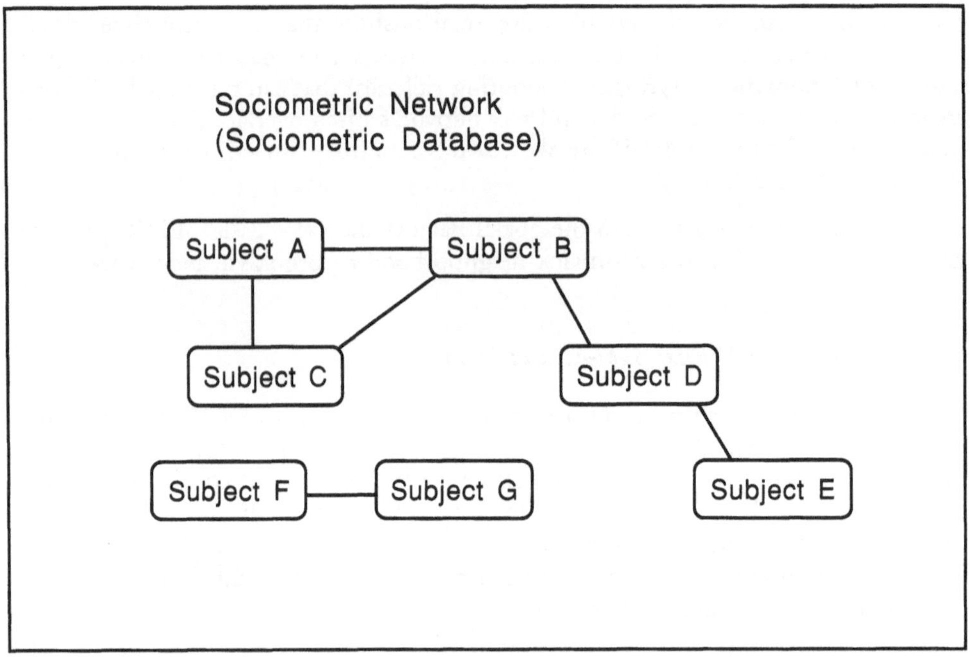

Fig. 7.4 Sociometric network among research subjects

tested. This restriction is because the analyses of sociometric structure were conducted using software–UCINET–that cannot conduct analyses on the entire 491 subjects.

Subjects are considered to be "linked" if one or both of them reported that, in the 30 days prior to the interview, they injected drugs together, had sex together, or had other non-casual interaction; and if these linkages were validated by face-to-face contact with research staff, by ethnographic observation, or by matching of identifying characteristics as is discussed in Neaigus et al. (In press.) Thus, the lines between subjects indicate that at least one of them named the other as part of their network of persons with whom they had injected drugs, had sex, or engaged in other non-casual interaction in the last 30 days. The data on sociometric ties among respondents comprise a "Sociometric Database" which is used for analyses of sociometric network properties. In the diagram, the subjects fall into two "connected components," one of which has 5 members and the other of which has 2 members. A connected component is a set of persons who all have direct or indirect links to each other, although these links may consist of paths through several other persons. Components are separate, therefore, if no members of either is linked to any member of the other. Within the 5-member component, there is a "core" (technically, a Seidman 2-core [Seidman, 1983]) of 3 members who are each linked to at least two other members of the core; and a two-member periphery. Note that although Subject D is linked to two other subjects, Subject D is not linked to 2 members of the core.

Units of Analysis:

These different databases provide the possibility of conducting studies based on different units of analysis. In studies of the predictors of personal attributes such as HIV infection or of risk behaviors as personal attributes, the unit of analysis will ordinarily be the individual. For such analyses, then, variables will typically be constructed that describe the social network and risk network characteristics of individual subjects. Sociometric network location (eg. being a member of the core of a large connected component) is derived from the sociometric database that describes the relationships among linked research subjects, and is also an individual attribute.

Another level of analysis is the larger-than-dyadic risk network. This level of analysis looks at the structures of sociometric linkages among the different subjects who are part of the sociometric database. Connected components are one kind of sociometric structure.

Data Validity and Reliability:

Comparisons among members of dyads who are both in the data set indicates that the self-report data about a number of personal characteristics and behaviors are of good to adequate reliability (Goldstein *et al.*, 1993, submitted; Neaigus *et al.*, in press). In addition, the fact that many analyses have found relationships between independent and dependent variables that were predicted by theory (Neaigus *et al.*, In press; Friedman *et al.*, 1994a; Friedman *et al.*, In press; Jose *et al.*, 1993; Curtis *et al.*, In press; Neaigus *et al.*, 1993a, 1993b) tends to provide construct validation for a number of these variables.

Limitations of Data:

Certain limitations of these data should be mentioned. First, as in all such studies, it is impossible to select a random sample of the population of drug injectors (Watters & Biernacki, 1989). Second, subjects may have underreported the number of persons with whom they had injected or had sex in the last 30 days as a way to shorten the interview or because they did not want to mention knowing certain other drug injectors or sex partners. Unknown biases may enter into the samples of egocentric dyadic relationships as a result. Since subjects recruited through snowball techniques had to be part of the list of subjects nominated by the index respondent, the sociometric database may also have limited representativeness. In all these limitations, the SFHR data essentially share the problems of what is a developing area of research. In spite of these limitations, as has been discussed above, the data have provided us with the opportunity to make a number of important discoveries.

Similarly, the interviews provide self-report data; like all such data, there is an element of imprecision in these self-reports. However, as has been discussed, we have been able to assess the reliability of these data through comparisons of self-reports with what other respondents report about subjects, and have shown that the data are quite reliable (Goldstein *et al.*, 1993, submitted; Neaigus *et al.*, in press).

Analysis:

In order to detect sociometric network structures, UCINET software was used to detect connected components–groups of subjects who are either linked to each other directly or who are linked to one or more other subjects who are directly or indirectly linked. UCINET also was used to detect Seidman 2-cores, where a Seidman K-core (Seidman, 1983) is a subset of a component in which each member is linked to at least k other members in the subset. Thus, in the 2-cores identified in this paper, each member is linked to 2 or more other members of the core.

Sociometric Results:

When analyzed to detect connected components, 90 components were detected. The sizes of the components varied between 2 members (dyads) and a large 187-member connected component. The numbers of components, by size of component, are presented in Figure 7.5. The k-core routine of UCINET was used to detect a 2-core within the large 187-member component.

Four structural categories were then defined on the bases of these analyses:

1) a core (all of whose members are linked to two or more other members) of 88 drug injectors within the 187-member linked component;
2) the periphery of this component, comprised of its other 99 members;
3) 217 IDUs who are members of 89 components ranging in size from 2 to 9 members; and
4) 283 unlinked IDUs.

These categories form a scale of decreasing social connection to other IDUs.

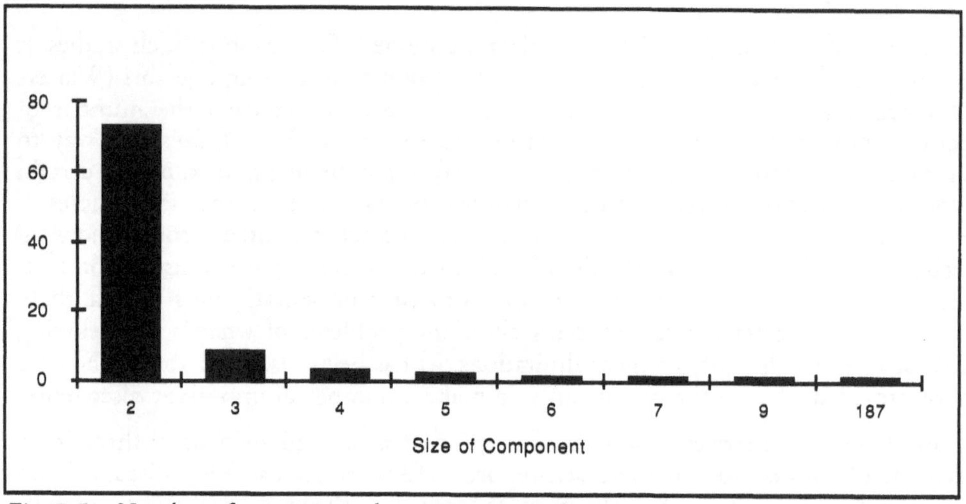

Fig. 7.5 Number of components by component size

This four-category measure of sociometric connections was then crosstabulated by HIV serostatus, hepatitis B core antibody, and a number of sociodemographic and behavioral variables. The results of these crosstabulations are given in Table 7.1. Thus, we can see that sociometric location is significantly related to a number of variables. Core location is associated with a considerably higher probability of HIV infection (55% vs. 36% to 39%). Hepatitis core antibody–an indicator of prior infection rather than of continuing infectiousness–increases with the degree of sociometric connection, being lowest in the unlinked and small-component members, and increasing for the periphery of the large component and the core. Several high-risk injecting practices which have been associated with higher probability of HIV

Table 7.1
Crosstabulations by Sociometric Category

	187-member Core	component Periphery	2 to 9 member component	Unlinked	p*
% HIV+	55%	36%	39%	37%	.019
% HBV CAb+	83%	78%	70%	69%	.022
Behaviors in last 2 years:					
Receptive syringe sharing	51%	47%	46%	36%	.008
Backloading	51%	32%	22%	16%	.001
Inject in outside places	72%	57%	39%	46%	.001
Injected in shooting gallery	43%	34%	18%	31%	.12
Injected cocaine or speedball	87%	85%	74%	65%	.001
Consistent condom use	19%	22%	13%	16%	.31
Commercial sex work	19%	19%	10%	15%	.35
Homeless	33%	22%	20%	16%	.001
Non-white	56%	52%	67%	77%	.001
Gender: % women	26%	27%	31%	30%	.44
Not in treatment	94%	80%	70%	80%	.018
Lack legal income	41%	23%	21%	23%	.006
Prior jail	69%	53%	53%	52%	.020
Sell syringes	31%	16%	13%	15%	.006
Sell drugs	15%	23%	13%	22%	.15
Program contact:					
Received in last 3 months any:					
Bleach	66%	58%	52%	53%	.049
Sterile syringes	51%	35%	29%	26%	.001
Condoms	66%	56%	57%	54%	.082
Medical treatment	2%	5%	4%	5%	.536

*Probabilities by Mantel-Haenszel test for trend.

infection, including injecting with syringes others have used (Anthony et al. 1991; Sasse *et al.,* 1989), backloading (Jose *et al.,* 1993), injecting in outside places (Neaigus *et al.,* 1993), and injecting cocaine or speedball (Chaisson *et al.,* 1989; Dasgupta *et al.,* In press; Novick *et al.,* 1989), are more likely to have been engaged in by drug injectors with more sociometric connection to other drug injectors. Condom use, on the other hand, is not associated with sociometric location. A number of measures of social stratification are also related to sociometric location: Homeless drug injectors, those who lack legal income, and, interestingly, white drug injectors are more likely to be in the core of the large connected component. Core members are also more likely to have been in drug abuse treatment and to have done time in jail or prison. HIV prevention programs seem to be reaching drug injectors in the core (and, to a lesser degree, in the rest of the large connected component) more effectively than those who are unlinked or in smaller components. This is indicated by the larger proportions of drug injectors in the core and periphery who had received bleach and sterile syringes from prevention programs in the 3 months prior to the interview.

Given that sociometric location is related to risk behaviors as well as to HIV, the question arises as to whether location is an independent risk factor for HIV. Table 7.2 presents the results of a logistic regression analysis in which previously-determined sociodemographic and behavioral risk factors for HIV among subjects in the SFHR project were entered simultaneously with sociometric location (core vs. non-core) as predictors of HIV. As can be seen, all of the variables, including sociometric location, remain independent significant predictors (with the exception that Black race/ethnicity loses significance, although remaining a strong trend).

Limitations of Data for Analyses of HIV Risk Factors:

In addition to the limitations discussed above, these data are somewhat limited for analyses of HIV risk factors. First, the network data are based on questions about links during the prior 30 days. The HIV epidemic in New York is over 15 years old. Social networks will have changed during this period, and seropositive subjects will

Table 7.2.
Logistic regression Predictors of HIV Serostatus

	Odds Ratio	95% C.I.
Core (vs. all other)	1.89	1.13, 3.17
Black (vs. White)	1.53	0.98, 2.39
Latino (vs. White)	1.96	1.30, 2.95
Years Since Started Injecting	1.06	1.04, 1.08
Behaviors in last two years:		
Any Backloading	1.56	1.05, 2.32
Speedball Injection Frequency (Scale = 10/month)	1.05	1.02, 1.07
Any Woman-to-Woman Sex	2.52	1.13, 5.63
Any Man-to-Man Sex	3.59	1.02, 12.6

almost certainly all have been infected with HIV prior to the last 30 days. Thus, it is impossible to be sure about the direction of causation. It could be that seropositive drug injectors gravitate towards the core of the large connected component. Somewhat more likely, it might be that the personal (egocentric) social networks of some drug injectors predispose them towards behaviors and patterns of social contact and social development that make them more likely to become infected with HIV early in their injection career and also predispose them to engage in interactions with core members. Of course, the third possibility – that drug injectors in the core are particularly likely to become infected – also undoubtedly operates for at least a number of drug injectors. This is because our data indicate that core members engage in a large amount of high-risk injection behavior, such as receptive syringe sharing, syringe-mediated drug sharing (backloading), injecting cocaine/speedball, and injecting in outside injecting locations. Furthermore, when they inject, they often do so in company with other members of the core – and 55% of these other members of the core are seropositive. Thus, although we cannot be sure of this until cohort studies using network techniques are conducted, it seems highly likely that the seroconversion rate among uninfected core members is a high one.

A second limitation on these analyses derives from our analytic limitations. The UCINET software[1] used for the sociometric analyses was not able to analyze all the members of the sociometric dataset, so we included only those members for whom we have HIV test results. This separation is artificial, since an infected subject who did not take the test is nonetheless able to transmit HIV to those who did. Thus, it would be more accurate to use a sociometric classification based upon the data for all 491 subjects for whom data on linkage are available (as well as the unlinked subjects).

Networks in Colorado Springs, a Low Seroprevalence City

Sociometric network data are also available for Colorado Springs, a city in which the HIV seroprevalence of drug injectors is much lower than in New York (Rothenberg *et al.*, in press[a]; Rothenberg *et al.*, in press[b]; Woodhouse *et al.*, in press; S. Muth, personal communication, April 1994). These data were collected by an El Paso County (Colorado Springs) Health Department project from 304 drug injectors who had injected drugs within the previous 6 months as part of a larger study that also collected data on commercial sex workers and the paying and non-paying sex partners of commercial sex workers and drug injectors. This project collected names and addresses of persons who were nominated by subjects as members of their risk networks, which aided them in seeking to recruit nominees for the study; and they were sometimes able to use other Health Department records to provide some data on nominees who were not recruited for the study.

The drug-injecting subjects reported that they had injected with 462 other drug injectors in the 6 months prior to their interview. 755 dyadic injecting relationships among these people are available for analysis, of which 183 involved people who had not only injected drugs together but who had also had sex with each other during

[1] UCINET is developing software that can handle larger matrices.

the prior 6 months. GRADAP software was used to detect connected components among all of these subjects. 97 connected components were detected, including one large component with 356 members (including some who were not "subjects" but for whom data were available from other sources) and 96 components of sizes 2 to 21. Thus, in spite of considerable methodological difference between the Colorado Springs and New York studies, both studies found that relationships among drug injectors fell into one large component and a large number of smaller components; furthermore, in both cities, most of the smaller components were dyads or triads.

In the larger study, of 595 respondents (including commercial sex workers and their clients as well as drug injectors), 341 fell into one large connected component and 254 fell into 146 smaller components. Seventeen subjects (including 16 present or past drug injectors) were HIV seropositive, 8 of whom were in the large component and 9 of whom were in smaller components. Thus, seroprevalence was 2.3% in the larger component and 3.5% in the set of smaller components. Within the large connected component, almost all (7 of 8) of the seropositive subjects had low centrality scores (on a number of different measures of centrality), which is similar to being on the periphery of this component.

Thus, the relationship between HIV and networks seems to be different in New York and Colorado Springs–although the methodological differences between the studies should be considered to limit our confidence in this conclusion. In New York, seroprevalence is high, and is highest in the core of the large connected component. In Colorado Springs, on the other hand, seroprevalence is low; and seropositive subjects seem either to be in the smaller components or among subjects who are of "low centrality" in the larger component (which means that they have relative weak linkages to other members of this component.) In sum, then, these data suggest that HIV transmission may remain low if the virus is restricted to persons in small components or to those on the peripheries of large components, but that rapid transmission may occur if it begins to spread in the core of a large component.

PERSONAL SOCIAL NETWORKS, RISK BEHAVIORS, AND HIV INFECTION

So far, the discussion has focused briefly on large-scale sociohistorical forces that affect the HIV epidemic, and then on the sociometric networks of drug injectors in communities. Next, we will briefly discuss the personal, or "egocentric," networks of drug injectors and how these affect their risk behaviors and the probability that new injectors are HIV-infected in Bushwick. First, however, it will be useful to discuss the nature of egocentric networks and of data about egocentric networks.

Diagram 6 presents "Subject's" egocentric network. The members of this network consist of four persons who did not take part in the study and one person ("Another Subject") who did. The social relationships and shared behaviors between the subject and the five members of subject's egocentric network are indicated as lines between boxes in the diagram. When studying the subject as an individual, characteristics of his or her egocentric network (such as whether any of its members inject drugs more than once a day) may be entered as an "attribute"–i.e., as a variable characterizing the individual subject. Such egocentric network attributes can be analyzed just as can other attributes such as subject's gender or frequency of injection. Several egocentric risk network factors are related to HIV serostatus among the SFHR project subjects: (1) For new injectors who have been injecting for 6 or fewer years, having a high-risk egocentric network increases the probability that women and those who engage in risk behaviors are infected with HIV (Neaigus *et al.,* in press). Examples of high-risk network characteristics include having a drug injector in one's network who (a) is 5 or more years older than the subject, and thus may have had more time to become infected; (b) whom the subject has known for a year or less (a measure of network turnover); (c) who injects more than once a day (a risk factor for HIV); or (d) who injects in shooting galleries (a risk factor for HIV). (2) Among women who have been injecting less than 10 years (but not for men), having a drug injector member who is 5 or more years older, having a drug injector in one's network whom one has known one year or less, and having a drug injector in one's network who injects daily or more are associated with higher seroprevalence (Friedman *et al.,* 1993b).

The dyadic social relationships (indicated by connecting lines in Figure 7.6) between subjects and the members of their egocentric networks can also be used as units of analysis. These data comprise our "Contact Database," which has 3,165 dyadic relationships as its components. The contact database contains information about subjects and each of the (up to 10) members of their personal social network about whom they answered detailed questions.

Egocentric social relationships and peer group culture are related to two risk behaviours – consistent condom use and receptive syringe sharing (that is, injecting with a syringe which an egocentric network member has previously used).

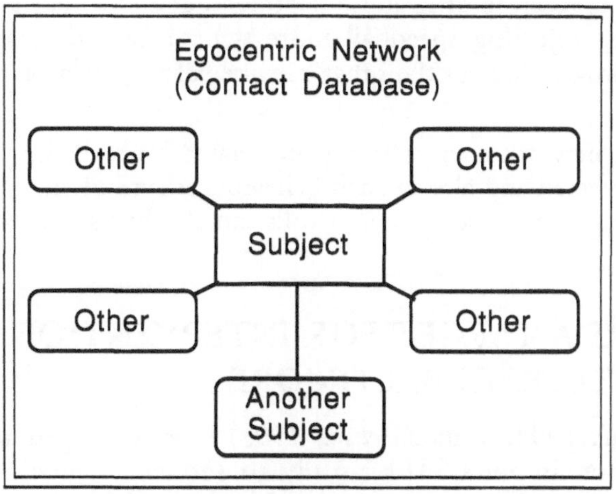

Fig. 7.6 Dyadic social relationships

In studying consistent condom use (Friedman *et al.,* 1994a), we found that: (1) Individual subjects may have consistent condom use with one partner but not with another. Thus, condom use is relationship-specific rather than being an individual characteristic. One implication of this is that data sets that treat condom use either as an individual characteristic or by asking about condom use with types of partners (such as primary partners, or with sexual clients) are unable to analyze how the relational characteristics of dyads predict condom use. (2) The extent of consistent condom use varies by drug injector subject serostatus and by whether the partner in a relationship is a drug injector or not. In particular, there are high levels of consistent condom use (68%) in relationships between seropositive drug injectors and non-injecting partners. (3) Independent significant predictors of consistent condom use in dyadic relationships include relationship characteristics (type, duration), perceived peer norms about condom use, subject characteristics (not being homeless, commercial sex work), partner characteristics (age 25), and the relationship's being between a seropositive drug injector and a non-injector.

In studying receptive syringe sharing (Neaigus *et al.,* 1993b), we found that: (1) Individual subjects may engage in receptive syringe sharing with one partner but not with another. Thus, injecting with a syringe someone else has used is relationship-specific rather than being an individual characteristic. One implication of this is that data sets that treat syringe sharing as an individual characteristic will be unable to analyze the relational predictors of receptive syringe sharing and will thus have limited ability to guide the development of intervention programs. (2) Independent significant predictors of receptive syringe sharing (in dyads) include (a) social characteristics of the dyads (daily or greater contact; injecting together more than one year; "very close" relationship; the relationship is also a sexual relationship; and the dyad members also steal together); and (b) peer culture (such that subjects who report that they and their peers "rotate who injects with a syringe first" are more likely to use syringes that others have used; but if they report that they think that "a shooting partner who refuses to share a syringe with you is a true friend," this is protective; (c) individual protective characteristics such as Black race/ethnicity, having received drug abuse treatment, and older age at first injection; (d) individual risks (injecting speedball more than once a day, and exchanging sex for money or drugs); and (e) the other member of the dyad being 30 years old or older.

Thus, egocentric network characteristics are related both to the probability that new injectors are infected and also to such behaviors as syringe sharing and condom use. As will now be shown, egocentric networks can also be used as targets for AIDS interventions.

NETWORKS AS A TARGET FOR INTERVENTIONS: THE "SAFE" STUDY IN BALTIMORE

Latkin (Latkin *et al.,* 1993; Mandell *et al.,* 1993) have developed an experimental network intervention in the "SAFE" study to influence the risk behaviors of individual drug injectors by working both with the individual and with persons with whom he or she did drugs. Sessions were held in which the subjects and the members of their networks were exposed to a self-help, peer-led group model based on a psychoeducational approach (Anderson *et al.*, 1986). This intervention was highly scripted and was facilitated by former heroin injectors who maintained contact with and were respected by active drug users in Baltimore. Their personal experience let the facilitators increase the relevance of the sessions for the subjects and their network members.

The intervention sessions focused on every member as an individual and also on the group as a whole. They aimed to provide an opportunity for participants to reconceptualize their HIV-related behaviors and to consider factors that might influence these behaviors. They were asked to choose among options to reduce their HIV risk behaviors and to make commitments to increase health-promoting behaviors. They were taught about social norms and social influence. Role-playing of problem situations allowed practice and further consideration of how to overcome difficulties in maintaining safer behaviors. Group exercises were designed to demonstrate the power of social norms on behavior.

The model was evaluated through comparison with a control group. All participants were recruited from among subjects in the AIDS Linked to Intravenous Experiences (ALIVE) study of the natural history of HIV infection among drug injectors in Baltimore. To enroll in the SAFE study, ALIVE subjects were required to have reported sharing drugs with other users.

Participants were randomly assigned to either an experimental or control group. Experimental "index participants" were asked to bring into the clinic their drug sharing network for the intervention. For an intervention session to occur, the index and half the nominated network members were required to be present. Index participants who attended three or more sessions were considered to have completed the study. Post-test interviews occurred, on average, 3 months after completion of the final intervention session. Controls received no additional intervention beyond the extensive counseling and testing that all participants in the ALIVE study undergo each time they are interviewed and give blood for HIV and other testing. Participants in the control and experimental groups were reinterviewed within the same time frame.

Of 189 potential index subjects, 42 (22%) had an initial interview but did not return with members of their drug network. Another 69 (37%) brought in at least some members of their drug network for initial interview but never started in the intervention. There were 78 (41%) index participants who started the sessions, and 66 of these completed the intervention. (The completion rate for those index participants who attended the first session was 85%). Altogether, 62 index experimentals and 90 controls completed the three-month follow-up interview. The indexes were significantly more likely than the controls to report that they always carried bleach ($p < 0.01$), always cleaned their needles before injecting ($p < 0.05$), had reduced their frequency of sharing needles ($p < 0.05$) and had reduced injecting in shooting galleries ($p < 0.05$).

Thus, it appears that group interventions with drug injectors' egocentric networks may be an effective way to reduce their risk behavior even among persons who have previously been exposed to considerable counseling, testing, and education. Additional research is needed to confirm this finding, to assess the extent to which it can be generalized to other social settings, and to further improve the intervention techniques. Furthermore, since only a limited number of persons who were assigned to the experimental condition actually succeeded in bringing network members to the group sessions, research is needed to determine the barriers to such participation and to develop ways to overcome these barriers.

DISCUSSION AND IMPLICATIONS

The first implication of this paper is simply that research, policy and prevention efforts should consider both sociohistorical factors and intermediate-scale factors – particularly including social and risk networks – to reduce the scope and impact of the HIV epidemic.

Issues of social structure and social policy clearly have an impact on AIDS. The failure of the United States to end racial/ethnic subordination has led to there being more AIDS cases among African-Americans and Latinos than among other population groups. Among drug injectors in New York, at least, HIV seroprevalence has been higher among African-Americans and Latinos than among whites for many years, and it appears as if the (partial) segregation of risk networks may be one contributor to maintaining this racial/ethnic differential. Elsewhere we have shown that Black Latino drug injectors (who are subjected to two forms of racial/ethnic subordination) are more likely to be infected with HIV, and less likely to receive drug abuse treatment and other medical treatment (Friedman *et al.*, in press).

Policies that focus on disrupting the drug trade and on penalizing drug users and dealers have failed to prevent injectable drugs from reaching users in the United States, Europe, and other economically developed areas. Furthermore, these policies have failed to prevent the spread of drug injecting in many developing countries. Indeed, it is likely that these policies may have contributed to the relocation of drug commerce routes and, as a consequence, to the spread of drug injecting and HIV to additional countries. Economic and urban policies (as well as "market forces") that lead to large-scale geographic movements of people have also helped to spread HIV both within countries and from country to country. Furthermore, in many cases, drug policies, economic policies, and urban policies are decided upon without consideration of their impact on the spread of HIV or other diseases. One prevention implication is that "AIDS impact statements" should be required as part of the decision-making process on a wide variety of issues and policies. Another is that research needs to be conducted to allow us to have a clearer understanding of how these policies and market forces affect HIV diffusion and transmission.

Social structures of smaller scale than these are also important. In particular, sociometric network structures have important consequences both on risk behaviors and on the probability of infection. For research, then, analyses of HIV epidemiology and of drug injection behaviors need to measure and analyze sociometric network location into account.

Egocentric networks also seem to have consequences for infection probabilities and for risk behaviors.

The central aim of research on HIV epidemiology, risk behaviors, social structures, and interventions is to use the analyses to suggest more effective techniques to reduce HIV spread. Here, we start from an observation about AIDS prevention efforts among drug injectors – and, although we are less familiar with these efforts, among other groups of people as well. Many, perhaps most, of the interventions that aim to prevent HIV transmission among drug injectors, or from drug injectors to their sexual partners, have been based on psychological and social-psychological perspectives on individual and small group behavior. Adding network-based interventions might considerably improve our efforts to reduce HIV spread. (A tentative typology of such interventions is presented in Table 7.3).

Table 7.3
Typology of Network Interventions*

Interventions can focus on

1. helping individuals navigate within & between network structures.
2 helping individuals re-shape their egocentric networks to be less dangerous.
3. using network pressures to change individual behavior, including getting them into contact with syringe exchanges or treatment.
4. using large-scale network pressures to change behaviors of small groups.
5. shaping the movement patterns within networks.
   a. reducing turnover
   b. helping new (& others) avoid cores etc.
6. changing network structures.
   a. before HIV becomes widespread in large components, maybe work with the members of it to (1) reduce its size; (2) change the intensity of relationships among members; (3) change the culture of risk within them; (4) become a center for outreach (and needle exchange) for others who come into contact with the core.
   b. before HIV becomes widespread in large components, change policy (away from suppression of users) so as to reduce pressures to be members of large components/cores.
   c. conceivably, before HIV becomes widespread in large components, use police to disrupt large components. There is, however, considerable reason to suspect that this will fail, and indeed will drive IDUs even further into large components/cores.
   d. after HIV becomes widespread in a component, it becomes a possible source of infection for others. Possible approaches include (1) helping component bifurcate by serostatus; (2) reducing interaction between component and other IDUs/network structures; (3) helping component reduce its behavioral risk.
7. Programs aimed at risk-reduction that are differentiated by network location. That is, maybe develop different approaches for cores & peripheries of large components; for small & large components; for unlinked.

* As we come to understand the population dynamics of recruitment to components/cores, of weak ties between cliques and other subgroupings, of the role of multi-user settings and the associated changes in use of these settings, of individual leavings and group secessions from network structures, of formation of egocentric networks, and so forth, we may be able to deepen this categorization and make it more processual.

Several issues need to be addressed:

1. Close social relationships between drug injectors (Neaigus *et al.*, 1993b) and between drug injectors and their sexual partners (Friedman *et al.*, 1994a) that have been associated with greater behavioral risk pose a dilemma for intervention–between the harm that might be done by weakening such relationships and the potential benefit in terms of reducing risk behaviors. This suggests that research demonstration projects might be conducted on the relative extent of risk reduction attained by the somewhat opposed approaches of (a) trying to weaken such relationships; (b) trying to develop and/or mobilize solidarity between drug and/or sex partners as a resource to motivate risk reduction; and (c) a "standard" intervention control condition.
2. There seems to be solidarity between infected drug injectors and their non-injecting sex partners that leads to high levels of consistent condom use (Friedman *et al.*, 1994a; Vanichseni *et al.*, 1993). Such solidarity might be a resource that can be used for risk reduction efforts.
3. The analyses presented here suggest the hypotheses that the cores of large connected components in high seroprevalence cities may be social locations particularly conducive to HIV spread; and that preventing widespread HIV transmission in low seroprevalence cities may depend on preventing the virus from reaching and/or being transmitted within such cores. These hypotheses suggest several possible intervention strategies: (a) new injectors should be reached and instructed about the desirability of minimizing their ties to "cores" and, additionally, to older injectors; (b) to the extent that contact with core members is dangerous to drug injectors who are not members of the core (or, in low prevalence cities, perhaps vice versa)–and this is suggested by our analyses of the ethnographically-defined core and the behaviors and infection levels of its inner and outer peripheries (Curtis *et al.*, in press), as well as having been implicitly suggested by the analysis of weak and strong ties among Houston drug injectors (Williams & Johnson, 1993)–methods should be developed to convert these same ties into risk reduction resources. One such method might be to recruit core members to act as voluntary or paid members of syringe exchange projects, who would both encourage their contacts to take precautions and provide them with sterile syringes and condoms to facilitate such risk reduction–which is already happening to some degree in some cities (Des Jarlais & Friedman, 1992a); (c) interventions that try to recruit core members as AIDS prevention agents should also reduce risk behaviors in the core (or cores). Nevertheless, drug injectors who remain in such cores may remain at high risk of infection with HIV (and other blood-borne pathogens) or of transmitting their already-existing infection to others. Research is needed on how the different roles, behaviors, and perceived peer norms of core members may provide clues for additional interventions that might reduce these risks.
4. Research is needed on the policy dimensions of why and how IDUs join cores. The ethnographic component of the SFHR project (Curtis *et al.*, in press) suggests that the structures of drug markets (which lack Durkheim's

non-contractual elements of contracts–i.e., which lack both normative and judicial mechanisms for enforcing contracts and mediating disputes) can mean that non-core IDUs seek relationships with core IDUs so they can successfully buy high-quality drugs and so they can find safe sites to inject them. Drug laws, police tactics, and gentrification that disrupt drug networks may increase this motivation. Such drug and social policies that encourage IDUs to join cores may need to be re-assessed.

5. We have shown that women injectors get infected with HIV earlier in their injection careers than do men, and that this is specifically true for women with high-risk egocentric networks. We have suggested that (Friedman *et al.*, 1993b; Friedman *et al.*, 1994b): (a) this means that there is an urgent need for interventions that target women who are at high risk of beginning to inject drugs and women who have recently begun to inject drugs; and (b), since these earlier infections among women may be a result of women having less power or status within drug scenes or local communities than men have, public policy and the efforts of drug users' organizations should develop programs to counteract such inequality while promoting risk reduction. Further research on why women become infected earlier is needed, and may suggest additional intervention possibilities.

   Finally, egocentric and sociometric social networks are an intermediate level of social structure, larger than the individual or the dyad yet smaller than the neighborhood, community, or world society. Clearly, all levels of analysis can contribute to our understanding of the spread of infectious diseases such as HIV. The almost exclusive emphasis of research funds and prevention programs on individual-level variables and interventions, and the over-emphasis even among sociologists on models based on the assumptions of methodological individualism (such as the health belief model, social learning theory, and the theory of reasoned action) should be ended.

Additions to our HIV prevention efforts should include a mixture of network-focused interventions–which should not be particularly controversial–and efforts to change those social policies and social structures that, as by-products, contribute to HIV spread. These last changes are likely to involve considerable debate, controversy, and conflict.

ACKNOWLEDGEMENTS

Support was provided by the National Institute on Drug Abuse grants DA05723 "Social Factors and HIV Risk"; DA03574 "Risk Factors for AIDS among Intravenous Drug Users"; DA08950 "HIV Risk Behaviors and Social Influence in IDUs' Networks"; and DA06326 "Prevention of AIDS in IV Drug User Networks."

The New York State Department of Health AIDS Institute assisted in drawing serum samples, HIV testing and referrals.

We would like to acknowledge assistance provided by Stephen Q. Muth, John J. Potterat, and Donald E. Woodhouse of the El Paso County Department of Health and Environment; Richard B. Rothenberg of Emory University School of Medicine; and Thomas Ward of National Development and Research Institutes, Inc.

REFERENCES

Anderson, C.M., Reiss, D.J., Hogarty, G.E. (1986) *Schizophrenia and the Family.* New York: Guildford.

Annual Report of the AIDS Prevention and Control Programme, Myanmar, 1992

Anthony, J.C., Vlahov, D., Nelson, K.E., *et al.* (1991) New evidence on intravenous cocaine use and the risk of infection with Human Immunodeficiency Virus type 1. *American Journal of Epidemiology* **134**,1175-1189.

Auerbach, D.M., Darrow, W.W., Jaffe, H.W., Curran, J.W. (1984) Cluster of cases of the acquired immune deficiency syndrome: Patients linked by sexual contact. *Am J Med* **76**,487-492.

Carvalho, H.B., Bueno, R., Paes, G., Mesquita, *et al.* (1994) HIV and infections with related transmission in an IDU community of Santos, Brazil. Tenth International Conference on AIDS, Yokohama, Japan, 7-12 August, 1994.

Chaisson, R.E., Bacchetti, P., Osmond, D., Brodie, B. *et. al* (1989) Cocaine use and HIV infection in intravenous drug users in San Francisco. *JAMA* **261**, 561-565.

Chitwood, D.D., Rivers, J.R., Comerford, M., McBride, D.C. (1993) A comparison of HIV-related risk behaviors of street-recruited and treatment program-recruited injection drug users. In: Fisher DG, Needle RH (eds.), *AIDS and Community-Based Drug Intervention Programs: Evaluation and Outreach.* Binghamton, NY: Harrington Park Press.

Curtis, R., Friedman, S.R., Neaigus, A., Jose, B., *et al.* (in press) Street-level drug market structure and HIV Risk. *Social Networks.*

D'Aquila, R.T., Peterson, L.R., Williams, A.B., Williams, A.E. (1989) Race/ethnicity as a risk factor for HIV-1 infection among Connecticut intravenous drug users. *J AIDS* **2**, 503-513.

Darrow, W.W. (1991) AIDS: Socioepidemiologic responses to an epidemic. In Ulack R & Skinner WF, *AIDS and the Social Sciences.* Lexington: The University Press of Kentucky. 83-99.

Dasgupta, S., Friedman, S.R., Jose, B., *et al.* (In press) Using retrospective behavioral data to determine HIV risk factors among street-recruited drug injectors. *Journal of Drug Issues.*

Des Jarlais, D.C., Friedman, S.R. (1992a) AIDS and legal access to sterile drug injection equipment. *Ann Am Acad Poli Soc Sci* **521**, 42-65.

Des Jarlais, D.C., Friedman, S.R., Choopanya, *et al.* (1992b) International Epidemiology of HIV and AIDS among Injecting Drug Users. *AIDS,* **6**, 1053-1068.

Des Jarlais, D.C., Friedman, S.R., Sotheran, J.L., Wenston, J., *et al.* (1994) Continuity and change within an HIV epidemic: Injecting drug users in New York City, 1984 through 1992. *JAMA* **271**,121-127.

Friedman, S.R., Sotheran, J.L., Abdul-Quader, A., Primm, B.J., *et al.* (1987) The AIDS epidemic among Blacks and Hispanics. *The Milbank Quarterly* **65**,455- 499.

Friedman, S.R., Sufian, M., Des Jarlais, D.C. (1990) The AIDS epidemic among Latino intravenous drug users. In: Glick, R., Moore, J. (eds.), *Drug Abuse in Hispanic Communities* (pp. 45-54). New Brunswick, NJ: Rutgers University Press.

Friedman, S.R., Young, P.A., Snyder, F.R., Shorty, V., *et al.* NADR Consortium. (1993a) Racial differences in sexual behaviors related to AIDS in a nineteen-city sample of street-recruited drug injectors. *AIDS Educ Prev* **5**,196-211.

Friedman, S.R., Jose, B., Neaigus, A., Goldstein, M., *et al.* (1993b) Female injecting drug users get infected with HIV sooner than males. 121st Ann. Meeting of the Am. Public Health Assoc., San Francisco, CA [session 3137].

Friedman, S.R., Des Jarlais, D.C., Deren, S., Jose, B., Neaigus, A. (1993c) HIV seroconversion among street-recruited drug injectors. In Harris L (ed.) *Problems of Drug Dependence, 1992.* Rockville, MD: National Institute on Drug Abuse Research Monograph #132: p. 124.

Friedman, S.R., Jose, B., Neaigus, A., Goldstein, M., *et al.* (1994a) Consistent condom use in relationships between seropositive injecting drug users and sex partners who do not inject drugs. *AIDS* **8**,357-361.

Friedman, S.R., Des Jarlais, D.C., Ward, T.P., Jose, B., Neaigus, A., Goldstein, M.F. (1994b) Drug injectors and heterosexual AIDS. In: L. Sherr (ed.), *AIDS and the Heterosexual Population* (pp. 41-65). Chur, Switzerland: Harwood Academic Publishers.

Friedman, S.R., Jose, B., Stepherson, B., Neaigus, A., Goldstein, M.F., *et al.* (in press[b]) Multiple racial/ethnic subordination and HIV among drug injectors. In: Singer M, Carlson R, Koester S (eds.), *The Political Economy of AIDS.* New York: Baywood Press.

Goldstein, M., Neaigus, A., Ildefonso, G., Jose, B., Mota, P., Friedman, S.R. (1993) Quality of data provided by IDUs about HIV risk network members. 121st Ann. Meeting of the Am. Public Health Assoc., San Francisco, CA [session 4042].

Goldstein, M., Neaigus, A., Jose, B., Ildefonso, G., Curtis, R., Friedman, S.R. (submitted) Self-reports of HIV risk behavior by injecting drug users: Are they reliable? *Addiction.*

Gould, P. (1993) *The Slow Plague.* Cambridge, MA: Blackwell.

Grund, J.P.C., Kaplan, C.D., Adriaans, N.F.P., Blanken, P. (1991) Drug sharing and HIV transmission risk. *J Psych Drugs* **23**,1-10.

Hahn, R.A., Onorato, I.M., Jones, T.S., Dougherty, J. (1989) Prevalence of HIV infection among intravenous drug users in the United States. *JAMA* **261**, 2677-2684.

Hunt, C.W. (1989) Migrant labor and sexually transmitted disease: AIDS in Africa. *J of Health and Social Behavior.* **30**,353-373.

Jose, B., Friedman, S.R., Curtis, R., Grund, J.P.C., Goldstein, M.F., *et al.* (1993) Syringe-mediated drug-sharing (backloading). *AIDS* 7,1653-60.

Koblin, B.A., McCusker, J., Lewis, B.F., Sullivan, J.L. (1990) Racial/ethnic differences in HIV-1 seroprevalence and risky behaviors among intravenous drug users in a multisite study. *Am J Epidemiology,* **132**, 837-846.

LaBrie, R.A., McAuliffe, W.E., Nemeth-Coslett, R., Wilberschied, L. (1993) The prevalence of HIV infection in a national sample of injection drug users. In: Brown BS, Beschner GM (eds). Handbook on Risk of AIDS (pp. 16-37). Westport, CT: Greenwood Press.

Latkin, C.A., Mandell, W., Oziemkowska, M., Celentano, D.D., Vlahov, D. (1993) A social network approach to AIDS prevention. Paper presented at the NIDA Technical Review on Social Networks, Drug Abuse, and HIV Transmission.

Lima, E.S., Bastos, F.I.P.M., Telles, P.R. & Ward, T.P. (1992) Injecting Drug Users and the Spread of HIV in Brazil. AIDS & Public Policy, 7, 170-174.

Mandell, W., Latkin, C.A., Oziemkowska, M., Celentano, D.D., Vlahov, D. (1993) Impact of social network intervention on HIV risk behaviors in injecting drug users. Paper presented at Annual Meeting of the American Psychological Association. San Francisco, August.

Marmor, M., Des Jarlais, D.C., Cohen, H., *et al.* (1987) Risk factors and infection with human immunodeficiency virus among intravenous drug abusers in New York City. AIDS **1**, 39-44.

Mesquita, F. (1991) AIDS and injecting drug users. In Vivendo em Tempos de AIDS (ed Paiva, V.) Sao Paulo, Editora SUMMUS: pp. 187-190.

Neaigus, A., Friedman, S.R., Jose, B., Goldstein, M., Curtis, R., Des Jarlais, D.C. (1993a) Latino race/ethnicity and injecting at outside settings are HIV risk factors among new injectors. 121st Annual Meeting of the Am. Public Health Assoc., San Francisco, CA.

Neaigus, A., Friedman, S.R., Jose, B., Goldstein, M., Ildefonso, G., Curtis, R., Des Jarlais, D.C. (1993b) Syringe sharing and the social characteristics of drug-injecting dyads. 121st Annual Meeting of the Am. Public Health Assoc., San Francisco, CA.

Neaigus, A., Friedman, S.R., Curtis, R., Des Jarlais, D.C., Furst, R.T., Jose, B., Mota, P., Stepherson, B., Sufian, M., Ward, T.P., Wright, J.W. (1994) The relevance of drug injectors' social networks and risk networks for understanding and preventing HIV infection. Soc Sci & Med **38**, 67-78.

Neaigus, A., Friedman, S.R., Goldstein, M., Ildefonso, G., Curtis, R., Jose, B. (in press) Using dyadic data for a network analysis of HIV infection and risk behaviors among injecting drug users. National Institute on Drug Abuse monograph on Social Networks, Drug Abuse and HIV Transmission. Bethesda, MD: NIDA.

Novick, D.M., Trigg, H.L., Des Jarlais, D.C., Friedman, S.R., Vlahov, D., Kreek, M.J. (1989) Cocaine injection and ethnicity in parenteral drug users during the early years of the human immunodeficiency virus (HIV) epidemic in New York City. Journal of Medical Virology **29**, 181-185.

Nwanyanwu, O.C., Chu, S.Y., Green, T.A., Buehler, J.W., Berkelman, R.L. (1993) Acquired immunodeficiency syndrome in the United States associated with injecting drug use, 1981-1991. *Am J Drug Alcohol Abuse,* **19**, 399-408.

Rothenberg, R.B., Woodhouse, D.E., Potterat, J.J., *et al.* (in press[a]) Social networks and disease transmission. National Institute on Drug Abuse monograph on *Social Networks, Drug Abuse and HIV Transmission.* Bethesda, MD: NIDA.

Rothenberg, R.B., Potterat, J.J., Woodhouse, D.E., *et al.* (in press[b]) Choosing a centrality measure: epidemiologic correlates in the Colorado Springs study of social networks. *Social Networks.*

Sarkar, S., Das, N., Panda, S., Naik, T.N., *et al.* (1993) Rapid spread of HIV among injecting drug users in north-eastern states of India. *Bulletin on Narcotics* **45**, 91-109.

Sasse, H., Salmaso, S., Conti, S., *et al.* (1989) Risk behaviors for HIV-1 infection in Italian drug users: report from a multicenter study. *Journal of Acquired Immune Deficiency Syndromes.* **2**, 486-496.

Seidman, S B. (1983) Network structure and minimum degree. *Social Networks* 5:269-287.

Stimson, G.V. (1993) The Global Diffusion of Injecting Drug Use: Implications for HIV Infection. *Bulletin on Narcotics,* **45**, 3-17.

Vanichseni, S., Des Jarlais, D.C., Choopanya, K., *et al.* (1993) Condom use with primary partners among injecting drug users in Bangkok, Thailand, and New York City, USA. *AIDS* 7, 887-891.

Waller, T. & Holmes, R. (1993) Hepatitis C. *Druglink* May/June, 7-9.

Watters, J.K., Biernacki, P. (1989) Targeted sampling: Options for the study of hidden populations. *Soc Problems* **36**, 416-430.

WHO Collaborative Study Group. (1993) An international comparative study of HIV prevalence and risk behavior among drug injectors in 13 cities. *Bulletin on Narcotics* **45**, 19-46.

Williams, M.L., Johnson, J. (1993) Social network structures: An ethnographic analysis of intravenous drug use in Houston, Texas. In: Fisher DG, Needle RH (eds.), *AIDS and Community-Based Drug Intervention Programs: Evaluation and Outreach.* Binghamton, NY: Harrington Park Press.

Woodhouse, D.E., Rothenberg, R.B., Potterat, J.J., *et al.* (in press) Mapping a social network of heterosexuals at high risk for human immunodeficiency virus infection. *AIDS.*

8

Amphetamine Injecting Women and their Primary Partners: An Analysis of Risk Behaviour

HILARY KLEE

INTRODUCTION

A review of trends in HIV risk behaviour among injecting drug users (IDUs) reported at the Berlin AIDS Conference in 1993 revealed considerable variations in patterns in different nations (Deren *et al.*, 1993). In general, however, there seemed to be an overall decline in the sharing of injecting equipment. Sharing now seems to be most pronounced among IDUs who have close personal relationships with other injectors and inject in their company (Barnard, 1993; Darke *et al.*, 1994; Klee *et al.*, 1993; Ross *et al.*, 1994). There is still little evidence of a decline in unprotected sex (Deren, 1993, op cit.). The use of condoms remains consistently low and this applies most particularly to IDUs in relationships with their primary sexual partners. The sexual transmission of HIV to the primary partners of the majority of IDUs is, therefore, still a major concern.

Because injecting male IDUs tend to have non-injecting or non-using partners (Donoghoe, 1992; Klee, 1993), there is a major risk of HIV transmission through sex to the wider, non-drug using population. However, there is little information about the behaviour of female injectors, particularly non-opiate injectors, who are in extended relationships with one primary partner. It is difficult to assess their vulnerability to HIV infection or their potential for passing this on. There is a view (Rosenbaum, 1981) that women may be at a disadvantage because of their dependence upon partners for drugs and for economic support, particularly if they have children. Hence, the emotional and social dynamics of primary relationships may be a major impediment to health protection. This paper explores the HIV-related risks for a group of women injectors in a primary sexual relationship, perceptions of risk and self-protection strategies.

THE PROJECT

The research context was a study (1) of the lifestyles of 200 amphetamine users carried out in the North-West of England (Klee *et al.*, 1992). Respondents were interviewed by research assistants about their injecting and sexual risk behaviours. Sampling was opportunistic and the majority of contacts were mediated by other drug users in networks across 35 different locations in the region. All of the interviews were recorded on audio tape.

Injecting amphetamine users who reported one close and continuous sexual relationship (n=70) were selected from the larger sample. Only 6 were receiving treatment for drugs, although 42% of them used a needle exchange regularly. The majority were, therefore, not in contact with specialist services that provided HIV education and counselling.

There were 24 women with regular partners and their average age was 24 years. Inevitably a small sample invites speculation concerning the generalisability of the observations. The respondents came from a wide area over the North West of England in which drug sub-cultures vary considerably. Nonetheless, the risks identified as important for this sample may not apply to women sampled in other studies.

Twenty-two (92%) of the sample had drug-injecting partners, compared with seven (15%) of the male amphetamine injectors (see Klee, 1993 for comparisons with opiate users). This asymmetry has considerable relevance for patterns of sharing injecting equipment. Injecting sexual partnerships provide more opportunities for HIV transmission to occur. There are 2 routes for HIV transmission between such partners: the sharing of injecting equipment and sexual intercourse without condoms. With non-injecting partnerships the disease can only be transmitted through sex. Quantitative statistical analyses of the data were used in conjunction with the qualitative analyses of transcripts and field observations. The emphasis in the presentation of these findings in this chapter is on the verbatim material provided by the women, with quantitative analyses used to provide a structural base for these 'insider accounts'.

RESULTS

Sharing Injecting Equipment

No statistical differences were found in the incidence of sharing injecting equipment between men and women but the characteristics of donors and recipients of the injecting equipment were different because of the differences in partners' drug status. The overall levels of sharing were typical of the total sample of injectors in the parent study (n=110), 55% of whom had received others' injecting equipment and 70% had passed theirs on. The presence of a regular partner neither enhanced nor reduced the incidence of sharing.

Gender differences in the donors and recipients of used needles and syringes were expected because of partner differences. Predictably, because more women had injecting partners, they shared more with their partners than their friends. In some cases this was because they preferred to be injected by their partner, this occurring after he had injected himself. Often the partner was the one who prepared the amphetamine for injection. A typical pattern was described by this woman:

Interviewer: *How does it work (injecting) with your boyfriend — does he always inject you?*

Respondent: *He does do it, yeah. I'll only let a couple of people do it who I trust — I've got to really trust them... there's only a couple. He does himself and then puts mine in the works, gets a vein up and puts it in.*

In most cases this was because the partner was seen as more expert:

Respondent: *I think if I didn't have him to look after me I'd have ended up dead years ago ... 'cos I didn't know what I was doing... I mean, I was full of bruises and all sorts (through attempting to inject herself).*

Sharing 'turns' was also dependent on physical factors however. Blunt needles were not only painful, they produced unsightly bruises on the arms – an important negative aspect of injecting for women. There was no spontaneous mention by any woman, either when describing sharing with partners or with friends, of the desire to go first because of the danger of infection. This is not to say that the implications of turn-taking were not known:

Respondent: *I would never go second because the needle's blunt and it's harder to get a hit... and it hurts and makes a mess of your arms... so I always use it first... but that's not out of cleanliness... it's just because the needle would be blunt.*

The typical use of the term 'sharing' by the women was with reference to drug-using associates, and it implied an acknowledgement of risk. It was not a term used willingly by them when talking about people who were close. Using this restricted definition, most women said that sharing was rare and unnecessary:

Interviewer: *Do you ever share with Rick (boyfriend)?*

Respondent: *Yes.*

Interviewer: *Have you had a test?*

Respondent: *No, I feel confident that the only people I do share with are clean enough for me to share with. They're as clean as I am.*

Interviewer: *So how many people is it that you generally share with?*

Respondent: *Not as many as you're thinking. Four of us who share if we have to.*

According to respondents, the equipment was always cleaned although this could be a cursory business. The majority (58%) of both men and women flushed equipment under an available tap. Some of the women were more watchful, however:

Interviewer: *Does he do anything with the works between hitting himself up and hitting you up?*

Respondent: *Yes, he always, like, puts it under boiling water.*

Interviewer: *Do you worry about using his needles?*

Respondent: *Yes, I worry about AIDS... he's very thin... and if he looks ill I think he's got AIDS you know, and it frightens me that, yeah.*

Thus, there were doubts about the safety of sharing with the partner among some of the women and this obviously created tension at times:

Respondent: *I said 'Have you been using in there?' He said 'No... do you want me to have me blood checked?' I was asking him to be honest to see if I had it... because if he's been checked then that means I haven't got it.*

Although some women were reticent about raising the issue with the partner, others were not:

Respondent: *Like my boyfriend — he's a digger (injector) as well...and thinking who's he shared a pin with, you know, well, he could have AIDS.*

Interviewer: *Have you talked a bout it at all?*

Respondent: *No, I just asked him if he'd got AIDS. He said no, he'd been tested.*

However, such doubts were not confined to the women. Suspicion and uncertainty was also expressed at times by the male partners:

Respondent: *I've shared with some of my friends... but I always use it first with them. My boyfriend says to me 'if there's a party and they start using speed and you want some... would you share the needle with them...' and I tell him I wouldn't use anyone else's.*

The high rates of sharing were largely due to the sociable nature of these amphetamine users and the long-standing friendships among them. Sharing was not contemplated with a stranger and there were particular rules about heroin addicts that were common throughout the whole sample, despite the fact that a high proportion of these women used heroin occasionally:

Interviewer: *How often would you do that (share)?*

Respondent: *Quite often.*

Interviewer: *What would cause you to do that.*

Respondent: *Because we've got no money to buy any more, or because that's the only one there. But I won't share a heroin addict's needles... they're just dirty to me.*

Interviewer: *Why's that?*

Respondent: *They don't give a shit whose works they use... I mean, as long as they've got their gear, they don't give a shit... so I'll not use theirs.*

Summary of Injecting Risk

Many factors combined to increase the probability that these women would share their injecting equipment. Deferring to the greater expertness of the partner, particularly at the early stage of injecting and being injected by him was common. Under these circumstances a woman was unlikely to be wholly in control of the order of injecting. The houses and flats of injecting couples are sometimes a convenient focus for group injecting and in this sort of environment, injecting became more chaotic and the order of injecting with shared equipment largely irrelevant, although some may attempt to be first in the queue. Since amphetamine is associated with sociability the norms governing sharing tend to encourage it between established friends. Nonetheless, the hazards were recognised, particularly by the women, whose partners disappeared for greater parts of the day to 'score' drugs and whose activities outside the home were unknown.

HIV Risk Through Sexual Transmission

There were no gender differences in the use of condoms and the attitudes to them. Sixteen (70%) of the women and 27 of men (60%) actively disliked condoms. The majority (13) of the women discounted the need for condoms since they were already sharing needles, or, alternatively, discounted the dangers of sharing needles because they were having unprotected sex. For example:

Interviewer: *How many times (shared) in the last 6 months?*

Respondent: *Not often. Only if we're really stuck and we haven't got any. It seems pointless not doing it because we've both been tested for HIV and we're both negative... we sleep together anyway and we don't use Durex so if we're gonna get something, we're gonna get it anyway... so sharing needles isn't gonna make any odds to us.*

The most common response to questions about condom use was that it simply never crossed their minds.

All females reported sex without condoms with their partners in the previous 6 months. All but 4 of the males had sex without condoms with their regular partners. Given that nearly half the men had shared needles and syringes with associates in that time, this indicates a high risk for their partners. Similar proportions of males (65%) and females (67%) said that they would not use condoms with their regular partners in future.

There were no significant differences in proportions who believed themselves at risk to HIV through sex — 50% of the women and 39% of the men voiced uncertainties about this. The main concern of the respondents was about their partners' sexual activities with other women. Perhaps it was because these could result in the break up of the relationship they were a more frequent source of complaint than suspicions about the partner sharing needles with others:

Interviewer: *Do you feel you might be at risk because you're not using condoms?*

Respondent: *I do in a way, because I think Pete's messed about behind my back... and I'm not doing anything. I mean... I haven't had an AIDS test... I don't know if I've got it or I haven't. Actually, I threw a packet at him yesterday. I said 'if you're doing anything... get hold of them'. I do worry about it because if Pete goes with someone... another drug user and they've shared needles... that would make me mad... to think he hadn't used one, do you know what I mean, and thought about me and not just himself.*

The fear of infection was inextricably bound up with a sense of potential betrayal that came across in accounts of the sexual relationships some of the women had with their partners. Drug users' personal relationships are often unstable and most women had a history of unhappy liaisons:

Interviewer: *Do you think you're at risk?*

Respondent: *No, 'cos I don't knock around with any Tom, Dick or Harry. I don't just jump into bed with anybody.*

Interviewer: *But what about him? (boyfriend)*

Respondent: *No, He's always with me. I've had it done on me too many times by other men. I've told him straight... if he does it on me I'll go out and pick a fella and bring him home and do it in front of him... but I'd be very wary who I'd pick.*

Summary of sexual risk

Sexual risk of HIV infection tended to be discounted by these women who were sharing injecting equipment with their partners since sharing was regarded as a much greater risk. However, the reputation of amphetamine as a stimulant that promotes casual sexual behaviour was fairly accurate for some males and aroused their partners' suspicions. The use of condoms with the regular partner was not normally considered; there was a desire to trust the other person and a reluctance to open up the issue of infidelity.

Changes in Drug Use

There were indications that the women's use of drugs may have increased as a consequence of their relationships with their partners. This has been noted in previous research (Hser *et al.*, 1987). Such an increase could, potentially, be injurious to health if it increased the probability of dependency. Table 8.1 shows that women tended to report an absence of influence or negative influence in contrast to the men (most of whom had non-injecting partners) who reported restraining influences that tended to keep drug use under control.

None of the women attributed their problems with drugs and feelings of psychological dependence to their partners, who rarely encouraged the women to use more:

Interviewer: *Does your partner affect how much whizz (amphetamine) you have?*

Respondent: *Well, he goes 'you've got to stop'. I mean, why should I stop... he smokes his gear (heroin)... I've got to have my enjoyment... he's having his. So I just tell him to get lost.*

It was claimed by some women that the influence was in the other direction. This was supported by observations made by research assistants of the partners together in their homes:

Table 8.1
Heroin use, dependency, perceived control and partner influence in male and female amphetamine injectors

	Females	Males
	n=24	n=46
No use of heroin	1 (4%)	9 (20%)*
INFLUENCE OF PARTNER		
Restrains use	4 (21%)	26 (72%)
Encourages use	6 (32%)	0
None	9 (47%)	10 (28%)**
DEPENDENCE		
Physical	10 (46%)	3 (8%)**
Psychological	17 (77%)	19 (49%)*
Control difficult	9 (41%)	4 (20%)*

** $p < 0.01$ * $p < 0.05$

Interviewer: *Does Dave influence how much speed (amphetamine) you take?*

Respondent: *I influence him. I tell him when he's had enough because he never knows when he's had enough. He wants to carry on until he ends up being ill.*

Among opiate users the strength of withdrawal tends to be a positive function of the amount of drug consumed and the frequency of administration. The urgency to avoid withdrawal is often cited as a reason for sharing injecting equipment among opiate users when drugs are available but sterile needles are not (Ross *et al.*, 1994, op cit.). In the case of amphetamine misuse however, there is little claim for physical addiction of the nature of opiate dependence (Klee *et al.*, 1992).

Although analyses revealed that dose levels were significantly associated with the use of others' injecting equipment in these data, no gender differences were observed. Both male and female respondents using high doses (4 grams or more of amphetamine in an average day) were more likely to use others' equipment — 75% compared with those using 2–3 grams (42%) and less than 2 grams (43%).

There were gender differences however in perceived drug dependence — with women feeling more dependent and less in control of their drug use than male respondents. Self-evaluated psychological dependency was a variable that proved independently predictive of the use of others' injecting equipment in logistic regression analyses of the whole sample of injectors (Klee & Morris, 1994, op cit.).

Perceptions of dependency among women may have been due, indirectly, to the ways they acquired drugs. It was fairly easy to increase the frequency of use of drugs through trading services or as recipients of gifts. For example, most of them 'scored' for friends and associates, and were given drugs in return:

Respondent: *I don't buy it... people just give it me because I do things for them. I'm handy... I set up scores (contacts with dealers) and I get rewarded with speed. They're my friends as well... they're not just business arrangements.*

Respondent: *We have people come round for works or dig here. The other night we had six in. They all had some and they give us a bit of theirs, you know, for letting them do it here.*

Several couples were small-time dealers and divided the amphetamine to sell to their network. An increase in drug use among the women was not, therefore, a consequence of any direct influence by partners but due to easy accessibility to drugs and an environment that was characterised by communal drug-taking. As a result, the women were potentially vulnerable to greater health risks through a lack of control of their drug use.

A closer examination of their use of heroin was instructive. Only 1 woman reported that she did not use heroin compared with 9 (20%) of the sample of

46 men. An analysis of the partner's use of heroin revealed that 14 (58%) of the women had heroin using partners, 10 of those partners were injecting the drug. Three partners of the 46 male injections used heroin, only 1 injected it. In addition to the greater probability of attracting only injecting males, the women were likely to risk increased dependency through the use of heroin. Compared with male amphetamine injectors, they and their partners seemed to be in transition to polydrug use or opiates:

Interviewer: *So you've been into smack (heroin) recently?*

Respondent: *There's a couple of people who score locally that can't use at home and they know they can use it here... so it stands to reason doesn't it. Unfortunately, those people have got habits... so they're coming round offering... and I've got myself a little habit.*

Summary of changes in drug use

The association of female amphetamine injectors with heroin users, either their partners or friends, suggested a trend towards polydrug use and greater drug dependency. Heroin is one drug that is used to attenuate the withdrawal from amphetamine, which induces severe depression in those using amphetamine frequently and in high doses. The lifestyle of those involved in attempts to balance the use of 'uppers' and 'downers' easily becomes chaotic and out of control with high levels of risk and consequent dangers for health.

DISCUSSION

It could be argued that these observations suggest the risk of HIV infection was rather similar for male and female amphetamine injectors since the proportion of women sharing their needles and syringes was no different from that of the men. However, because of the injecting status of their partners, women tended to share with their partners and men with friends or associates.

Irrespective of gender, the reality of the risk depends first on how accurately people detect previous or current risk behaviour in the person donating the injection equipment, and second, whether they feel able to adopt self-protective strategies. There was occasional suspicion by both members of an injecting and sexual partnership that sharing outside the partnership was leading to risk for themselves.

A prevailing view across the whole sample was that there was no need to share now that equipment was so readily available. The high rates of sharing were, therefore, a matter of choice or convenience and normally not regarded as risky with partners and close friends. Despite the feelings of dependency, there was no suggestion of desperation in their need for a 'fix' that would drive them to share with others. Even within close relationships, whether partners or friends, it was usually avoided for purely physical reasons of damage caused by blunt needles. Sexual risks were similarly ignored. The use of condoms was low and attitudes towards them largely negative for both men and women.

However there were some important differences that could increase the risk for women. Their control over their use of drugs was diminished by their relationship with a partner, though this did not emanate from direct encouragement to use more. The use of heroin and increasingly higher doses of amphetamine seemed to occur mostly through environmental factors. Injecting couples lived in houses which served as meeting places for others to congregate to inject, or to obtain drugs. They were likely to have injecting equipment on hand, often through contact with needle-exchanges and could provide either sterile or used equipment for their visitors. Why so many women and their partners were using heroin in this sample is difficult to say. In several cases it seems that among the visitors were heroin users who offered heroin in exchange for the use of a 'safe house' in which to inject or for the services of the woman or her partner in obtaining drugs for them. This also seemed to be a major source of amphetamine for these women and their partners and was likely to increase their use.

In other cases the partner of the woman was already using heroin prior to the relationship and it may be that these women injectors, not tolerated by male amphetamine users, received a more sympathetic reception from heroin users. The move to heroin for the women may have been facilitated by their partners (Parker *et al.*, 1988). The argument here is that such environmental and social pressures towards increased use of drugs will have similar effects on men and women, but women are more exposed to them because their partnerships are more likely to be restricted to injecting drug users. One hypothesis that was rejected fairly early in the analyses was that the women were dominated by their partners, that they were led or driven by them. In fact, it was soon apparent when pursuing this theme of interpersonal influence, that the majority of the women were very strong characters. Only 2 women reported that, at the start of their drug careers, they were unwilling victims of pressure to inject. The rest had actively sought the 'buzz' from injecting.

Although there were exceptions among the younger women, they could be forceful in their dealings with their partners. The overwhelming impression of the majority of these women was that they were active initiators in the use of drugs and in their relationships with their partners. They were concerned about the path their drug use was taking but did not lay the blame with their partner (for similar findings, see Taylor, 1993, op cit.). Some were concerned about the behaviour of their partner, and whether this put them at risk to HIV infection, but this was also true for some of their partners.

A form of empowerment that could lead to greater self-protection from HIV would have to acknowledge the mutual risk to both parties if it were not to induce alienation in one of them. Both partners need to be convinced of the advocacy of a health-protective practice since allegiance by only one individual has the effect of jeopardising the relationship by implying a lack of trust. Trust has to be separated from the practice of only and always using your own needles and syringes. An excellent argument for not sharing is the practical one of ensuring a better 'hit' with a sharp needle, that risks less damage to tissue and hence preserves veins. This approach to the empowerment of drug injectors of either sex who share unwillingly could save face and preserve relationships. It seems to be a strategy already used by injectors who need a convincing excuse to desist.

The respondents who shared as a matter of course tended to be ones in which the woman, often a novice, was injected by her partner or an expert friend. Most drug users find this too inconvenient to sustain for long and start to inject themselves. The early stage of initiation into injecting is particularly risky since ignorance is high and the novice is dependent on the good will and greater experience of the injector. The power imbalance makes it difficult to insist on sterile needles or thorough hygiene when being injected by others.

Ease of access to injecting equipment has meant that the majority of amphetamine injectors believe that it is unnecessary to share. They are not driven to inject their drug to the extent reported by heroin users. Sharing is chosen as a solution to a temporary problem, and is made easy by the belief that it is safe with certain people in an environment in which HIV infected people are virtually unknown. It is also a social act of solidarity in a group in which social relationships are very important. Exposing something of the pressures inherent in interpersonal dynamics and group behaviour to amphetamine injectors through educational materials could help to accelerate normative changes.

With respect to protection from sexual transmission of HIV infection, the task remains problematic. These amphetamine injecting women did not like the thought of using condoms with their primary partners. The association between condoms and HIV is strong among drug injectors and their use therefore is laden with implications. They are acceptable for use with casual or new partners, but not for more long-lasting relationships. Because the women tend to have injecting partners with whom they frequently share injecting equipment, the use of condoms is irrelevant. No-one has arrived at a solution to this problem. This rationale for not using a condom means that the problem of HIV transmission by sharing or sex cannot be separated. The women were well aware of the danger of undisclosed acts by partners with others. It was preferable to close the mind to them unless the evidence became pressing. The source of the impasse lay in the fear of losing a valuable relationship or the support it offered. There will be little further progress in reducing risk behaviour in close relationships until a strategy is devised that circumvents the destructiveness that could occur following open acknowledgement of the need for self-protection.

ACKNOWLEDGEMENTS

Funded by the Economic and Social Research Council. The contribution of colleagues Julie Morris and Brian Faragher, and research assistants Barbara Nodwell and Alex Howie to the research are gratefully acknowledged.

REFERENCES

Barnard, M. (1993) Needle sharing in context: patterns of sharing among men and women injectors and HIV risks. *Addiction*, **88**, 805-812.

Darke, S., Swift, W., Hall, W. & Ross, M. (1994) Predictors of injecting and injecting risk-taking behaviour among methadone maintenance clients. *Addiction*, **89**, 311-316.

Deren, S., Paone, D., Friedman, S.R., Neaigus, A., Des Jarlais, D.C. & Ward, T.P. (1993) IDU's and HIV/AIDS: interventions, behaviour change and policy. *AIDS Care*, **5**, 503-514.

Donoghoe, M. (1992) Sex, HIV and the injecting drug user. *British Journal of Addiction*, **87**, 405-416.

Hser, Y., Anglin, M.D. & Booth, M.W. (1987) Sex differences in addict careers 3: Addiction. *American Journal of Drug and Alcohol Abuse*, **13**, 231-251.

Klee, H. (1993) HIV risks for women drug injectors: heroin and amphetamine users compared. *Addiction*, **88**, 1055-1062.

Klee, H. & Morris, J. (1994) The impact of needle exchanges on sharing behaviour: cross-study comparisons 1989-1993. (Submitted for publication).

Klee, H., Morris, J. & Faragher, B. (1992) *Amphetamine misuse: Implications for HIV Transmission.* Final Report, UK: The Economic and Social Research Council.

Klee, H., Morris, S. & Ruben, S. (1993) Polydrug *Misuse: Health Risks and Implications for HIV Transmission.* Final Report, UK: Department of Health.

Parker, H., Bakx, K. & Newcombe, R. (1988) *Living With Heroin*, Milton Keynes: Open University Press.

Rosenbaum, M. (1981) *Women on Heroin*, California: Rutgers University Press.

Ross, M.W., Wodak, A., Stowe, A. & Gold, J. (1994) Explanations for sharing injection equipment in injecting drug users and barriers to safer drug use. *Addiction*, **89**, 473-479.

Taylor, A. (1993) *Women Drug Users*, Oxford: Clarendon Press.

9

Recognizing and Countering the Psychosocial and Economic Impact of HIV on Women in Developing Countries

CATHERINE HANKINS

From the psychological distress of infected individuals and their families to the social disruption in affected communities, from the microeconomic level, the HIV/AIDS epidemic is undermining significant improvements in health indicators and compounding prexisting economic difficulties onto which structural adjustments programmes have already been imposed. Until a clearer understanding is achieved of the potential and real impact of HIV/AIDS at the individual, community, and societal level, efforts to prevent further HIV transmission and its consequences for women as well as to provide appropriate care, treatment, and support for those who are living with HIV/AIDS in developing countries will provide sub-optimal results. Action-oriented research and programme development involving women infected and affected by the epidemic and aimed at enhancing the responses of families and communities to the HIV epidemic combined with efforts to sensitize and engage decision makers are the first steps to countering the potentially devastating psychological and economic impact on women of HIV in developing countries.

Elizabeth-Kubler-Ross has stated "We are solely responsible for our choices and we have to accept the consequences of every deed, word, and thought throughout our lifetime." Whereas women with HIV infection are clearly living with the consequences, it can be cogently argued that they are not solely responsible for their choices. Keeping on the front burner this issue of choices and consequences for women, let us consider HIV and vulnerability in women, the importance of education for girls and young women, the unequal burden of care, and the potential impact of HIV on the status of women in developing countries.

If prevention of transmission of HIV infection to women is to be effective, we must critically examine societal forces and gender-based power inequalities that put women at risk. Socialized concepts of masculinity and femininity as well as gender and power relations limit the capacity of young women to negotiate the boundaries of sexual encounters so as to ensure both their safety and their satisfaction (Holland *et al.*, 1992). This is true to a greater or lesser extent in all societies. But in developing countries, poverty further interacts with gender imbalances to prevent women from protecting themselves from HIV.

The lack of economic and educational ooportunities for women in developing countries can lead them to resort to entering into sexual relationships for economic reasons. In this context extra-marital sexual encounters almost always involve the transfers of material resources, such as cash, clothing, as gifts from a man to his female partner. Vos (1994) has argued that these gifts have to be seen as a contribution to a woman's survival and that the term commercial sex should be reserved to describe a straight forward transaction of money for sex. For many women commercial sex work is an occupation born of necessity – cold, stark economic necessity – and directly related to a woman's survival. But these survival strategies have been turned into death strategies (Schoepf *et al.*, 1991). The vulnerability of prostitutes in many developing countries is amplified by personal and societal poverty. They provide sexual services in social contexts which are ripe for transmission of HIV, have limited education and hence choice, are frequently exposed to STD and receive wholly inadequate STD care, provide vaginal intercourse to large numbers of clients, and seldom use condoms (Wilson, 1993).

We need, as Gill Seidel (1993) has argued, to deconstruct the category of prostitution, and understand better the contexts of sexual servicing where few jobs are available to women and where women have limited access to the cash economy. Not only may there be different types of work in this context, all survival strategies for women, but often there may be no dichotomy between marriage and other relations which imply sexual-economic exchange, but rather a continuum of forms of sexual service. And in fact, delegates from 14 African states at the first Society of Women and AIDS in Africa meeting held in 1989, unanimously agreed the 'forces ranging from early childhood training to state laws governing marriage, divorce and property rights prepare women to defer to male partners, not to instruct or oppose them, especially in the context of marriage' (Mahmoud *et al.*, 1989).

Social structure limits the ability of women to become independent social actors and those who perceive themselves to be powerless often may erect psychological defences against the pain of risk assessment (Schoepf, 1993). For example, fear of losing one's status may motivate even highly educated women, with the financial means to afford an HIV test, to avoid being tested for HIV. Women that I have spoken to in East Africa who themselves are actively involved in AIDS education and counselling have told me that they would not consider being tested for HIV unless they themselves became sick.

These women find the medical arguments about the possibility of increased life expectancy and better quality of life with the treatment of tuberculosis and other opportunistic infections convincing, but, they told me, the major reason that they would not be tested was that the sole source of the infection would have had to have been their own husbands. Perceiving themselves to be powerless to either demand fidelity or negotiate marital condom use, they would prefer not to confront the issue of male infidelity and not to have to face the possibility of rejection by their husbands if they were found to be HIV-positive themselves. As the policy of the community-based AIDS Support Organisation, TASO, in Kampala, Uganda states. the test should not be taken unless the answer is going definitely to help you (Kaleeba, 1992). And for many women the test cannot help them. On the contrary, a positive HIV test result may cause a premature social death years before the biological one.

Increasingly it is being argued that short term solutions to women's vulnerability to HIV infection and other sexually transmitted diseases lie in the development of clandestine, woman-controlled, methods of HIV prevention that do not require male complicity or agreement and that only the empowerment of women to achieve economic autonomy will provide protection in the long term. It is also evident that reducing the impact of the HIV epidemic for women and girls in developing countries will also involve strategies that focus on educational opportunities, on careful review of the impact on women of changing models for the care of people living with HIV/AIDS, and vigilant analysis of the impact of the HIV epidemic on the status of women.

STATUS OF WOMEN

The link between the education of women and health has been clearly documented throughout the developing world. The lack of educational and economic opportunities for young girls can and does act to encourage early partnership formation and early sexual activity and can affect child mortality rates in their children. Demograpic and health surveys in 25 developing countries have shown that even one to three years of maternal schooling reduces child mortality by about 15% and when mothers have 7 or more years of schooling child mortality risk are reduced nearly 75% (World Bank, 1993, p. 42).

Education strengthens women's ability to perform their vital role in creating healthy households. It increases the chance that they will make good use of health services, increases their access to income, and enables them to make healthier choices. Continuation of schooling appears to have a retardant effect on the onset of sexual activity in young women, helping girls move beyond the heightened biological vulnerability of adolescence, caused by cervical ectopy or lack of maturity of the genital tract, and increasing the chances that healthy sexual choices will be made. In developing countries, better educated women marry later and start their families later (World Bank, 1993, p. 42).

Furthermore, improving the access of girls and women to formal education, not only helps to equalize the age of partnership formation which can reduce the risk of HIV but it also increases women's competitiveness in urban economies which could positively affect the unequal gender mix seen in many cities (DeCosas & Pedneault, 1992). The uneven gender ratio created by the movement of a mainly male labour force to urban environments has combined with a lack of economic resources other than the commercial sex trade for women who are not married to create conditions for rapid spread of HIV in cities.

A study by Over and Piot (1992) revealed a strong correlation between female to male school enrolment ratios at the secondary school level and HIV prevalence in the general adult population. Their results suggeset that significant decreases in seroprevelance could be achieved if the urban sex ration and the secondary school sex ratio could move steadily toward parity.

To increase the chance that girls will receive schooling we must address the link between poverty, education, cultural constraints, and gender factors. The World Development Report 'Investing in Health' (World, Bank, 1993) argues that lowering the barriers to schooling for girls can be done through scholarships, by offering free textbooks or free exemptions, with safeguards to prevent diversions to males, and by sitting schools close to people's homes so that parents are less worried about their daughter's safety. Investing in women through improved education is not simply a desirable end in itself, it is a key not only to reduced HIV transmission but also to higher productivity and growth for developing country economies in the long term.

BURDEN OF CARE

The second topic is that of changing models of care and the potential of increased burdens on women and girls. As one woman stated: "if there is ever any talk of anyone replacing another and doing the work, it is always the woman, never the man". Or as Margaret Mshana of the KIWAKKUKI Women's group in Tanzania (personal communication, 1994) said: "Women are everything to everybody". And it is often female children who are required to spend less time in school and more time at home performing tasks normally carried out by adults when someone in the family has advanced HIV disease.

Meeting the medical needs of those affected by HIV alone is a great challenge in sub-Saharan Africa due to the large and rapidly growing demand in the context of extremely severe resource constraints. In order to reduce costs, countries have moved rapidly towards provision of hospital-based or community-based home care services for patients with HIV disease. However, as Sue Foster has pointed out, "planning the care of patients with HIV disease and AIDS must be understood as an exercise in damage limitation, balancing the provision of a humane standard of care for patients with HIV with the needs for care for other patients" (Foster, 1994). But in the effort to relieve pressure on acute care hospital beds, home-based care can so easily become a method for dumping patients back into an unprepared home setting. It is increasingly being asked whether this is humane in the absence of resources. It has been noted that volunteers who had received special training, were highly motivated to participate in programmes because of their own experience with a person living with AIDS in their own family. However, these volunteers found themselves visiting families which had dying family members without even being able to provide soap to bathe the patient with, let alone foodstuffs or medicines.

For women who are the traditional nurturers and caregivers both in the home in the community, having a sick person in the home without adequate support services may mean major changes in activities which could influence the health of other family members. For example, caring for someone in the home may mean one has less time available to tend crops and as a result decisions may be made to switch to less labour-intensive crops which may not be as nutritious or income-generating. Livestock may be sold to compensate for loss of income and remaining animals may have lower levels of care with resultant sickness and loss.

Distance from portable water supplies may become an additional strain for women coping with the demands of caring for someone in the home, increasing the chances of skin diseases related to water scarcity. But if the sick family member has chronic diarrhoea, as many AIDS patients do, the situation may become intolerable for most families who do not have convenient toilet facilities or running water. Finally, women who are employed outside the home may jeopardize their continued employment or their small business by missing too many work days caring for their sick loved one.

WOMEN IN DEVELOPING COUNTRIES

What is the impact of HIV on the status of women in developing countries? It is broadly recognized that the pandemic has catastrophically costly consequences since it affects mainly people in the economically productive adult years. The heavy macroeconomic impact of AIDS comes partly from the high costs of treatment which divert resources for productive investments and partly from direct effects on productivity due to illness and the loss of skilled adults. These macroeconomic effects are superimposed on a depending crisis associated both with the effects of structural adjustment policies and with employment structures inherited from colonial times that have contributed to the weakening of the extended family and to the feminisation of poverty (Seidel, 1993).

On the microeconomic level, the death of an adult can tip vulnerable households into poverty. A study conducted among affected rural households in Tanzania indicated that these families spent roughly the equivalent of the annual rural income per capita on treatment and funerals (World Bank, 1993, p. 20). Other studies are now showing that the effects of losing an adult in a house-hold persist into the next generation as children, and particularly female children, are withdrawn from school because school fees cannot be paid and because their help is needed at home. School attendance of young people aged 15 to 20 years is reduced by half if its household has lost an adult female member to AIDS in the previous year (World Bank, 1993, p. 20).

In Thailand today, one in 50 adults is infected. In Sub-Saharan African, 1 in 40 adults is infected and in certain parts of Africa, the prevalence of infection is as high as

1 in 33 (World Bank, 1993, p. 99). In some of these high prevalence communities, AIDS is already starting to reverse long term declines in child mortality and increases in life expectancy.

In Sub-Saharan Africa, life expectancy at birth had reached 50 years by the early 1980s (World Bank, 1993, p. 23). Projected life expectancies for males and females in a hypothecated sub-Saharan country explored in a World Bank Development report on health, indicate a major impact of AIDS on life expectancy. the trend to increasing life expectancy is reversed with life expectancy at birth declining steeply before it levels off and then recovers somewhat. Without the AIDS epidemic and under standard assumptions, the gap in life expectancies between women and men would gradually increase, with women living longer than men. But the trend is reversed in the AIDS scenario with women having a shorter life expectancy than men after the yar 2000. By the year 2020, life expectancy for males at birth in this scenario is 17 years below projected life expectancy in the no AIDS scenario. And for women, the loss is life expectancy is even greater - 21 years (Armstrong & Bos, 1992, p. 207).

A commitment to ongoing research is required to evaluate the specific impact of the community HIV/AIDS crisis on women's status as measured by standard indicators of status, health, and well-being and on the division of labour in the care of increasing numbers of sick family and community members and orphaned children. Questions remain about the potential for the HIV/AIDS epidemic to have a negative impact on the status of women in developing countries given the current context in which the status of women is already acting as a major inhibitor to the success of individual and collective efforts to prevent HIV transmission. Women account for half of the world's population, perform two-thirds of the hours, worked, receive one-tenth of the world's income, and have one hundredth of the world's property registered in their name (CEG, 1989).

Reid, of UNDP's HIV and Development Programme, argues that because so many facets of the HIV epidemic are gender speficif experience and knowledge must be made accessible so it can shape and reshape theory and practice. She highlights the importance of two major approaches to the challenge of obtaining information that can help identify new research areas and programme needs which are of concern to women (Reid, 1992). These are first-person narratives (Berer & Ray, 1993), which can increase our understanding of women's experiences, and systems level analysis, which helps us see the relationships between structural adjustments programmes, poverty, and the tragedy of being infected with HIV. An excellent example of the attempt to get as full a perspective as possible is Barnett's summary analysis of a series of case studies undertaken to examine the effects of HIV/AIDS on farming systems and rural livelihoods in Uganda, Tanzania, and Zambia, which includes the personal stories of several women (Barnett, 1994). Only if concrete detailed information like this is collected about the real impact of the epidemic at both the individual and at the systems level will we be able to begin to counter the devasting economic effects of this epidemic for women.

GENDER ISSUES

If we put on our gender spectacles to look at the issues surrounding the status of women, it is clear that the legal status of women which in many countries does not allow them to inherit land has several repercussions. It means that women lack collateral for financial services and this combined with low levels of education constitutes a clear gender-based constraint to economic activity. Inheritance laws also mean that widows are particularly vulnerable to making sexual decisions which are influenced by economics. This may mean accepting the levirate or traditional marriage to a brother-in-law, a social safety net with a distinct risk of encouraging HIV transmission, or it may mean becoming involved is some form of prostitution to support themselves and their children.

In order to address educational inequities, increasing health burdens being placed on women, and the impediments of the current status of women, a multi-pronged strategy will be required. At all levels of the strategy, women, both infected and affected, must be implicated if this is to be effective. These strategies should be aimed at enhancing the responses of families and communities to the HIV epidemic in such a way that they enhance women's status. Only by doing so will women's vulnerability to HIV transmission be reduced and the possibility that women will play full roles in society enhanced.

Both Joseph DeCosas (1992) and Jonathan Mann (1992) have proposed subjecting development programmes to an AIDS impact audit in the same way that environmental impact audits are becoming increasingly routine. Clearly we need to ensure that the concept of an AIDS impact audit includes serious gender analysis. As the HIV/AIDS epidemic intensifies, we are seeing increasing stigmatisation of women, and change in women's social and political position.

IMPLICATIONS

What does this mean for the industrialized world? Although recipient countries must retain the right to determine local orientations and approaches, donors can encourage the integration of HIV impact audits and gender impact analyses into overall thinking on economic development and development co-operation, ignoring the broader social conditions makes effective programmes impossible. To ignore the economic impact of AIDS in agriculture and in industry, with its resultant impact on the status of women, and to ignore the impact of requirements to provide care in the home on access to education for young girls and on access to other sources of income among adult women is to ignore some of the root causes of the psychosocial and economic impact on women of HIV in developing countries.

Solutions are not simple but the seeds of those solutions are found in the conventional wisdom to be found in communities. And they are found in systems level analysis that should inform the creation of gender-sensitive HIV and development policies. We must sensitize and engage decision makers at local, national and international levels about these imbalances and about these issues if we are to avoid the potentially devastating psychosocial and economic impact on women of HIV in developing countries. As citizens of the world we all have this as both a duty and a responsibility to our sisters in those countries that are most vulnerable to HIV and its effects.

REFERENCES

Armstrong, J., & Bos, E. (1992) The demographic, economic, and Social impact of AIDS. In. J. Mann, D.J. M. tarantola & T. Netter (Eds.), *AIDS in the World* (pp. 195-226). Cambridge, MA. Harvard University Press.

Barnett, T. (1994) *The Effects of HIV/AIDS on Farming Systems and Rural Livelihoods in Uganda, Tanzania and Zambia.* Overseas Development Group, University of East Anglia, Norwich, U.K. Project TSS/1 RAF.92/TO/A.

Berer, M. & Ray, S. (1993) *Women and HIV/AIDS - An International Resource Book.* London, England: Pandora.

CEG (Commonwealth Expert Group) (1989) *Engenderning Adjustment for the 1990s* (Report of a Commonwealth Expert Group on Women and Structural Adjustment). London, England; Commonwealth Secretariat, London.

DeCosas, J. (1992) The impact of underdevelopment on AIDS. *Eighth International Conference on AIDS*, Amsterdam, The Netherlands.

DeCosas, J. & Pedneault, V. (1992) Women and AIDS in Africa: Demographic implications for health promotion. *Health Policy and Planning*, 7, 227-233.

Foster, S. (1994) *Cost and Burden of AIDS on the Zambian Health Care System*: Policies to Mitigate the Impact on Health Services. (USAID/ZAMBIA Report ICQ PDC-5929-I-0109-00).

Holland, J., Ramazanoglu, C., Scott, S., Sharpe, S. & Thomson, R. (1992) Risk power and the possibility of pleasure; young and safer sex. *AIDS Care* 4, 273-283.

Kaleeba, N. (1992) Adapted from: "Community-Based Care in an LDC: The AIDS Support Organization." In Jonathan Mann, Daniel J.M. Tarantola and Thomas Netter (Eds). *AIDS in the World* (pp. 458-459) Cambridge, MA: Harvard University Press.

Mahmoud, F.A., de Zalduondo, B.A., Zewdie, D., Williams, E. *et al.* (1989) Women and AIDS in Africa. issues old and new. Paper presented at the *1989 Annual Meeting of the African Studies Association*, Atlanta, GA.

Mann, J. (1992) Plenary address. *Eighth International Conference on AIDS.* Amsterdam, The Netherlands.

Over, M., & Piot, P. (1992) HIV infection and sexually transmitted disease. The World Bank health sectors priorities review. In D.T. Jamison & W.H. Mosley (Eds.), *Disease control priorities in developing countries.* New York, NY: Oxford University Press for the world Bank.

Reid, E. (1992) Gender, Knowledge, and responsibility. In J. Mann, D.J. M. Tarantola & T. Netter (Eds.) *AIDS in the World.* (pp. 657-667) Cambridge, MA: Harvard University Press.

Schoepf, B.G., Engundu, W., Mkera, R.W., Ntsomo, P. & Schoepf, C. (1991) Gender, power and risk of AIDS in Zaire. In *Gender and Health in Africa* (pp. 187-204) Trenton, NJ: Africa World Press, IUC.

Schoepf, B.G. (1993) Women at risk: case studies from Zaire. In M. Berer & S. Ray *Women and HIV/AIDS*: An International Resource Book (pp. 249-254) London, England: Pandora.

Seidel, G. (1993) The competing discourses of HIV/AIDS in Sub-Saharan Africa: discourses of rights and empowerment vs discourses of control and exclusion. *Social Sciences and Medicine*, **36**, 175-194.

Vos, T. (1994) Attitudes to sex and sexual behaviour in rural Matabeleland, Zimbabwe. *AIDS Care*, **6**, 193-203.

Wilson, D. (1993) Preventing Transmission of HIV in Heterosexual Prostitution. In L. Sherr (Ed.) *AIDS and the Heterosexual Population* (pp. 67-81) Chur, Switzerland: Harwood Academic Publishers.

World Bank. (1993) *World Development Report 1993*. New York, NY: Oxford University Press.

10

Caregiving and the Natural Caregiver of the Person Infected With HIV

MARY REIDY

THE NATURAL CAREGIVER AND FAMILY

In time of illness, despite professional intervention, the primary source of care or support in most cultures remains the family. One person, by habit or inclination, usually becomes the primary health agent or natural caregiver within the family. However, AIDS, like any fatal or chronic illness, imposes a stress which may have long term disruptive effects on the family system or which may stimulate the family to reorganize its structure or to increase the cohesion of its members (Durham & Cohen, 1987; Flaskerud & Ungarski, 1992).

When young infected adults require care, they may either return to the nuclear family, or through ties of commitment call upon other "family" members, such as lovers, friends or committed volunteers to assume the caregiver role. The legal definition of family no longer seems to be sufficient within the reality of AIDS, as the natural caregivers of persons infected by HIV are frequently found outside the traditional nuclear family unit. Family, then, must be defined within the parameters of mutual obligation based on devotion, rather than on law (Reidy & Taggart, 1995).

Nevertheless, even with roles changed, relationships modified and families restructured, natural caregivers are called upon to care within the context of a social paradox. Despite the development of primary health care, the focus on health care decentralisation, adherence to a philosophy of "responsibilization" of the population in health matters, the greatest value and the greater part of any health budget are still accorded to acute professional care within the hospital setting. Further, the explosion of expensive, sophisticated medical technology and the value accorded to technical medicine directly denigrates the worth accorded to caregiving. The commitment of a natural caregiver, to the quality of life of the person with AIDS, between hospitalizations, is often ignored or taken for granted (Reidy & Taggart, 1995).

Social scientists and health professionals agree on the relationship between social support and health, as well as, on the primary role of the "family caregiver" in such support. However, exaggerated fears fed by social taboos and supported by customs and institutional regulations, contribute to the feelings of powerlessness of many caregivers in the face of social and therapeutic decisions. Natural caregivers frequently feel powerless, not only, because of their inability to meet the needs of the infected person, but also, because of the health professional's control of information. Preventing or distorting the flow of information may occur when the creditability or the legal, social and moral acceptability of the caregiver is held in doubt by the health care team. Natural caregivers, such as the grandmother, who is not given information, or the lover, who is excluded from decision making, neither being legally "next of kin", become diminished as caregivers. Their attitudes toward health and social services may well become passive, fatalistic or hostile, influencing negatively their commitment to care and compliance with medical regimen (Stulberg & Buckingham, 1988).

Experiences of health, illness and care, and the family role in caregiving are framed within a cultural context. Within such a context, health may be defined as those beliefs, values and ways of acting which are generally known, culturally accepted and which are employed in order to preserve and to maintain the wellbeing of the individual or the group (Leininger, 1991). The meaning of AIDS, takes the form of a mental representation devolving from the perceptions of those who are infected, as well as, from those who care for them. The significance of being infected by HIV is determined by the individual's perceptions, values and opinions as a family member and as a member of a larger cultural and social aggregate. The sick person presents signs and symptoms, emotional states and social behaviour which provoke actions and reactions structured by the customs and norms of his society.

Further, the values and customs of sub-cultures, which may be in conflict with or marginal to the prevailing culture, influence the importance and meaning of health and care. Many HIV infected persons are culturally marginal, socially alienated or profess sexual orientations, values or customs which are far different from those of mainstream society or of their natural caregivers. Membership in distinct ethnic groups or the belonging to groups with high risk behaviour influences self-care and the type of care that is both offered and accepted (Carmack, 1992; Perreault & Savard, 1992).

ROLES AND TASKS OF THE NATURAL CAREGIVER

The success of the care regimen of persons infected by HIV depends in great part on the attitudes, activities and committed participation of their natural caregivers.

While the role of the natural caregiver is attributed almost naturally to women by the social and political organization of most societies, the partners and gay friends of infected men have been known as active caregivers since the beginning of the epidemic (Cowles & Rogers, 1991; McCann & Wadsworth, 1992).

A recent study about natural caregivers of men infected by HIV - III & IV[1], describes the factors which influence and are influenced by their caregiving. The method of this study is descriptive/associative, with an availability/representative sample (n = 102). Variables include Psychological Distress, Quality of Life, Burden, Coping and Social Support. Data was collected by an interview/questionnaire and analyses include descriptive statistics and correlation techniques.

Analyses indicate that the relationship between caregiver and infected person, was more or less equally divided between that of lovers or spouses, parents or family members and friends. Their mean age was 43.1 years (range: 25-60 years); more than half were men; more than three-quarters had post-secondary education and more than one-half earned over 20 000$ (Canadian). Most had managerial positions or blue or white collar jobs, which they maintained during the process of caregiving. These caregivers reported having been close to the infected person for 45 years. Less than half shared living accommodations with the infected person.

A review of the antecedent literature (Flaskerud and Ungarski, 1992; McCann & Wadsworth, 1992; Mansour, 1990; Speigel & Meyers, 1991) indicated that the role of the natural caregiver, at home or when the sick person is in hospice or hospital, includes such tasks and actions as: a) emotional, logistical and financial support; b) direct physical care; c) help with treatments; d) help with activities of daily living; e) mediation with health, social and community services; e) participation in complementary social roles; f) sharing of living accommodations and g) sharing in social and recreational activities. These responsibilities demand not only time, energy and financial resources, but also, a possible redefinition of family roles and responsibilities (Meyers & Weitzman, 1991). While these may be shared among several family members, they have a tendency to fall on the shoulders of a "designated" caregiver. For example, the infected mother of an infected child may continue to work in order to support the family, continue her usual domestic and maternal duties and care for the child, as well as for her symptomatic husband (Reidy *et al.*, 1995).

In the study of Taggart & *al.* (cited above) of the natural caregivers of men with AIDS (living at home but not yet considered to be in the terminal phase), the caregivers enumerate diverse tasks, other than therapeutic intervention: accompanying the person with AIDS (59.8%); budgeting or managing their affairs (23.6%); light house work (59.1%); preparing meals (65.1%); aid with dressing or undressing (19.9%); aid with bath or shower (29.8%); and aid moving about the house (21.5%).

[1] Principal investigators: M.E. Taggart, M. Reidy & S. Jutras; funding: FRSQ-CQRS, Quebec, Canada 1993-94

QUALITY OF LIFE

The role played in caregiving both influences and is influenced by the caregiver's quality of life. Perceptions of quality of life varies according to culture, personal world view, aims, habits and resources and it evolves with life cycles, age and career advancement. The age (20-40 years), at which most infected persons show the first signs and symptoms of AIDS, falls during the period in which they, and many of those caring for them are demonstrating their status as adults, through financial and emotion independence from their family of origin, as well as, consolidating career or new family patterns. The appearance of symptoms and the need for care requires changes in the role of partners or friends, or a return to dependence on their family of origin (Reidy & Taggart, 1995). Whatever the choice, it results in modification in aims, resources and life habits which will affect the quality of life of both the person infected and his natural caregiver. The multiple losses associated with AIDS reduces the amplitude ofplans, aims and life projects of both the infected person and his caregiver (Carmack, 1992).

Quality of life is much discussed by clinicians and researchers alike, giving rise to various conceptual and operational definitions even within the domain of AIDS research (Marchette *et al.*, 1991; Lamping *et al.*, 1992). An appropriate conceptual framework would be one sensitive to the effects of a chronic, fatal illness such as AIDS on the life situation, but at the same time, free from the parameters imposed solely or principally by pathology and symptomology.

The quality of life of an individual depends on great part on the adoption of behaviour which is appropriate to the accomplishment of his life goals and his day to day projects. Quality of life encompasses various dimensions of life: physical health, psychological health, social relations, life as a couple, recreation, work/career and home care. The essence of the quality of life, however, rests in one's perceptions of the congruence between one's goals and one's actual situation (Dupuis *et al.*, 1989). The maintenance of a high quality of life of the infected person is dependent on the care and support of his natural caregiver, whose ability to continue to give care and support is, in turn, interrelated with his own quality of life (Reidy & Taggart, 1995). Mental health, coping abilities, perception of burden and ongoing social support are primary factors which determine not only the caregiver's response to situational distress caused by the evolution of the illness, but also his ability to maintain normality and quality in daily life for himself and for the person for whom he is caring.

Mariun and Boyd (1990), in their review of the literature on the impact of mental illness on the family, and Brown (1993), in her qualitative study of families of persons with HIV/AIDS, reported that all spheres of the caregivers' lives were affected and the impact was cumulative with time. The effects ranged from having less energy for work, to losing time and energy for "quality of life" activities, to the tasks and demands related to caregiving. These demands were so extensive that many caregivers felt that they were being "managed by AIDS" rather than "managing the disease".

DISTRESS AND THE IMPACT OF CAREGIVING

On the one hand, the natural caregiver suffers stress from the social stigma associated with AIDS and from the demands of caregiving. On the other hand, change or poor definition of roles, inapplicability of usual decision making processes, conflict in obligations and financial pressures also generate stress which threaten physical and mental health. This stress can be heightened by the uncertainty of the future, particularly if the infected person and his caregiver were exposed to the same risks or share the same life style (Pearlin *et al.*, 1988).

Incertitude is lived by the natural caregiver as hope gradually erodes and powerlessness increases with the progression of the illness. As symptoms appear, the caregiver shares in the infected person's anxiety, fear of the future, sadness, guilt and a deterioration of self-esteem. Such incertitude provokes anger and anxiety and tends to exacerbate existing relational problems (Cowles & Rodgers, 1991; Mansour, 1990; Mercier & Reidy, 1995; Ross & Rosser, 1988; Speigel and Mayers, 1991). Caregiving can also provoke conflict in other roles and disrupt other areas of life (i.e. financial, occupational and social) which in turn become further sources of stress.

Prolonged caregiving with plateau or deterioration in the disease process without promise of improvement, coupled with "roller-coaster" evolution of certain types of chronic illnesses, produces a cumulative negative emotional effect (Brown, 1993; Gaynor, 1990). Moreover, in their qualitative grounded theory study of 53 natural caregivers (lovers, spouses, parents, siblings and friends) of persons with AIDS, Brown and Powell-Cope (1991) reaffirmed the distress engendered by the social-psychological state of uncertainty. Uncertainty, here being defined as the care givers inability to predict the future and difficulty in making decisions about care or life situations. Transitions (major changes) in the development of the disease, negotiations in relationships, in learning to live with loss and death and in managing and being managed by the illness all contributed to the impact and the challenge for care givers and families affected by AIDS.

Distress is manifested by feelings of perturbation, isolation, loss, distress, powerlessness and intense emotional reactions. High levels of stress coupled with a forced reorganization of life can lead to physical and psychological burnout. The caregivers, in the preliminary analyses (n = 50) of Taggart's study (cited above) reported:

> *It is difficult to find an equilibrium between taking care of him and meeting my other responsibilities – family, work, etc.* (64%).
>
> *I feel overcome by the responsibility of taking care of him* (62%).
>
> *It seems to me that he needs care that I cannot give him* (60%).
>
> *I feel that I have lost control of my life since I began taking care of him* (44%).

While relatively little has been written about the impact (positive/negative) for someone with AIDS, it is clear that the negative impact, or burden, as it is often termed, is as much associated with the perceptions (subjective burden) of the natural caregiver as with the actual demands and the care (objective burden) required by the infected person (DeMontigny & Lapointe, 1989; Fletcher & Winslow, 1991; Perreault & Savard, 1992).

The principal determinants of the impact of caregiving have been found to be: 1) the level of incapacity or dependency of the sick person; 2) the previous emotional relationship and pattern of interpersonal communications between the sick person and the caregiver; 3) the state of health of the caregiver; 4) the fatigue caused by caregiving; 5) the presence or absence of other sources of aid and support and 6) the conflict of the caregiving role with other roles (Reidy & Taggart, 1995).

In the terminal phase of AIDS, the demands of caregiving in the home increase and the burden on the caregiver becomes extreme. Even the most devoted of caregivers are not necessarily well equipped to deal with the effects of the illness at all levels of its evolution: at diagnosis with the agony of acceptance and disclosure and during periods of latency with incertitude and hope; at the symptomatic stage when living life and compliance with medical regimen may well be in conflict; or in the near terminal or terminal phase when comfort and symptom management are so elusive. Persons with AIDS suffer from, or anticipate the onset of a multi-symptom, progressive debilitating disease, that is infectious and fatal. Moreover, the differential signs and symptoms of AIDS relate to virtually every body system and are accompanied by the secondary effects of medications which can be both toxic and unexpected. It requires skill, knowledge, as well as expert advice, and social and logistical support (all of which are difficult to obtain), in order to respond appropriately to severe pain, frequent diarrhoea, skin breakdown, perceptual and sensory deficits, anxiety, dementia, debilitating fatigue or fever. In addition to emotional support, care must be directed toward comfort and security: turning and positioning, massage of bony prominences, skin lubrication, cooling, soothing foods or liquids for mucosal lesions, reality orientation to reduce confusion, the use of prosthetic equipment, chemical or physical restraints and the giving of medications.

Moreover, natural caregivers, must often face the death of their loved one in the context of social rejection. Implicated in an affective relationship which will culminate in death, they frequently suffer from isolation, disorganization, stress and possibly employ mechanisms of adaptation which are inefficient or inadequate. Many caregivers find it becoming more difficult to give care as they suffer a gradual using up of their physical, emotional and financial resources (Carmack, 1992; Perreault & Savard, 1992). Such a situation may render the relation between caregiver and the sick person less and less satisfying and may even provoke premature disengagement and abandonment by family and natural caregivers leaving the dying person abandoned emotionally or physically, and the mourner guilty with unresolved grief (Fontaine & Reidy, 1995; Rando, 1988; Régnier, 1990).

Nevertheless, the literature has identified strategies employed by natural caregivers to cope with stress and alleviate burden. These include acts which 1) change the situation; 2) change the negative connotation or reduce feelings of fear or threat; 3) maintain or control anxiety; 4) find solutions for problem situations; 5) encourage self-affirmation or participation in social or political action, rather than support of a conspiracy of silence; and 6) reaffirm spiritual or religious beliefs (Greif & Porembski, 1988; Pearlin *et al.*, 1988, Reidy & Taggart, 1995).

More importantly, it should be remembered that the impact of caring can also be positive. The natural caregiver's values, commitment, habits of daily life, his energy and mental health maintain the tissue of his daily life. The effects of burden are even balanced by the rewards of caregiving. In the preliminary analyses (n = 50) of the study by Taggart *et al.* (cited above), these caregivers affirm the positive impact of caring for someone with AIDS:

> *I find that taking care of him gives sense to my life* (94%).
>
> *I feel reassured to know that when I take care of him he receives the care he needs* (100%).
>
> *I feel happy to contribute to his wellbeing* (98%).
>
> *I feel useful in taking care of him* (92%).

SOCIAL SUPPORT

The impact of caring for someone with AIDS is believed to be alleviated by social support (McGough, 1990; Hart *et al.*, 1992). Social support rests on a multitude of interrelationships and interactions in a great variety of daily activities: family life, work, recreation, use of health and social services, etc. Such support can be instrumental or relational and may be provided by family friends, volunteers or health and social welfare professionals (Lieberman, 1988; Kristjanson & Chamers, 1991).

With the social disruption caused by the diagnosis of HIV, the natural caregiver and the infected person often are denied the closeness of family support, available to those suffering from other chronic illness. Because of their proximity to the person who is infected and to the disease process, natural caregivers also suffer from stigmatization and various forms of rejection and harassment. Characteristicly, they often hide the situation from family friends and neighbours, further decreasing their social support and increasing in their isolation and burden (Fortin *et al.*, 1989; Perrault, 1995). Moreover, social support available at the onset of the illness may become reduced in size and quality, auxiliary caregivers becoming burned out and incapable of giving the care required by both (Thomas, 1989; Turton, 1992).

Preliminary results (n = 50) of the study by Taggart *et al.* (cited above) indicate that while caring for the person with AIDS, less than 25% (range: 8%-22%) of the caregivers received either formal or informal help, in terms of finance, arrangement of the home or the loan of equipment, respite care for the infected person, or personal care, housekeeping tasks and personal care for themselves. Further, 26.53% of these caregivers did report the provision of nursing care in the home from a formal agency and another 14.29% from informal sources. However, the greatest source of support came from other caregivers like themselves: nearly three quarters of these caregivers participated in and were supported by self-help groups.

It should not be forgotten, however, social support also has a "dark side" which can distort the efforts of caring (Tilden & Galyen, 1987). Tilden (1985) notes that social support encompasses the dimension "conflict", as well as the dimensions "interpersonal relationships" and "reciprocity". A number of the caregivers of Taggart *et al.* (cited above) complained that others in the extended family care group "took too much place" or failed to repay as much as they were given. Further they reported that their loved ones presented certain problems or behaviours which provoked conflict or complicated the care role. These include: aggressive verbal or physical behaviour (62%), physical symptoms or deficits (54%), confusion or loss of memory (36%), incontinence (30%), psychiatric problems (16%).

CARE FOR THE CAREGIVERS

Future research, and inter-related clinical interventions are in great part dependent on the clarification of the concept "impact" and differentiation of positive and negative subjective impact (perceived burden-perceived benefits) and from the "load" or "weight" of the demands, tasks and activities of caregiving (objective burden). More important would be the theoretical grounding of this work and the syntheses of a family impact conceptual framework possibly based on certain aspects of role theory, family stress or stress and coping (Lazarus & Folkman, 1984; McCubbin & Patterson, 1983).

Uncertainty as a theoretical concept with its social and cultural features plays a role in any conceptual framework devoted to the natural caregiver. Development of the theoretical base for the process of anticipatory guidance could lead to the refinement of important strategies to help the caregiver live with the uncertainties of AIDS caregiving. Learning to identify, expect and accept uncertainty leads to definition of those life circumstances which should and could be changed. Anticipating caregiving as a period of transition marked by burden and by positive sentiments as well as with the realization of a new perspective on life could reduce the distress engendered by the care process (Brown & Cope-Powell, 1991).

Current research efforts in the domain of family caregiving or the aged person have found both group support interventions and respite care to be effective in alleviating the impact of long term caregiving (Neundorfer, 1991). Groups for AIDS caregivers which are also becoming available particularly in various large cities in North America and Europe are an important complement to professional care. Further, while Neundorfer (1991) also found that respite care, which provides temporary relief and rest away from the impact of constant care demands, tended to have little effect on health or mental health, but did tend to improve emotional wellbeing and reduce feelings of distress. However despite the efforts of volunteer groups, providing volunteers who "fill-in", relatively little aid is available to the permanent natural caregiver, who, being reponsible for up to two thirds of the care and help required by the person with AIDS, becomes the cornerstone of society' response to this illness (Harque, 1989; Raveis & Siegel, 1991).

In order to care for the natural caregiver, professional caregivers, who by tradition and perhaps by inclination tend to be non-political, must become sensitive to approaches not necessarily viewed favourably by professional caregivers and to issues which touch upon the power structure of the health care establishment. Tension may be introduced into the care process between natural and professional caregivers with the adoption of "alternative" approaches directed toward the natural caregiver himself, the infected person or both of them. With a disease process such as AIDS, which is without cure, many such approaches must be viewed as complementary to the medical regime, rather than as a threat. With the collaboration and cooperation of the natural caregiver, certain alternative methods or therapies for pain control and stress management can be integrated into the multidisciplinary HIV/AIDS team care plans. These might include behaviourally oriented group interventions, imagery, relaxation and breathing exercises, music therapy or therapeutic touch (Tappan, 1988; Reidy, 1995).

Strategies such as advocacy, empowerment, self-efficacy and the use of "alternative" approaches to care, may well require change in values and attitudes of health professionals. The professional caregiver, in the role of social advocate, may assist the natural caregiver to find the means to manage difficult situations and to use the health system appropriately, or may encourage him to clarify his values and aims and to make informed decisions (Fahy, 1992; Griffin-Francelle, 1993; Ngansurian, 1992). The empowered natural caregiver, through social participation and negotiation, counters social isolation, extends social networks, increases control in interaction with health professionals and accesses available resources (Gibson, 1991). If his perception of self-efficacy (expectations of success) is improved, by vicarious or direct experience, he is more likely to engage in appropriate health behaviours, to promote a healthier lifestyle for himself and for the infected person, and to help the infected person maintain his medical regimen (Bandura, 1977, 1982).

In conclusion, whatever the theoretical base and engendered strategies, intervention for the natural caregivers of persons living with AIDS must be directed toward maintaining their emotional and social integrity and to promoting their health and general wellbeing (Gaynor, 1990). This can be done by reducing the impact of the care process or by increasing their abilities to deal with the impact. Caring will almost necessarily change the lives of natural caregivers; it can increase their knowledge and develop their sensitivities. Their roles, functions and self-esteem will grow and their status will improve if the care process forces mediation of relationships with health care professionals in a substantial way; negotiated care partnerships can only improve the care and the quality of life of those for whom they care.

REFERENCES

Bandura, A. (1977) Self-Efficacy: Toward a Unifying Theory of Behavioral Change. *Psychol Rev*, **84**, 191-215.

Bandura, (1982) Self-efficacy Mechanisms in Human Agency. *American Psychology*, **37**, 122-147.

Brown, M.A. (1993) Caregiver Stress in Families of Persons with HIV/AIDS. *The Nursing of Families*, 211-223. S.R.Meister, J.M.Bell & C.L.Gilless (Eds). California: Sage Publications.

Brown, M.A. & Powell-Cope (1991) AIDS Family Caregiving: Transitions Through Uncertainty. *Nursing Research*, (Nov.-Dec.), **40**, 338-345.

Carmack, B.J. (1992) Balancing Engagement/Detachment in AIDS-related Multiple Losses. *IMAGE: Journal of Nursing Scholarship*, **24**, 9-14.

Cowles, K.V. & Rodgers, B.L. (1991) When a Loved One Has AIDS: Care for the Significant Other. *Journal of Psychosocial Nursing*, **29**, 6-12.

De Montigny, J. & Lapointe, B.J. (1989) Les contours d'un nouveau symbole de mort. *Frontières*, **2**, 18-22.

Dupuis, G., Perreault, J., Lambany, M.C., Kennedy, E. & David, P. (1989) A New Tool to Assess Quality of Life: The Quality of Life Systemic Inventory. *Quality of Life and Cardiovascular Care*, **15**, 36-43.

Durham, D.J. & Cohen, L.F. (1987) *The Person with AIDS: A Nursing Perspective*, 192-210. D.J.Durham & L.F.Cohen (Eds). New York: Springer.

Fahy, K. (1992) Reflections on the Risks and the Rewards. *Aust Nurses J*, (June) **21**, 12-14.

Flaskerud, J.H. & Ungarski (1992) *A Guide to Nursing Care.* 2nd ed. Philadelphia, W.B. Saunders Co.

Fletcher, K.R. & Winslow, S.A. (1991) Informal Caregivers: A Composite and Review of Needs and Community Resources. *Family Community Health*, **14**, 59-67.

Fontaine, G. & Reidy, M. (1995) L'anticipation du deuil chez les soignants naturels de sidéens en phase invalidante: une analyse et un programme d'intervention. Section III: Les familles, les soignants naturels et le sida. *VIH/SIDA: une approche multidisciplinaire.* Gaëtan Morin Editeur Ltée, 173-195.

Fortin, M.F., Côté, J. & Taggart, M.E. (1989) Répercussions bio-psychosociales du SIDA et piste d'intervention et de recherche. *Santé mentale au Québec*, **14**, 96-102.

Gaynor, S.E. (1990). The Long Hawl: The Effects of Home Care on Caregivers. Image: *Journal of Nursing Scholarship*, **22**, 208-212.

Gibson, C.H. (1991) A Concept Analysis of Empowerment. *Journal of Advanced Nursing*, **16**, 354-361.

Greif, L.G. & Porembski, E. (1988) AIDS and Significant Others: Findings from a Preliminary Exploration of Needs. *Health and Social Work*, **23**, 259-265. National Association of Social Workers Inc.

Griffin-Francelle, C. (1993) Advocating for Seriously Emotionally Disturbed Children and their Families: An Overview. *Journal of Child and Adolescent Psychiatric and Mental Health Nursing*, (March) **6**, 33-37.

Harque, R. (1989) A Families Experiences with AIDS. J.H.Flaskerud (Ed.). *AIDS/HIV infection A Reference Guide for Nursing Professionals*, 230-240. Philadelphia, W.B. Saunders Co.

Hart, G., Mann, K. & Stewart, M. (1992) Les conséquences du sida dans la vie des hémophiles et de leurs soignants familiaux au Québec: stress, réponse au stress et soutien social. *Santé mentale au Québec*, **17**, 97-110.

Kristjanson, L.J. & Chalmers, K. (1991) Preventive Work with Families: Issues Failing Public Health Nurses. *Journal of Adv Nursing*, **16**, 147-153.

Lamping, D.L., Joseph, L., Ryan, B. & Gilmore, N. (1992) Détresse psychologique chez les personnes atteintes du VIH à Montréal. *Santé mentale au Québec*, **17**, 73-96.

Lazarus, R.S. & Folkman, S. (1984) *Stress, Appraisal and Coping.* New York: Springer Pub. Co.

Leininger, M. M. (1991) *Culture Care Diversity and Universality: A Theory of Nursing.* New York: National League for Nursing Press.

Lieberman, J.E. (1988) Home Health Care and Hospice for People with HIV Infection. C.Gayling & T.A.Moran (Eds.). *AIDS: Concepts in Nursing Practices,* chap. 14. Baltimore: Williams and Wilkins.

Mansour, S. (1990) Les retentissements psychologiques de l'infection à VIH sur l'enfant et la famille. Centre international de l'Enfance (Ed). *SIDA, enfant, famille.* Paris.

Marchette, L., McFarlane, M. & Padilla, G. (1991) Relationship Among Quality of Life and Other Variables in People with AIDS. *Florida Nurse.* (Nov./Dec.).

Maruin, J.T. & Boyd, .B. (1990) Burden of Mental Illness on the Family: A Critical Review. *Archives of Psychiatric Nursing,* 4, 99-107.

McCann, K. & Wadsworth, E. (1992) The Role of Informal Carers in Supporting Gay Men who have HIV Related Illness: What do They do and What are Their Needs? *AIDS Care,* 4, 25-34. Institute for Social Studies in Medical Care, London.

McCubbin H.I. & Patterson, J.M. (1993) Family Stress and Adaptation to Crisis: A Double ABCX Model of Family Behaviour. D.H.Olson & B.C.Miller (Eds.). *Family Studies Review Book.* Beverly Hills. CA: Sage Publications. 87-106.

McGough, K.N. (1990) Assessing Social Support of People with AIDS. *Oncology Nursing Forum,* 17, 31-35.

Mercier, L. & Reidy, M. (1995) L'incertitude et l'espoir chez les personnes vivant avec le VIH. Section VI: Les enjeux et les problèmes entourant l'infection par le VIH. *VIH/SIDA: une approche multidisciplinaire.* Gaëtan Morin Editeur Ltée, 479-490.

Meyers, A. & Weitzman, M. (1991) Pediatric HIV Disease: The Newest Chronic Illness of Childhood. *Pediatric Clinics of North America,* 38, 169-194.

Neundorfer, M.M. (1991) Family Caregivers of the Frail Elderly. *Community Health,* 14, 48-56.

Ngansurian, W. (1992) Stress and Its Management Thought Research. *Senior Nurse,* (July-August) 12, 40-43.

Pearlin, L.I., Semple, S. & Turner, H. (1988). Stress of AIDS Caregivers: A Preliminary Overview of Issues. *Death Studies,* 12, 501-517.

Perreault, M. (1995) La stigmatisation du sida. Section VI: Les enjeux et les problèmes entourant l'infection par le VIH. *VIH/SIDA: une approche multidisciplinaire,* Gaëtan Morin Editeur Ltée, 423-429.

Perreault, M. & Savard, N. (1992) Le vécu et l'implication d'aidants naturels de personnes vivant avec le VIH. *Santé mentale au Québec,* 17, 111-130.

Rando, T. (1988) *Grieving. How to Go on Living When Someone You Love Dies.* Lexington: Lexington Books.

Raveis, V.H. & Siegel, K. (1991) The Impact of Caregiving on Informal of Familial Caregivers. *AIDS Patient Care,* 5, 39-43.

Régnier, R. (1990) Soins palliatifs et travail de deuil. *Frontières,* 2, 34-37.

Reidy, M. (1995) Le principe de "caring" dans les soins. Section I: La prise en charge de la santé de la personne infectée par le VIH. *VIH/SIDA: une approche multidisciplinaire.* Gaëtan Morin Editeur Ltée

Reidy, M. & Taggart, M.E. (1995) La famille, le soignant naturel et la personne infectée par le VIH. Section III: Les familles, les soignants naturels et le sida. *VIH/SIDA: une approche multidisciplinaire.* Gaëtan Morin Editeur Ltée, 89-112.

Reidy, M., Robinette, L. & Deslongchamps, A. (1995) Les résultats de l'application du modèle auprès de deux familles d'ethnie différente. Section III: Les familles, les soignants naturels et le sida *VIH/SIDA: une approche multidisciplinaire.* Gaëtan Morin Editeur Ltée, 153-172.

Ross, M.W. & Rosser, B.S. (1988) Psychological Issues in AIDS Related Syndromes. *Patient Ed and Counselling,* **11**, 17-28.

Speigel, L. & Mayers, A. (1991) Psychosocial Aspects of AIDS in Children and Adolescents. *The Pediatric Clinics of North America,* **38**, 153-169.

Stulberg, I. & Buckingham, L. (1988) Parallel Issues for AIDS Patients, Families and Others. *Social Casework,* 355-359.

Tappan, F.M. (1988) Healing Massage Techniques: *Holistic, Classic, and Emerging Methods.* Norwalk, Conn.: Appleton & Lange.

Thomas, B. (1989) Supporting Carers of People With AIDS: How Can Carers of People with AIDS Receive the Support they Need? *Nursing Times,* 85.

Tilden, V.P. (1985) Issues of Conceptualization and Measurement of Social Support in the Construction of Nursing Theory. *Research in Nursing and Health,* **8**, 199-206.

Tilden, V.P. & Galyen, R.D. (1987) Cost and Conflict: The Darker Side of Social Support. *Western Journal of Nursing Research,* **9**, 9-18. Sage Publications Inc.

Turton, P. (1992) Families and HIV, United We Stand: With Care and Support, Nursing a Relative or Loved One with HIV/AIDS Can Help Overcome the Rifts that May Occur. *Nursing Times,* **88**, 29-31.

11

Children Born to Mothers with HIV/AIDS: Family Psycho-Social Issues

ROBYN L. SALTER GOLDIE, DALE J. DEMATTEO AND SUSAN M. KING

By the year 2000 more women than men will be infected with HIV (human immunodeficiency virus) even in many developed countries (Hankins, 1992). Women of childbearing age who are infected with the virus are increasing and adding to the complexity of issues this condition generates for families. The multigenerational aspect of this disease makes HIV/AIDS particularly devastating for both the nuclear and extended family affecting the viability and stability of whole communities.

There has not been a national surveillance of HIV infection in women and infants in Canada. Researchers report (Schechter *et al.*, 1992) that although Canadian women constitute 5% of all persons with AIDS, they comprise 10% of the 30,000 people in Canada estimated to have been infected with HIV since June, 1989. During the decade from 1982 to 1992, women accounted for 5.7% of all persons with AIDS; in 1992 that proportion rose to 6.3% (Hankins, 1993). The majority (70%) of Canadian women diagnosed with AIDS are of childbearing age, that is between 20-39 years of age at diagnosis (CQCS, 1992). The routes of HIV transmission documented for women were heterosexual contact for 63%, contaminated blood or blood products for 21%, and intravenous drug use for 9% (Hankins, 1993). According to the Laboratory Centre for Disease Control in Ottawa, men who have sex with women represent 21.5% of the total number of persons with AIDS in Canada (Hankins, 1993).

In a 1991 survey of pediatric centres across Canada, the cumulative number of children identified with confirmed or suspected HIV infection through vertical transmission of the virus from their mothers was 160 (King, 1992). A follow-up study completed in 1992 confirmed a rising case load of HIV-exposed infants born to infected mothers with 28% of the cumulative cases identified in the last year of the surveys (Duff *et al.*, 1994).

Epidemiological studies serve as an indicator of present and future incidence of vertical transmission of HIV but they do not begin to address the psycho-social, interpersonal, economic, health, reproductive and sexual issues specific to families. We are just beginning to identify that HIV-infected families require the attention of politicians and health and social service agencies, and the input of families themselves, if we are to learn how best to meet their needs.

METHOD

The biopsychosocial stages of illness model applied to the experiences of people living with HIV/AIDS (Tiblier, Walker & Roland, 1989) and a grounded theory approach provided the theoretical paradigms for this study. The concept of predictable stages of illness (Tiblier, Walker & Roland, 1989) associated with HIV and AIDS was useful for documenting parents' self-identified service needs and identifying appropriate social service responses.

Population

A total of 25 parents (18 mothers and 7 fathers) were individually interviewed for 2-3 hours by the clinical social worker between March 1992 and February 1993.

Materials

The questionnaire collected both qualitative and quantitative information. Closed questions provided standardized, quantitative information. Open-ended questions elicited qualitative data that was rich and contextual. Importantly, open-ended questions provided research participants with an opportunity for narration. Parents received an honorarium of $50 for their participation.

Information gathered from the questionnaire included: 1) demographic and socio-medical information; 2) parent-identified issues or concerns and parent ratings of interviewer-generated issues; 3) parent-identified social support networks and patterns of disclosure within those networks; 4) Parent-identified supports or services needed and parent ratings of interviewer-generated supports and services.

Data analyses included frequency calculations for quantitative information and techniques associated with a grounded-theory approach to qualitative data, including theme development, content analysis, and triangulation techniques for additional validity. A number of biopsychosocial variables were developed, specific to the population, for analyzing primarily, but not exclusively, the quantitative data. These included time since diagnosis, HIV classifications of parents and children, and level or burden of family illness.

RESULTS

Socio-medical family demographics

A total of 25 parents from 18 families were interviewed. There were 18 (72%) mothers and 7 (28%) fathers. Ten of 18 (56%) mothers were single parents. Husbands or male partners of seven women were interviewed providing us with data on seven couple relationships. The mean age of mothers and fathers was 30 and 33 years (range 20-52 years). Nearly half (44%) of parents were recent immigrants to

Table 11.1
Socio-medical Characteristics of Parents and Children

Socio-medical variables n for parents=25, n for children=36	n	%
HIV status of parents		
HIV-negative	5	20
HIV-asymptomatic	11	44
HIV-symptomatic	7	28
AIDS	2	8
HIV status of children		
HIV-negative	22	61
HIV-indeterminate	4	11
HIV-asymptomatic	5	14
HIV-symptomatic	1	3
AIDS	4	11
Place of parental origin		
Canada	13	52
Central/South America	4	16
Caribbean	3	12
Europe	2	8
Africa	2	8
United States	1	4
Time since family diagnosis		
<6 mos	1	4
6 mos to 1 yr	6	24
>1 yr to 2 yrs	5	20
>2 yrs to 3 yrs	7	28
>3 yrs to 4 yrs	3	12
>4 yrs to 5 yrs	3	12
Self-reported annual income		
<$10,000	1	4
$10,000-$14,999	14	56
$15,000-$19,999	5	20
$20,000-$39,999	4*	16
≥$40,000	1	4

* two parents were about to lose unemployment benefits which will result in a substantial loss of family income

Canada. Only one parent had a professional occupation. Single mothers (60% vs. 40% of all parents) dominated among parents who continued to work full-or part-time. Family incomes were low (84% of families had an annual income of less than $20,000). Only one parent had an income and benefit package to provide adequately for the family's needs in case of parental incapacitation.

Family HIV Configurations (patterns of HIV infection within families)

There are as many as 18 different possible patterns or configurations of family HIV, that is, combinations of family members who have tested positive, negative or are indeterminate for the virus. Families in this study represented 8 of these configurations.

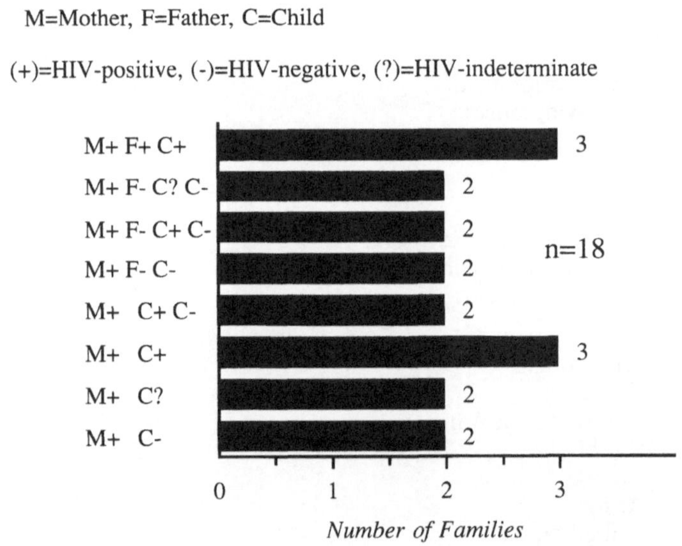

Fig. 11.1 HIV family configurations

The 25 parents involved in this study had 36 children who lived with one or both parents; of these children 14 (39%) were HIV-positive or -indeterminate, and 22 (61%) were known to be HIV-negative. Ten of 18 families had children diagnosed with HIV. A slightly higher percentage of single mothers (60% vs. 55% for all parents) had a child who was HIV-positive. Generally, at the time of their interview, the majority of parents and children were relatively healthy.

Emerging Themes

Using content analysis with open-ended, parent-generated issues and concerns we identified four major parental themes: isolation, secrecy and disclosure; coming to terms with the family infection; preparing for the family's future; and couple tension and sexual relationships.

1) Isolation, secrecy and disclosure: The predominant and interrelated psycho-social concerns of parents involved secrecy, isolation and disclosure. All parents spoke about the difficulties they experienced living with the secret of HIV and its effects on the family, including self-imposed isolation. Some parents came to accept "living with the secret." The personal reasons parents gave for not disclosing the family HIV diagnosis followed three patterns: 1. fear of social rejection and discrimination, especially for children; 2. fear of judgment resulting in personal rejection or the disapproval of family members and friends; 3. non-infected fathers who felt disclosure was singularly the infected mother's decision. Factors affecting a parent's ability to disclose included trust that the person would keep the secret and be supportive, loyalty – or a sense of duty – to family, level of personal acceptance of the diagnosis, coping styles (parent's and others') physical distance from family, quality of past relationships, and the level of shared intimacy before the diagnosis.

2) Coming to terms with the family's HIV infection: Parents commonly identified a feeling pattern of intense emotions including anger, grief, sadness, despair, multiple loss, uncertainty, guilt and hope. Woven throughout parents' narratives was a pervasive sense of stress. In addition to the stress of parents whose child has a catastrophic illness and for most parents their own stress of living with a life-threatening disease that has no cure, were the stresses associated with parenting, including economic stress. Mothers' own needs for emotional support and health care usually were secondary to the needs of the children, their partner, and the global needs of the family. Often mothers were additionally stressed by personal feelings of guilt or shame.

Parents demonstrated important differences in their coping styles. Some parents gained control of their situation by choosing to be vigilant about the disease and learning everything about the virus and actively participating in treatment decisions. For other parents, the thought of HIV weighed so heavily on their hearts and minds that they chose to not think about the infection and avoided people or situations that made them feel negative about themselves or their future to take in order to control of their lives and fulfill daily responsibilities.

The majority (83%) of parents spoke about the difficult task of learning to cope. They described various personal and social strategies for getting on with their lives which included: avoiding thinking about HIV, living day-to-day, maintaining a positive attitude, finding spiritual meaning for their lives, developing new priorities, reconnecting with or growing closer to extended family members and friends, finding solace and support in their children, learning to work with health care and service systems, and taking greater control when dealing with bureaucracies and professionals. Qualities such as hope, emotional strength, and achieving a sense of peace were valued and mentioned by some parents who felt they were coping fairly well. Often these qualities were associated with strong spiritual beliefs.

3) Preparing for the family's future: Most (75%) parents talked about needing to make preparations for the family's future, yet among mothers, only 56% made such a reference. Nearly all parents acknowledged the impact on the family of the mother's loss of health or possible death. A serious concern for both parents was preparing fathers for the work and responsibility of caring for the children. Fathers expressed feelings of inadequacy about their parental and household abilities, so much so, that several anticipated a need for foster care. Single mothers were much less likely to talk about planning for the future which may be related to the lack of a co-parenting partner; parents in a couple relationship said they especially relied on a partner for guidance and support. Non-infected children, often referred to in the literature as "the forgotten group" rated considerably lower in parents' level of concern for their well being and future care (Gibb *et al.*, 1991). It was our sense this was related to parents' belief and trust that family members could more easily care for healthy children than parents' lack of concern for these children.

4) Couple tension and sexual issues: For parents involved in couple relationships, tension between partners and issues of sexuality were common themes. For most couples (82% of partners) sexual issues – especially practicing safer sex, were of serious concern and a source of considerable stress. Fewer (28%) parents indicated that pregnancy decisions were a high concern and nearly all (86%) were women. There were several male partners at risk for transmission of HIV through unprotected sex who appeared quite unconcerned and were choosing not to be retested. Several women were ambivalent about sexual risk-taking; they were fearful, but at the same time flattered their partner accepted them as they were.

In response to closed questions initiated by the interviewer, parental concerns that received the highest ratings are shown in the following graph (Figure 11.2).

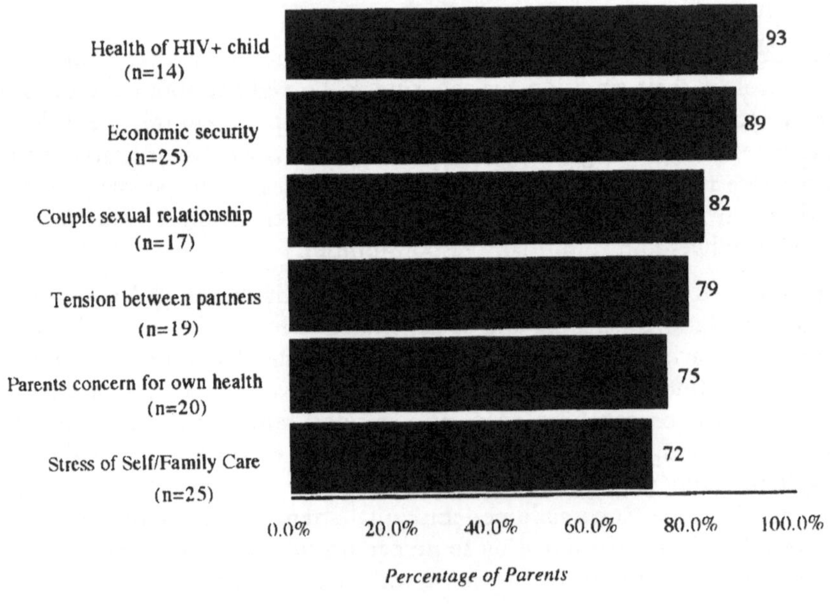

Fig. 11.2 Highest ratings of parental concerns

Services Parents Use or Want in the Future

The most valued support or service parents identified was continued access to financial resources including an opportunity to work for as long as possible. Additional supports and services parents identified wanting currently or in the future (in order of need and perceived value) included day care, individual counseling, parent support group, couple counseling, help with transportation, access to housing, respite care for infected and non-infected children, and legal guidance.

Social Supports and Disclosure Experiences

Parents were asked who provided them with emotional and practical support and to categorize these people as a partner, family member, friend, work mate, neighbour, volunteer, professional or other person. Parents reported they received support primarily from partners, family, or professionals, with support also coming from friends and volunteers. At time of diagnosis, professionals were often the only people to provide parents with emotional support and guidance. The number of people parents relied upon for social support ranged from 0 to 8 persons with a mean of 4 supportive persons per parent. Parents from families experiencing the highest level of illness (of parents or child) reported relying on the greatest number of support persons (5.3); the next highest were parents dealing with the crisis of a recent diagnosis (an average of 5 support persons – sometimes only professionals). Single mothers – especially those who worked, immigrant parents, and male partners reported relying on fewer (an average of 3) supportive persons. There was no difference in average number of social supports reported by parents with low- or high-family support (average of 4), although who provided the support (i.e., from formal or informal social network) was often different.

The majority (56%) of families had disclosed to less than half the people in their informal social network; several had disclosed to no one. Some parents told their extended family soon after diagnosis – for support, out of loyalty, or to maintain the integrity of family relationships. Out of the total of 36 children, only one teen-aged sibling had been told about HIV in the family.

When parents made the decision to disclose, in 91% of 127 individual cases they reported the relationship become closer or stayed the same. Three patterns of negative changes in relationships after diagnosis or disclosure emerged; these include: 1) parents who reported more distant relationships with their spouse or partner after diagnosis (11 of 16, 69%), 2) mothers whose sisters-in-law reacted negatively presumably out of fear for their children (3 of 11, or 27% of relationships described as more distant), and 3) males who more often than females reported a negative relationship change (57% vs. 33%) after diagnosis or disclosure. Mothers with no or few disclosures often said they feared the judgment or reaction of others especially that of their mothers. Telling one's mother was often the first (and described as either the easiest or most difficult) disclosure step. Unplanned disclosures were reported when couples separated and loyalties were broken.

DISCUSSION

The biopsychosocial model that provided the philosophical framework for this study is dynamic and one based on transitional change (i.e., in family or individual levels of health, in social functions of family members and the family as a unit, in levels of social support required by individuals and family as a unit). Although we attempted to quantify the biopsychosocial model using variables based on different stages of illness we did not find these tools particularly useful for this exploratory study. We believed this was related to several factors including: small sample and sub-sample populations, the static nature of a one-time survey, and the fact that family members were relatively well at the time of the parent interviews regardless of HIV classification.

When we examined the data there was an unusual, but consistent, pattern of parental response that neither the usual social variables (i.e., gender, age, marital status, etc.) or measures on biopsychosocial stages of illness (i.e., time since family diagnosis, current HIV classification(s), family burden of HIV/AIDS illness) could explain. An additional theoretical model of coping styles helped explain this unusual pattern of parental response (Weitz, 1989). This model identified vigilance and avoidance as coping styles that people living with HIV tend to choose between to reduce the stress of uncertainty by enabling them to normalize and retain control over their lives. Weitz recommends that health care providers holistically view these different coping styles – that is to appreciate both vigilance and avoidance as valid strategies that can help people cope with stress and maintain a sense of dignity and control in their lives. With this conceptualization comes the parallel responsibility for professionals to develop or adapt programs and services for families with HIV that are easily accessed when members of families move from chronic to acute stages of illness (and sometimes back again).

Parents participating in this study varied in family structure, number of children, HIV family configurations, ages of parents, ethnicity and first language spoken. They held various world views and they lived in both rural and urban settings. Given such diversity, the similarities in their experiences were quite remarkable. They considered maintaining an adequate income their primary concern and a source of stress.

Present or future social and familial implications of this infection which may hold for the 18 families participating in this study include: 18 mothers and 2 fathers who face premature death of themselves and possibly their child; 36 children who face the premature death of one or both parents; 36 children whose future care and guardianship must be planned; children who may become orphaned or the only surviving family member; grandparents, aunts and uncles who may be called upon to care for infected and non-infected grandchildren, nieces and nephews; establish the need to guardianship for some children which may require international negotiations and travel; seven couples who face a statistically higher risk of parental separation or divorce; non-infected male partners who may be at risk of transmission of HIV; additional planned or unplanned pregnancies; a number of HIV-infected children soon entering day care or public school; 35 of 36 children who have yet to be told their own or their families HIV diagnosis; non-infected fathers who are feeling inadequate to care for their children and maintain a household; mothers who may be ignoring their health needs – ironically to care for their children for as long as possible; and, infected mothers and fathers who may require a variety of supports to continue to care for their families, or to be cared for themselves, in the family home.

This complexity of family configurations and the multigenerational effect of HIV infection highlight the need for intergenerational coordination of care, and services that are flexible and accessed quickly and easily by families.

Although our data are limited there was evidence to suggest that a pattern of avoidance coping style may be more common among fathers and single mothers. Parents' coping styles (whether the same or different) appeared to have serious implications for the couples' sexual lives, especially for safer-sex practices and pregnancy decisions. Many important questions remain about parents with HIV and the coping styles and strategies chosen by or available to these individuals, including the influence of personality, sex, early family experiences, depression, a history of addiction, and stigma and resulting isolation associated with HIV. Parental coping styles can be a challenge for health and social service providers, especially when parents need to consider difficult issues including possibility of illness and death of parents and children, future guardianship of children, and disclosure of family HIV to children. Providing professionals with regular opportunities to learn and update counseling and helping skills should be integral to all HIV/AIDS health and social services. With sensitive and supportive counseling, health providers and social workers can validate parents' coping styles and strategies while helping them understand how their own coping style and those of others in their social network, may affect their decision-making and ability to plan for the future.

Guiding principles for services to families with HIV include that they be: family centered and when possible community based, responsive to cultural and language diversity, of high quality, coordinated, comprehensive and flexible, available early and continuously, respectful and protective of family privacy and autonomy, and conducive to normal living patterns (The Children and Family AIDS Task Force, 1993).

CONCLUSION

Identifying family configurations of patterns of HIV within a clinic population can be a useful way to visualize HIV as a complex multigenerational disease. This type of visual representation serves to help clinicians identify potential psycho-social issues and needs unique to individual families and those more common to whole clinical populations.

The structured interview format used with this study was a valuable clinical tool for the social worker/interviewer. As a result of the interviews, partnerships with parents were strengthened, important issues were identified and clarified, the clinical care team's understanding of parents coping styles and strategies increased, and importantly, parents expressed satisfaction in having the opportunity to educate others and voice their concerns without disclosing their identities.

REFERENCES

CQCS (1992) Mise â jour des données. *Surveillance des cas du SIDA,* Canada: Centre québécois de coordination sur le SIDA.

Duff, F., King, S.M., Lapointe, N., Read, S.E., Forbes, J., Allen, U., et al. (In press). Canadian national survey of perinatal HIV infection 1991-1992. *Canadian Journal of Public Health.*

Gibb, D., Duggan, C., Lwin, R., (1991) The family and HIV. *Gentourinary Medicine,* 7, 263-366.

Hankins, C. (1993) Gynaecological manifestations in women with HIV infection. *The Canadian Journal of Obstretrics, Gynaecology & Women's Health Care,* **5**, 385-389.

King, S.M.(1992). Survey of perinatally HIV-infected infants and children in pediatric centres in Canada. *Canadian Journal of Infectious Diseases* (supplement), **3**, 43A-44A.

Schechter, M., Marion, S., Elmslie, K., Ricketts, M. (1992) How many persons in Canada have been infected with HIV? An exploration using back calculation methods. *Clinical Investigative Medicine,* **15**, 331-345.

The Children and Family AIDS Task Force. (1993) *HIV/AIDS in Children and Families in Massachusetts Recommendations for Policy and Program.* Report to the Commissioner of the Massachusetts Department of Public Health.

Tiblier, K., Walker, G., Rolland, J., (1989) *AIDS and Families.* New York: Haworth Press.

Weitz, R. (1989) Uncertainty and the lives of persons with AIDS. *Journal of Health and Social Behaviour,* **30**, 270-281.

12

Young Women and HIV: The Role of Biology in Vulnerability

MIKE BAILEY

Attention has recently been drawn to the role of a biological factor in the high rates of HIV infection seen amongst young women (Reid & Bailey, 1992; Merson, 1993). This biological factor acts in addition to, and is amplified by, socio-economic influences on adolescent sexual behaviour. This discussion presents a biological mechanism whereby the cervix may be a target area for HIV infection during adolescence; as a result of infection by other sexually transmitted pathogens and; during and after pregnancy. Policy implications for sexual health and HIV prevention programming are discussed and key questions for further investigation identified. Whilst the emphasis is on women of developing countries where HIV infection rates are highest, the mechanism is relevant to young women everywhere.

Epidemiological analysis shows that HIV infection rates are highest in adolescent women, particularly in women in developing countries. Figure 12.1 shows age and gender disaggregated AIDS cases from Zaire showing that infection rates peaked in adolescent women (Quinn *et al.*, 1986), the first report of this profile which has been repeated since in epidemiological data from around the world. Figure 12.2 (MoH Uganda, 1992) shows the same profile from Uganda as an example. Sadly, whilst the vulnerability of young women has been clearly shown since 1986 it took six years to get this onto the agenda of policy makers. Even now the unique degree of risk faced by women in their adolescence is seldom, if ever, allowed to command a priority place in policy or resource allocation.

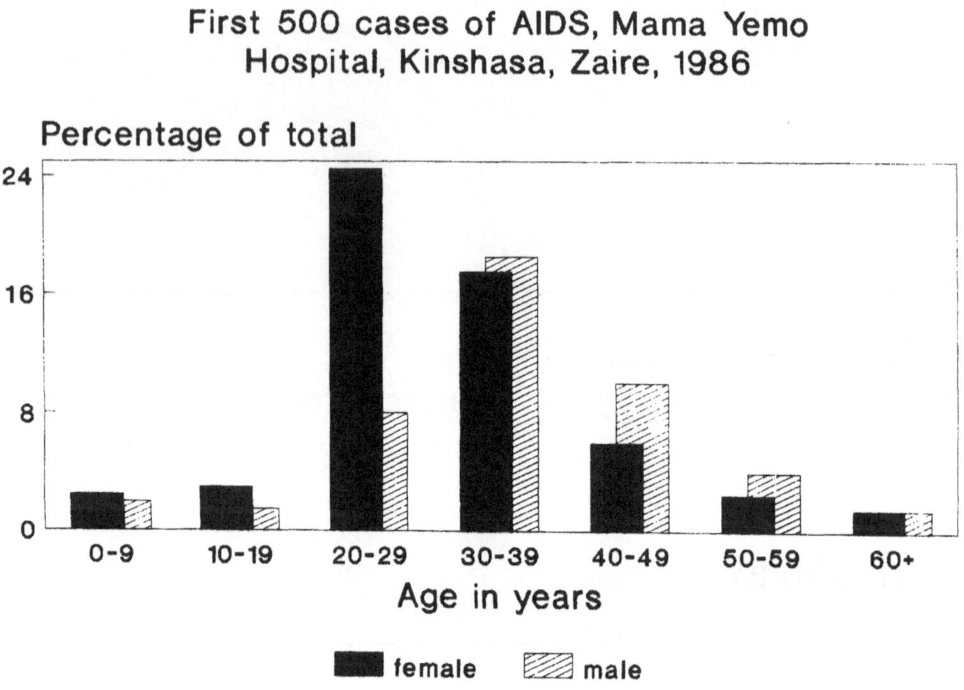

Fig. 12.1 Age and gender disaggregated AIDS cases from Zaire

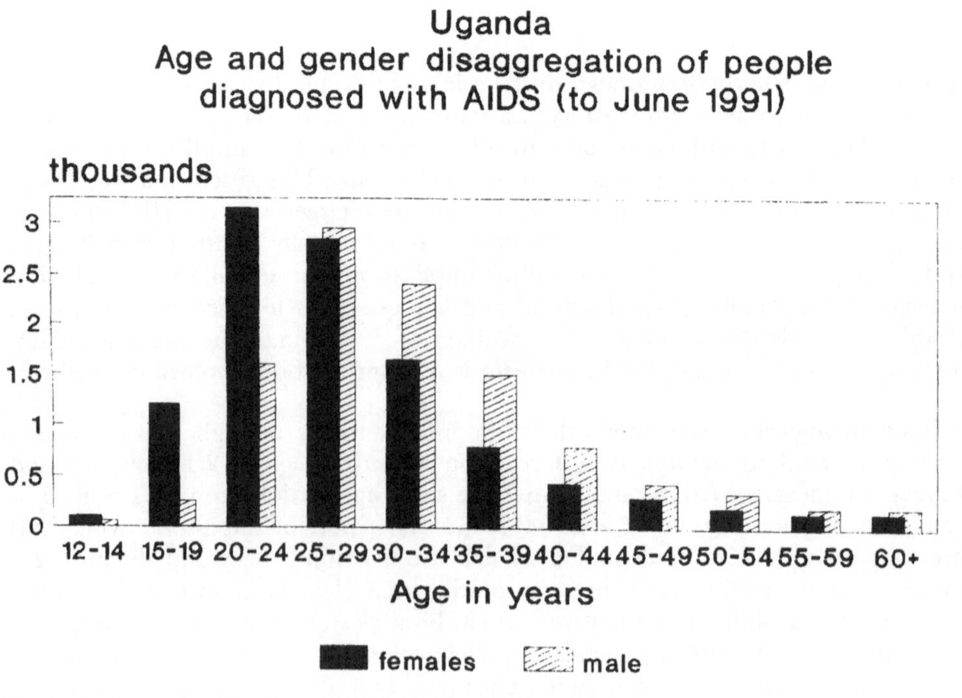

Fig. 12.2 Age and gender disaggregated AIDS cases from Uganda

THE PASSAGE OF ADOLESCENCE

Adolescence is a passage of opportunity and risk, frequently negotiated by trial and error. It is when the biological, psychological and social transitions from childhood to adulthood take place. The pace of these changes is uneven, at times rapid. Accompanying the changes are transient but critical periods of social, economic and physiological vulnerability.

The passage of adolescence is becoming no easier as secular trends are decreasing the age of menarche (Wyshak, 1982) and the age of sexual debut (Ankomah & Ford, 1994) whilst the age of first marriage is increasing. Sex in the bio-social gap between menarche and first marriage is starting earlier and leads to high rates of sexually transmitted infection and unwanted pregnancy (Erhardt & Wasserheit, 1991). One example comes from Ghana, where the economic pressures of structural adjustment have been accompanied by social changes whereby some families are no longer able to support their unmarried adolescent daughters and expect them to find their own means of support once they are old enough to have sexual partners (Ankomah & Ford, 1994).

During adolescence the health and social prospects of individuals may be compromised by the consequences of debut adult activities. This is not simply the adolescent experimenting with behaviours for which he or she is not prepared, the adolescent is also passing through a period of increased biological vulnerability.

Sexual maturation is central to adolescence. Physically it takes from as little as 18 months to as long as six years. It begins earlier and is completed faster in women than in men. It is triggered and controlled within the body by the endocrine system. The timing of puberty, in particular menarche, may be affected by lifestyle with under-nutrition (Henley & Vaitukaitis, 1985) and excessive energy expenditure delaying sexual maturation.

Psychological and social maturity proceeds in the wake of physical changes and continues longer, to less well defined end points. It is more dependent on environmental circumstances than on physiology (Erhardt & Wasserheit, 1991). Thus, the physical capacity for sexual intercourse and reproduction arrives ahead of the development of related decision making skills. For this reason sexual health advice to people in early adolescence often concentrates on delaying sexual debut whilst for late adolescence it deals with the avoidance of sexually transmitted infection and unwanted pregnancy.

Global trends of urbanisation, cultural transition and economic recession erode the traditional mechanisms which guide young women and men through the transition from childhood to adulthood. Weakened family networks leave a vacuum in the supply of information about sexuality and family life (International Labour Office, 1992). These pressures are most extreme in countries experiencing economic and social transition.

ADOLESCENT VULNERABILITY TO SEXUALLY TRANSMITTED INFECTION

Sexually active adolescent women and men experience the highest rates of sexually transmitted infections (World Health Organization, 1993), including HIV infection (Reid & Bailey, 1992). Furthermore, because fewer women are sexually active at this age than in the older age groups the infection rate amongst the sexually active is even higher than it first appears (Bell & Hein, 1984). Further support comes from the observation that young women with cervical invasive neoplasia began menarche later but started sex no later than their peers (Moscicki, 1989). The long term consequences of these infections are frequently severe, particularly for women (Aral, 1992), they include pelvic inflammatory disease, ectopic pregnancy, infertility, cancer and AIDS.

Sexual activity also influences adolescent well-being through teenage pregnancy which is the key determinant of inequality between adolescent males and females and is the mechanism for the intergenerational transmission of poverty. Worldwide, large numbers of children are born to adolescent women, for every 100 women reaching the age of 20 there are; in Africa 90 births; in Latin America 40; in North America 25 and in Asia and Europe 15 (International Labour Office, 1992). These high rates of teenage parenthood are markers of unprotected sexual activity as well as indicators of social pressures for young women to begin childbearing.

The high rate of sexually transmitted infection in adolescents has two separate causes. First, a greater risk of exposure to pathogens. The first years of sexual behaviour often involve the greatest number of partner changes particularly for men and for sexually active unmarried women. Sexually active adolescents are more likely to have partners who have sexually transmissible infections. Also, it is common for the male partner in heterosexual pairs to be older by some years. This means that newly sexually active (often newly married) women are immediately exposed to a sexually transmitted infection risk arising from the accumulation of sexual contacts from their partner, this is termed the male factor (Skegg, 1982). In North America, for example, for every woman who is at risk of sexually transmitted infections from her own multiple sexual partners, there are two at risk only from their partner's sexual contacts (Kost & Forrest, 1992).

The second cause is that adolescent exposure to sexually transmitted pathogens may carry a greater risk of infection because transmission is enhanced by damage to genital membranes during sex or because of an age-related biological susceptibility to infection, particularly in women. Trauma to genital or anorectal membranes during sexual contact is most likely for the receptive partner. It happens most often when lubrication is inadequate, when the sex is forced or otherwise violent and at the time of sexual debut. This has been sufficient to permit HIV transmission during a woman's first, and only, sexual intercourse (Bouvet *et al.*, 1989). Adolescent women may have sex without adequate lubrication because first sexual encounters are often a time of inexpertise and emotional ambivalence which may interfere with the vaginal lubrication response. For social and economic reasons adolescents may most often find themselves in unwelcome sexual encounters such as commercial sex selling, rape and sexual assault (Reid & Bailey, 1992; Heise, 1993; MacDonald *et al.*, 1994).

THE CERVIX, A SITE OF CHANGE IN CHANGING TIMES

An age-related biological susceptibility to sexually transmitted pathogens arises from the transformation zone of the adolescent cervix. In early to mid adolescence this susceptibility is exacerbated by the absence of protective cervical mucus which is not present until regular ovulation is established (Duncan, M.E., *et al.*, 1990). During adolescence the cervix is more likely to comprise cells which are susceptible to infection by *Chlamydia trachomatis* (Hobson *et al.*, 1980), human papilloma virus, *Neisseria gonorrhoea* (Draper, 1980) and HIV (Reid & Bailey, 1992). An increased risk of precancerous morphological changes in the cervix of sexually active adolescent women has also been noted for some time (Terris, 1960). The cervix is also regarded as a prime site of *Treponema pallidum* and herpes simplex virus-2 infection (Holmes *et al.*, 1990).

The cervix forms a channel between the uterus and the vagina. It secretes cervical mucous which plugs the channel during the follicular and luteal phases of the menstrual cycle and which facilitates the passage of sperm into the uterus during ovulation. The external surface of the cervix may have three types of cells, columnar and metaplastic squamous cells which are vulnerable to attachment by pathogens and mature squamous cells which are not (Draper, 1980). In adults, the junction between these cells in the cervix, called the transformation zone, is usually within the cervical canal and only mature squamous cells are exposed on the outer surface. The cervical transformation zone in adolescents is frequently exposed on the outer surface of the cervix and initially comprises a simple junction between columnar cells and squamous cells.

THE ONSET OF PUBERTY

The onset of puberty and of menarche is related to growth which is dependent on nutrition, the adequacy of which is related to energy expenditure (Goldfarb, 1977; Baker, 1985). The delaying influence of childhood malnutrition has been reported as has the difference between rural and urban populations (Wilson & Sutherland, 1950; Kulin *et al.*, 1982) and variation with socioeconomic status (Roberts *et al.*, 1977; Dare *et al.*, 1992).

Puberty in women follows a general sequence beginning at age eight or so with the opening of the endocervical canal. Prior to menarche oestrogen triggers maturation of the epithelial cells of the lower genital tract, progesterone stimulation of these vaginal cells causes them to fill with glycogen, this supports lactobacilli which create a lower pH environment. A year or so before menarche, the glycogination of squamous cells in the vaginal epithelium leads to lower pH in the vagina because of lactobacterial colonization. This provokes squamous cell growth to cover the columnar cells which are sensitive to low pH (Reid & Campion, 1989; Singer, 1975; Coppleson, 1976). This is a process of cellular response to a newly hostile environment. At this time, the vaginal lubrication mechanism begins to mature. Menarche marks the beginning of menstruation but regular cycles including ovulation may take some months to become established. At this stage cervical mucous production begins to play its role fully in creating a periodic barrier to the egress of sperm and pathogens into the uterus.

I propose that the cells of the reparative response which takes place in the transformation zone are significant target cells for HIV infection. The metaplastic cells of the transformation zone are growing squamous cells. A range of inflammatory cells are recruited to the area of active metaplasia and will comprise a distinct part of the cell population of the transformation zone. Many of these cells will be rich in HIV attachment sites. Examination of cervical cells from women with HIV infection women reveals HIV infection in many of the inflammatory cells associated both with the epithelium and the endothelium but none in the epithelial cells themselves (Pomerantz, 1988).

As women age, the position of the transformation zone migrates into the cervical canal and cells sensitive to low pH are no longer exposed in the vagina. In one study, the transformation zone was noted on the outside surface of the cervix in 74% of 16-20 year olds, 50% of 26 year olds and in none of the over 60's (Ostergard, 1977).

Migration of the transformation zone into the cervical canal may be inhibited by adolescent sexual activity (Reid & Champion, 1989). In one study, the transformation zone persisted on the outside of the cervix in twice as many sexually active women seven years after menarche as in sexually inactive women of the same gynaecologic age, the difference having arisen over the previous four years (Gottardi, 1984). This delay is probably the result of infection events. For example, *C. trachomatis* infections of the cells of the transition zone may perpetuate the presence of active metaplasia on the external surface of the cervix (Moscicki *et al.*, 1989).

Women may experience a further period of enhanced vulnerability to infection if they become pregnant. When the first pregnancy is established the cervix becomes everted and columnar cells in the cervical canal are exposed to a lower than normal vaginal pH (Hobson, 1980; Draper *et al.*, 1980). This triggers a further inflammatory response and more metaplasia. Figure 12.3 shows a comparison of the size of the transformation zone in women at different stages of the reproductive spectrum. The transformation zone is most often wide and has leucocyte involvement (cells of the inflammatory process) during pregnancy (Fluhmann, 1959). This mechanism could be behind the vulnerability implied in findings from Rwanda (Chao *et al.*, 1991). Figure 12.4 shows an increased risk of HIV infection in women who have not been pregnant and in those who have had only one or two pregnancies and an increased risk in relation to the age at which they first became pregnant. It has also been suggested that pregnancy is a period of increased risk for human papilloma virus infection (Schneider *et al.*, 1987).

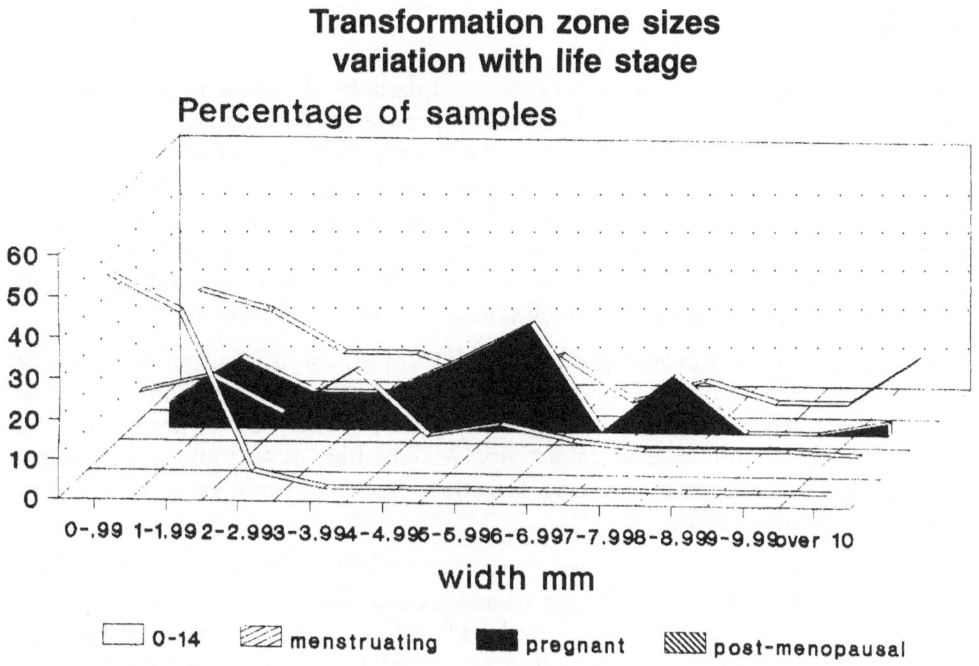

Fig. 12.3 Transformation zone sizes variation with life stage

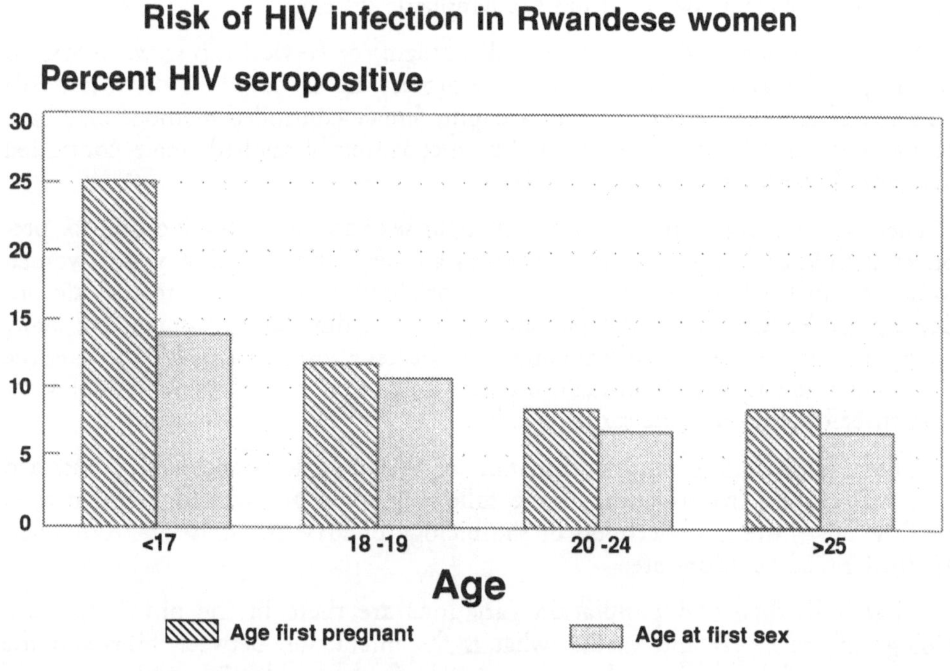

Fig. 12.4 Risk of HIV infection in Rwandese women

DISCUSSION

The evidence suggests that the process of metaplasia in the transformation zone is accompanied by recruitment of inflammatory process cells which are susceptible to HIV infection. This occurs whether metaplasia is triggered by exposure of columnar cells to low vaginal pH at puberty and pregnancy or by infection by HPV and HSV-2 or *C. trachomatis.* These risk amplifying factors may act synergistically further increasing the risk of HIV infection for young women with human papilloma virus, herpes simplex virus or *C. trachomatis* infections of the cells of the transformation zone because of prolonged exposure of susceptible cells on the cervix.

In developing countries susceptibility to HIV transmission is amplified in young women whose puberty, including menarche, is delayed by poor nutrition and calorie wastage. They have an increased risk that susceptible cells will be present on the cervix when they commence sexual activity. Malnutrition is also known to depress immunological competence, making infection easier to establish and harder to suppress (Chandra, 1983).

The biological vulnerability of young women to HIV infection has implications for policy which promotes the health of adolescents. We do not know how much protection against sexually transmitted pathogens, including HIV, is enough. Condoms protect men but do not effectively protect women because they are not used consistently enough to address the magnitude of the risk women face. Barriers which cover the cervix would offer protection to women but not to men as the female genital secretions to which the penis is exposed come predominantly from the vaginal transudate derived from the lymphatic system.

Will microbicide (with or without a diaphragm) or cervical cap serve women as well in practice as a condom because they protect the cervix where the susceptible cells are? If compliance is taken into account, female controlled methods may have greater efficacy than more efficient, but inconsistently applied, male controlled methods (Rosenburg & Gollub, 1992).

There are also urgent policy questions about sex and life skills education for pre-pubertal children; social and cultural norms and legislation to allow young women to delay sexual debut and; changes in the socialisation of children so they do not develop gender identities which perpetuate the subordination of women. For many young women, whatever is offered after they become sexually active is too late; the critical question is what information, advice and support is available to adolescent women before they become sexually active?

Fuller understanding and confirmation of the biological mechanism described here will require investigation of the following questions which, in themselves confirm how little is understood of the biology of HIV transmission (Alexander, 1990). Critical questions are:

What individual and population variations are there in the physiology and biology of the cervix and vagina, what is the interaction between HIV and the various cells of the vagina and cervix and what further epidemiological evidence is there for increased HIV infection rates in adolescent women and primigravidae? Understanding this will help to determine how many young women are at increased risk due to the exposure of readily infected target cells on the cervical face. It may allow women at increased risk to be identified and counselled on ways to reduce their risk. More knowledge should lead to more information being available to women and to more choices for them on means to achieve and sustain sexual health.

How does nutrition, energy expenditure and illness affect the timing of puberty and of the critical events of vaginal and cervical maturation in populations in developing countries? If nutrition does play a critical role then this will add to the arguments for improving the access of young women to adequate nutrition.

How does sexual activity affect the timing of puberty and of the critical events of vaginal and cervical maturation? Information on this will guide young women and the sexual health educators and counsellors who work with them. If early sexual debut is shown to raise the risk of HIV substantially then delaying sexual debut should be adopted as a priority for HIV prevention by young women, their parents, communities and governments.

Finally, if pregnancy brings an increased vulnerability to HIV infection, the interpretation of HIV surveillance data based on serotesting of pregnant women will need to be reviewed.

REFERENCES

Ankomah, A., Ford, N. (1994) Sexual exchange: understanding premarital heterosexual relationships in urban Ghana. In Aggleton P, Davies P, Hart, G. (Eds.), *AIDS: foundations for the future.* pp. 123-135. University of London.

Alexander, N.J. (1990) Sexual transmission of human immunodeficiency virus: virus entry into the male and female genital tract. *Fertility & Sterility* **54**, 1-18.

Aral, S.O. (1992) Sexual behaviour as a risk factor for sexually transmitted disease. In: Reproductive tract infections, Germain *et al.*, (Eds.), pp. 185-198. Plenum Press, New York.

Baker, E.R., Body weight and the initiation of puberty. *Clin Obst & Gynae,* **28**, 573-79.

Bell, T.A., Hein, K. (1984) Adolescents and sexually transmitted diseases. In: Holmes KK *et al.* (Eds), *Sexually transmitted diseases,* McGraw-Hill, New York. 73-84.

Bouvet, E. *et al.* (1989) Defloration as a risk factor for heterosexual HIV transmission. *Lancet.* p. 615.

Chandra, R.K. (1983) Nutrition, immunity and infection: present knowledge and future directions. *Lancet.* p. 688-690.

Chao, A. *et al.*, (1991) Risk factors for HIV-1 among pregnant women in Rwanda. Poster MC3097, VII International Conference on AIDS, Florence.

Coppleson, M., (1976) The new coloscopic terminology. *J Rep Med* **16**, 214-219.

Dare, O. *et al.* (1992) Biosocial factors affecting menarche in a mixed Nigerian population. *Cent Afri J Med,* **38**, 77-81.

Draper, D.L. *et al.* (1980) Scanning electron microscopy of attachment of Neisseria gonorrhoeae colony phenotypes to surfaces of human genital epithelia. *Am J Obstet Gynaecol*, **138**, 818.

Duncan, M.E. *et al.* (1990) First coitus before menarche and risk of sexually transmitted disease. *Lancet*, **335**, 338-40, 1990.

Ehrhardt, A.A., Wasserheit, J.N. (1991) Age, gender and sexual risk behaviours for sexually transmitted diseases in the United States. In: Research issues in human behaviour and sexually transmitted diseases in the AIDS era, Wasserheit, Aral, Holmes and Hitchcock, (Eds.), 97-121. American Society for Microbiology, Washington.

Fluhmann, F.C. (1959) The squamocolumnar transitional zone of the cervix uteri. *Obst & Gynae*, **14**, 133-148.

Goldfarb, A.F. (1977) Puberty and menarche. *Clin Obst & Gynae*, **20**, 625-31.

Gottardi, G. *et al.* (1984) Coloscopic findings in virgin and sexually active teenagers. *Obstet Gynecol*, **63**, 613.

Heise, L. (1993) personal communication.

Henley, K.M., Vaitukaitis, J.L. (1985) Hormonal changes associated with changes in body weight. *Clin Obst & Gynae*, **28**, 615-631.

Hobson, D. *et al.* (1980) Quantitative aspects of Chlamydial infection of the cervix. *Br J Vener Dis*, **56**, 156-162.

Holmes, K.K. *et al.* (Eds.) (1990) Sexually transmitted diseases, McGraw-Hill, New York.

International Labour Office. (1992) Equal opportunities for women: the implications of adolescent pregnancy and childbirth in SubSaharan Africa for ILO policies and programmes.

Kost, K., Forrest, J.D. (1992) American women's sexual behaviour and exposure to risk of sexually transmitted diseases. *Fam Plann Pers*, **24**, 244.

Kulin, H.E. *et al.* (1982) The effect of chronic childhood malnutrition on pubertal growth and development. *Am J Clin Nut*, **36**, 527-36.

MacDonald, N.E., Fisher, W.A., Wells, G.A., Doherty, J.A.A., Bowie, W.R. (1994) Canadian street youth: correlates of sexual risk taking activity. *Paed Inf Dis J*, **13**, 690-697.

Merson, M. (1993) The HIV/AIDS pandemic: Global spread and global response, plenary address at IX International Conference on AIDS, IV STD World Congress, Berlin.

Ministry of Health Uganda. (1992) NACP AIDS figures.

Moscicki, A.B. *et al.* (1989) Differences in biologic maturation, sexual behaviour and sexually transmitted disease between adolescents with and without cervical intraepithelial neoplasia. *J. Pediatr*, **115**, 487-93.

Ostergard, D.R. (1977) The effect of age, gravidity and parity on the location of the cervical squamocolumnar junction as determined by colposcopy. *Am J Obstet. Gynecol*, **129**, 59.

Pomerantz, R.J. *et al.* (1988) Human immunodeficiency virus infection of the uterine cervix. *Ann Int Med*, **108**, 321-327.

Quinn, T.C. *et al.* (1986) AIDS in Africa, an epidemiologic paradigm. *Science*, **234**, 957.

Reid, E., Bailey, M.R. (1992) Young women: silence, susceptibility and the HIV epidemic, Issues paper, UNDP HIV and Development Programme.

Reid, R., Campion, M.J. (1989) HPV associated lesions of the cervix: biology and coloscopic features. *Clin Obst & Gynae*, **32**, 157-79.

Roberts, D.F. *et al.* (1977) A study of menarcheal age in India. *Ann Hum Biol*, **4**, 171-77.

Rosenberg, M.J., Gollub, E.L. (1992) Commentary: Methods women can use that may prevent sexually transmitted disease including HIV. *Am J Public Health*, **82**, 1473-1478.

Schneider, A. *et al.* (1987) Increased prevalence of humanpapilloma virus in the lower genital tract of pregnant women. *Int J Cancer*, **40**, 198-201.

Skegg, D.C.G. *et al.* (1982) Importance of the male factor in cancer of the cervix. *Lancet*, **ii**, 581-83.

Singer, A. (1975) The uterine cervix from adolescence to the menopause. *Br J Obst & Gynae*, **82**, 81-99.

Terris, M., Oalmann, M.C. (1960) Carcinoma of the cervix: an epidemiologic study. *JAMA*, **174**, 1847-1851.

Wilson, D.C., Sutherland, I. (1950) Age at menarche. *BMJ*, **i**, 1267.

World Health Organization. (1993) Adolescent Health Programme, Sexually transmitted diseases amongst adolescents in the developing world.

Wyshak, G. *et al.* (1982) Evidence for a secular trend in age of menarche. *NEJM*, **306**, 1033-1035.

13

HIV Testing in the Antenatal Clinic: Setting up a Counselling and Testing Service

JEAN MEADOWS, TRACEY CHESTER, PAUL LEWIS AND JOSE CATALÁN

BACKGROUND

Heterosexual transmission of the Human Immunodeficiency Virus (HIV) to women, in the UK., continues to increase. 38% of cumulative reported HIV cases in women to April 1987 were as a result of heterosexual contact. By April 1994, this figure had risen to 62% (CDSR 1986, 1994). Amongst antenatal clinic attenders in London, the overall seroprevalence rate in 1992, as determined by unlinked anonymous screening of maternal blood, was 0.24% (range 0.05% to 0.54%) (CDSR, 1993). In the Riverside Health District in Central London, the seroprevalence rate was 0.16% in 1992 and 0.24% in 1993. HIV, therefore is becoming of increasing concern in the antenatal clinic. Current opinion considers it desirable for a woman to be aware of a positive serostatus so that she may make an informed decision about her pregnancy, and receive care and support for herself and her child (Holman, 1992; Sperling & Stratton, 1992).

To this end, it has been advocated that voluntary HIV testing should be offered in the antenatal clinic. There is still debate, however, as to whether this offer should be to women living in a high prevalence area, as has been put forward in the Department of Health guidelines (D.O.H., 1992), or to those with a history of behaviour putting them at risk of HIV infection, or to all women. There is good evidence that many parturient women who are HIV positive are not aware of, or unwilling to disclose, a history of risk behaviours (Landesman *et al.*,1987; Krasinski *et al.*, 1988;Wenstrom and Zuidema, 1989). Also offering the test to all women, rather than to a selected group, with adequate pre test counselling, appears to be a more effective way of identifying HIV positive women than selective testing (Barbacci *et al.*,1991). Findings from the Royal College of Obstetricians (RCOG) study showed that in 46% of women who are HIV positive, the infection was identified by antenatal testing. For the majority, pregnancy was the factor that led to the discovery of their serostatus (Davison *et al.*, 1989).

In 1987, the Riverside Health District commenced a policy of offering HIV testing to all women booking for antenatal care in two hospitals, St Stephen's and Westminster. The uptake rate of the test in that year, following pre test counselling by a midwife practitioner at the 'booking' appointment was 87% (Howard *et al.*, 1989). This policy was extended to a further hospital, the West London, in 1988. In 1991, only the West London Hospital continued to provide maternity care. The uptake rate was, at this time, 17% (Meadows *et al.*, 1991). At this point a study began of the issues around HIV testing in Riverside.

Interviews with midwife practitioners revealed that the majority were in favour of offering the HIV test to all women in the antenatal clinic. However, they did not feel adequately trained to be able to offer pre and post test counselling particularly concerning the practical and psychological implications of being HIV positive (Meadows *et al.*, 1992) It also became apparent that whether a woman was tested depended largely on which midwife practitioner she saw. Uptake rates varied across midwife practitioners from 82% to 3% (Meadows *et al.*, 1990) suggesting a difference in counselling approach which possibly reflects the midwife practitioner's differing beliefs about the value of HIV testing.

Whilst the women attending for antenatal care felt that the test should be offered to all mothers, many felt that they themselves did not need the test (Meadows *et al.*, 1993a). Their reasons for accepting or declining the test were many and varied, the former being largely out of concern for the baby's health and the latter from assumption of being at no risk of infection. Being in a stable relationship or not wanting to think about HIV when pregnant were other reasons that were given (Meadows *et al.*, 1994). The women's knowledge of HIV and its transmission was very poor, some believing HIV was transmissible by sitting on a toilet seat or by drinking from a contaminated glass. Women's knowledge was shown to be a predictor of testing intention (Meadows *et al.*,1993b). They also felt that they had been given insufficient information by the midwife practitioner to make an informed decision about the test and they had been generally unsatisfied with the pre test counselling they had received.

As a result of this study, a specialist HIV counsellor was appointed in March 1992 to establish a counselling and testing service for all maternity clients, which includes improving the provision of health education information to all women and offering the HIV test to partners. This allows heterosexual men who otherwise might not come into contact with services to have access to HIV counselling and testing.

It is important to note that the purpose of the service is not to increase the uptake of the test but to increase the number of seropositive women identified. It is now even more important to identify seropositivity given the new developments in studies of vertical transmission: AZT has been shown to reduce in vitro transmission by up to two-thirds (ACTG 076, Boyer *et al.*, 1994), caesarean section halving the rate of transmission during delivery (European Collaborative Study, 1994), and avoidance of breastfeeding reducing the risk of postnatal infection by 14% (Dunn *et al.*, 1992). Now that vertical transmission can be reduced, it becomes ethically sounder to promote testing for an infection that has no cure when one rationale is prevention of spread to the child (Sharf 1993). Previously we could only be concerned with prevention of spread to partners, which cannot be guaranteed in a population who, by definition, are engaging in unsafe sex.

We would suggest that it is not for the service to test the majority of the women, the cost of which is prohibitive in itself, but to provide women with appropriate health education information in a format and a context that gives seropositive women the opportunity to identify themselves by voluntary testing.

SETTING UP THE SERVICE: APPOINTMENT OF COUNSELLOR

As a response to the recommendations of the research findings the post of HIV specialist counsellor was created with a remit of developing a comprehensive HIV counselling and testing service. The post has six integral parts which are:

1. Establishing an HIV counselling and testing service. The service provides pre and post HIV test counselling for women and their partners. Also, short and long term counselling is offered to those either diagnosed HIV positive through the testing service or those who are HIV seropositive prior to pregnancy. Counselling and support is also offered to those who are frequently tested HIV negative but for whom the subject of HIV remains a cause of anxiety.
2. Liaising with other professionals both in statutory and non statutory services.
3. Training of midwife practitioners and medical staff.
4. Providing support for the specialist counsellor, midwife practitioners and medical colleagues.
5. Providing a resource base for the unit with relevant and up to date information pertaining to HIV and pregnancy.
6. Auditing to ensure a quality service.

The counselling and testing service was established as a rapid response service, which is easily accessible and initially available at the booking clinic. Raising the issue of HIV and AIDS can be difficult given the intricacy of the issues and the emotive nature of HIV infection which can sometimes be overwhelming. As previously outlined, it is essential that the women attending the antenatal clinic are given the opportunity to discuss these issues with either the midwife practitioner, medical staff or specialist counsellor (Chester and Lewis,1994). To encourage this within our maternity unit women are sent a leaflet which gives information regarding the HIV test and HIV and pregnancy prior to their first appointment and included with their booking letter.

However, written information in lieu of counselling may not be enough (Sherr & Hedge,1990). The leaflet is therefore used as a device to create an opportunity for discussion. Provision is made for the woman and her partner to have the HIV test with counselling either from the midwife practitioner or the HIV specialist counsellor. The results are available 24-48 hours later. Those women who wish to further consider the implications of being tested for HIV before agreeing to be tested may contact the counsellor by telephone and arrange a mutually convenient appointment. A uniform approach to the information given and the offering of the HIV test has been established and a systematic approach to this is used.

One of the major issues involved in setting up an HIV counselling and testing service is the question of confidentiality and the argument of who 'needs to know' versus who 'wants to know' a women's serostatus. The concern of staff who felt the 'need to know', largely in order to protect themselves, when the service was first established, has now noticeably diminished. The majority of midwife practitioners now acknowledge that the HIV status of a woman has little or no relevance to their daily working practices (Chester & Lewis,1994): the adoption of universal precautions within our service has resulted in both the midwife practitioners and obstetric staff becoming strong advocates of such practices. However, consultant obstetric staff are informed of an HIV diagnosis, with the woman's consent, as there is a need to discuss treatment and obstetric intervention, such as caesarean section, and follow up care for the baby.

There is a multi-ethnic mix of women attending our services. Taking account of the needs of non-English speaking women is important when establishing an HIV counselling and testing service: within our service we have access to interpreters who provide a range of over 20 languages.

Another important aspect of establishing a service is liaison with all midwife practitioners and obstetric staff during the development and evolution of the service. Involving the staff has resulted in the development of a consistent approach which, because of their input, they have more inclination to adopt. Links also need to be established with virology departments to ensure rapid HIV testing and return of results. As a result of the departments working closely together, a system has been developed in which all of the HIV results are returned to the HIV counsellor. A coding system has been introduced which offers confidentiality to the women and their partners. Each midwife practitioner has an individual code and this, along with a code number for the woman, is the only information that is recorded on the testing form. No names are used and identification is only known to the person having the test and the member of staff who carried out the HIV pre-test counselling.

Liaison with Genito-Urinary Medicine departments is essential for medical follow up if an HIV diagnosis has been made. Involvement of the general practitioner, with the woman's consent, is also important to ensure continuity of care. Also involvement of statutory and non statutory services is important for long term support and help.

KEY MIDWIVES

The key midwifery system was developed as a concept within our unit to ensure a comprehensive approach to HIV/AIDS. Key midwife practitioners work closely with the HIV specialist counsellor and maintain continuity of the HIV counselling and testing service in her absence. They provide pre and post HIV test counselling and support to other midwife practitioners within their team around the issues related to HIV.

Within our unit there are ten hospital teams and four community teams with six midwife practitioners in each. A key midwife is identified within the team and is responsible for disseminating information by using the cascade approach to training.

The key midwives meet on a regular basis, providing a forum for support and discussion on issues that may have arisen. The development of the key midwifery system is an invaluable and integral part of the HIV testing and counselling service within the maternity setting.

STAFF SUPPORT

When a key midwife, midwife practitioner or member of the obstetric staff is confronted with giving an HIV positive diagnosis, additional support and guidance is needed from the HIV specialist counsellor, as this can often be emotionally demanding. The HIV specialist counsellor offers supervision to monitor, develop and support the individual in their counselling role. She in turn, has support and supervision both clinically and managerially. These are essential requirements and should not be overlooked when setting up a service of this nature (Dryden & Thorn 1991).

TRAINING PROGRAMME

The initial study (Meadows *et al.*, 1992) highlighted the need for regular training for midwife practitioners regarding HIV/AIDS in relation to women and pregnancy to enable them to feel more confident in offering the HIV test and discussing the implication of a seropositive result. The training takes place on a six monthly basis and has been approved by the English National Board. It is expected that all staff attend these sessions and provision is made to accommodate that. Before the HIV testing and counselling service commenced, all midwife practitioners attended a training day which focused on how the service would operate. The day also focused on building up confidence in approaching the subject of HIV and offering the HIV test.

The areas that are covered in the study days are:

- counselling skills, particularly pre and post HIV test counselling.
- Recent research developments in relation to HIV, women and pregnancy.
- The importance of universal precautions and their relevance to midwifery and obstetric practice.

As obstetric staff also conduct booking interviews, the above training is made available to them also.

AUDIT

An integral part of a developing service is to monitor effectiveness of the service provided and to maintain quality standards. This has been achieved by auditing all aspects of the HIV counselling and testing service. Initially all midwife practitioners were given individual guidelines regarding HIV transmission and offering the HIV test. An evaluation of this was carried out in which 48 women were surveyed. The results indicate a significant change in the provision of the service since the introduction of structured counselling and training. Findings show that 90% of midwife practitioners offered the test, 87% discussed the option of using the HIV counselling service but only 74% of midwife practitioners discussed the implications of the HIV test and what the results mean. Finally, only 37% addressed any aspect of risk behaviour.

a) Audit Form

From these findings, and changing research information regarding HIV and pregnancy, it was decided to implement a much more systematic approach to giving HIV health education information and offering the HIV test. A document is placed in all booking notes which midwife practitioners/obstetric staff sign when information has been given.

The midwife practitioner/obstetric staff determines with the woman whether her command of English makes it difficult to understand the information. If so, the information should be given through an interpreter which can be arranged for her next appointment. If not, the following information is given:

HIV is the Human Immunodeficiency Virus, and is considered to be the virus which causes AIDS, Acquired Immune Deficiency Syndrome.

HIV infection is thought to be transmitted in four ways:

1. Through unprotected vaginal or anal sex with an infected partner, as HIV is present in both vaginal and seminal fluid.
2. Through unscreened blood and blood products. This is usually through sharing needles and equipment during intravenous drug use. Blood transfusion in the United Kingdom is considered relatively safe as since 1985 all blood has been screened. However in other countries this may not be the case.
3. HIV can be transmitted from mother to unborn baby through the placenta or during childbirth. This is known as vertical transmission and is currently estimated to be 14-25% in the U.K.
4. HIV can be transmitted by infected mothers through their breastmilk and the transmission rate is currently estimated to be 14%. While breastfeeding is method of choice for most mothers, for the HIV infected mother avoidance of breastfeeding will reduce post partum transmission.

At this point it is ascertained whether the woman is considering having the HIV test or whether she requires any further information or referral to the specialist counsellor. If the woman wants the midwife practitioner/obstetric staff to continue with pre test counselling, they then discuss the following issues: the confidentiality policy, implications for life insurance and mortgages, and the meaning of a negative or a positive HIV test result. The client expectation of the HIV test result is then ascertained, and the psychological and practical implication of both a negative and positive HIV result are explored. The midwife practitioner then describes the procedure of the test, obtains written consent and arranges a post test counselling session.

The completed forms are stored by the HIV specialist counsellor. Test decision is not recorded in the obstetric notes.

Preliminary findings from this audit, commencing February 1994, suggest that midwife practitioners/obstetric staff take a mean of 9 minutes to impart HIV transmission information only and a mean of 23 minutes to give full pre HIV test counselling. From 151 audit forms, 127(84%) women received HIV transmission information only, 11(7%) went on for full pretest counselling with the midwife practitioner/obstetric staff. Of those 11 women, 6 went on to be tested. The remaining 13(9%) women were referred to the HIV specialist counsellor and, of those, 12 decided to have the HIV test, giving an overall uptake rate of 12%.

b) Midwife Practitioner Training

Evaluation by the HIV specialist counsellor after training sessions revealed that consistently 80–90% of the midwife practitioners were more confident in offering pre test counselling.

CONCLUSIONS

As a result of the service set up by the specialist counsellor:

a) More women are now satisfied with the counselling they receive.

b) Midwife practitioners are now regularly trained and updated on developments in the HIV field.

c) Women are now given the necessary information to make an informed decision about HIV testing and about the issues associated with HIV seropositivity.

ONGOING ISSUES

Obstetric staff training

This has not been evaluated but the training sessions are not well attended. Future research intends to address this problem with a view to appointing a specialist medical trainer.

Midwives approach

There is still a wide variation in uptake rates across midwife practitioners with 10% still not mentioning the HIV test at the booking interview. Future research intends to investigate this anomaly.

The use of the audit form has improved the method of giving health education information and offering the HIV test. However, the method needs to be constantly monitored and modified accordingly.

Women's knowledge and attitudes to testing

1 Preliminary findings show that the majority of women are declining the HIV test, primarily because they considered HIV to be of no relevance in their life. Reasons for declining testing will continue to be monitored.

2. Future research will re-evaluate women's knowledge about HIV transmission and attitudes to HIV testing as this has been found to predict testing intention (Meadows & Catalan, 1993a).

Uptake rate

Preliminary findings suggest that the uptake rate has been consistently 10-12% during the last three years (1992-4). We are still investigating the discrepancy between the RCOG reported figures and the figures from unlinked anonymous testing to establish accuracy of identification. In 1992, all seropositive women were identified in the antenatal clinic (Davison & Nicoll,1994).

e) Cost effective service

Future research aims to monitor the cost effectiveness of offering voluntary named HIV testing in the antenatal clinic, the aim being to maximise the number of seropositive identified whilst minimising the number tested.

SUMMARY

The establishment of a Key Midwife system and co-ordination of HIV services within Riverside, which is now located within the Chelsea and Westminster Health Care Trust, has led to a marked improvement in provision of care. More women acknowledge satisfaction with the information, advice and care they receive in relation to HIV disease. Midwife practitioners receive regular, ongoing training and up-dating about all aspects of HIV. It is evident that women are receiving the necessary information to make informed decisions about testing and feel better placed to make such decisions in relation to pregnancy and care.

However, some issues remain unresolved and these require further study. Whilst training sessions for obstetric staff have been put in place, their uptake is poor and, as yet, doctors appear to remain apart from developing consensus about maternity care provision in respect of HIV disease. The messages from obstetricians can differ markedly from those of midwives and debate can often rage around the issues of consent, testing and the 'need to know'.

A wide variation in the uptake of the test is also evident and it is recognised that some 10% of midwives still fail to mention HIV disease and its implications at booking. Why this occurs is still unclear and further research into this area is imperative. Future research is also required to monitor the cost effectiveness of offering voluntary named HIV testing in the antenatal clinic.

Nevertheless, in spite of advances in the knowledge, treatment and provision of care related to HIV disease, a not inconsiderable number of women still feel that it has little relevance to their own particular situation. Preliminary findings indicate that a majority of women attending for pregnancy care decline an HIV test in spite of receiving information about vertical transmission and the implications of breastfeeding for HIV seropositive mothers. The reasons for this remain unclear and relate to many factors. What is clear however, is that there is a fundamental failure of the health education message which requires further evaluation and study.

REFERENCES

Barbacci, M: Repke, J.T; Chaisson, R.E. (1991) Routine Prenatal Screening for HIV Infection. *Lancet* **337**,709-711.

Boyer, P.J; Dillon, M; Navaie, M *et al.* (1994) Factors Predictive of Maternal-fetal Transmission of HIV-1: preliminary analysis of zidovudine given during pregnancy and/ or delivery, *JAMA* **271**,1925-1930.

Chester T, Lewis P. (1994) HIV testing and support; Keying in the midwives. *Modern midwife* vol. 4 no.2;8-10.

Communicable Disease Surveillance Centre/Communicable Diseases (Scotland) Unit (1986) Report 87/22 June 1987.

Communicable Disease Surveillance Centre/Communicable Diseases (Scotland) Unit (1994) vol 4 no.15 April.

Communicable Disease Surveillance Centre/Communicable Diseases (Scotland) Unit (1993) Unlinked Anonymous Monitoring of HIV Prevalence in England and Wales: 1990-92 vol. 3 Review no.1 January 1993.

Davison, C.F; Hudson, C.N; Ades, E *et al.* (1989) Antenatal Testing for Human Immunodeficiency Virus. *Lancet* **2**,1442-1444.

Davison, C.F; Nicoll, A (1994) Estimated Rate of Clinical Diagnosis of HIV Infection in Pregnant Women in 15 London Centres: Data to end 1992. Institute of Child Health, London and Public Health Laboratory Service.

Department of Health Guidelines (1992) PL/CO(92)5: Appendix 2 Offering Voluntary Named HIV Antibody Testing to Women Receiving Antenatal Care, HMSO.

Dryden, W; Thorn, B; (1991) Training and supervision for counselling in action. SAGE Publications.

Dunn, D.T; Newell, M.N; Ades, A.E; Peckham, C.S. (1992) Risk of Human Immunodeficiency Virus Type 1 Transmission through breastfeeding. *Lancet* **340**,585-588.

European Collaborative Study (1994) Caesarean Section and Risk of Vertical Transmission of HIV-1 Infection. *Lancet*, **343**, 1464-1467.

Holman, S. (1992) HIV Counselling for Women of Reproductive Age. Balliere's Clinical Obstetrics and Gynaecology, **6**, 53-68.

Howard, L.C; Hawkins, D.A; Marwood, R. *et al.* (1989) Transmission of Human Immunodeficiency Virus by Heterosexual Contact with Reference to Antenatal Screening. *British Journal of Obstetrics and Gynaecology*, **96**, 135-139.

Krasinski, K; Borkowsky, W; Bebenroth, D *et al.* (1988) Failure of Voluntary Testing for HIV to Identify Infected Parturient Women in a High Risk population. *New England Journal of Medicine*, **318**, 185.

Landesman, S; Minkoff, H; Holman, S. *et al.* (1987) Serosurvey of HIV Infection of Parturients. *Journal of American Medical Association*, **258**, 2701-2703.

Meadows, J; Jenkinson, S; Catalan *et al* (1990) Voluntary HIV Testing in the Antenatal Clinic: differing uptake rates for individual counselling midwives. *AIDS Care*, **2**, 229-233.

Meadows, J; Catalan, J; Gazzard, B *et al.* (1992) Testing for HIV in the antenatal clinic: the views of the midwives. *AIDS Care*, **4**, 157-164.

Meadows, J; Catalan, J; (1993a) I Plan to have the HIV test: predictors of testing intention in women attending a London antenatal clinic. *AIDS Care*, **5**, 239-246.

Meadows, J; Catalan, J; Gazzard, B (1993b) HIV Antibody testing in the Antenatal Clinic: the views of the consumers. *Midwifery*, **9**, 63-69.

Meadows, J; Catalan, J. (1994) Why do antenatal attenders decide to have the HIV Antibody Test? *International Journal of STD and AIDS*, **5**, 400-404.

Scharf, E. (1993) HIV Prevention as a Rationale for Antenatal HIV Testing Programmes: a Critical Analysis Poster C25-3210 presented at the 9th International Conference on AIDS, Berlin.

Sherr, L; Hedge, B. (1990) The impact and use of written leaflets as a counselling alternative in mass HIV screening. *AIDS Care,* **2**, 235-245.

Sperling, R.S; Stratton, P. (1992) Treatment Options for Human Immunodeficiency Virus-Infected Pregnant Women. *Obstetrics and Gynaecology,* **76**, (3) 443-448.

Wenstrom, K.D; Zuidema, L.J. (1989) Determination of the Seroprevalence of HIV Infection in Gravidas by Non-Anonymous Versus Anonymous Screening. *Obstetrics and Gynaecology* 74, 558-561.

14

Bridging the Gap between Science and AIDS Service Provision

EDWARD KING

Since the late 1980s there has been an important trend towards a truly multidisciplinary approach to the day-to-day medical and psychosocial management of HIV infection, and this has been reflected in the scope of major AIDS-related meetings. International conferences such as this one on the Biopsychosocial Aspects of AIDS have brought together social scientists, medical researchers, psychologists, doctors and nurses, service providers, health educators and people living with HIV, to update each other and learn from each other's expertise.

In many respects two-way communication now takes place very effectively between scientists on the one hand and those responsible for planning and providing AIDS services on the other. However, substantial failures of communication still exist. This paper focuses on two problematic cases in different areas of AIDS service provision. First, I shall explore how the planning and prioritisation of HIV prevention interventions often fails to take account of the realities of the epidemic as revealed by epidemiological science. Secondly, I shall examine the neglect by many AIDS service organisations of the provision of treatment information to people living with HIV as an example of a failure to equip those facing treatment choices to make truly informed decisions. In each case, we could and should do much more to ensure that service provision is firmly based on the realities of the epidemic and the needs it engenders.

HIV PREVENTION

First let us focus on primary HIV prevention work, a field in which the gap between science and service provision has been horrifying. Consider the following snapshot of the epidemiology of HIV infection. By the end of September 1994, there had been a cumulative total of over 22,500 cases of HIV infection reported in the UK. Of these, 61% were in men who are believed to have become infected through sexual intercourse with other men. Even if one just looks at infections that were newly detected during the first nine months of 1994, the proportions are not very different: 62% were among gay or bisexual men. Of the 10,000 people who have developed AIDS, three-quarters have been gay or bisexual. Finally, 76% of all AIDS deaths in Britain up to end of 1993 were among gay or bisexual men, while the next largest toll was among men or women infected through heterosexual sex with a partner abroad, just 7% of the total (Gay Men Fighting AIDS, 1994).

Compare this evidence of the epidemic's continuing disproportionate impact upon gay men with the results of a 1992 survey of HIV prevention activities in the United Kingdom (King *et al.*, 1992). Out of 226 agencies with an HIV prevention remit, two-thirds reported that they had never undertaken any kind of work with gay men, even though all had targeted heterosexuals. Only 4% of the sample – a total of 8 agencies – had undertaken work that could be defined as substantial. In explaining this neglect, workers commonly said that they simply did not know how to contact gay men, or that they were opposed to targeting gay men in case this was seen as stigmatising. Nearly one in ten actually believed that there were no gay men in their area.

That survey was conducted as a direct consequence of the concerns of a small number of gay men working in the AIDS sector, that prevention priorities were being determined more on the basis of dogma and myth than in response to real, demonstrable need. This was an astonishing turn-around, given that early responses to AIDS had come almost exclusively from the gay community. The early safer sex campaigns, which resulted in the most extensive health-related behaviour changes in history, were the result of gay community organising, as were pioneering services for people living with HIV or AIDS such as buddying, counselling and legal and welfare rights advice (King *et al.*, 1992; King, 1993a). It was only in 1986, when there were fears that an explosion of HIV infection among heterosexuals was imminent, that the UK Government embarked on its high-profile public information campaigns for heterosexuals.

From then on, the new urgency in AIDS policy was based primarily on an intention to prevent a heterosexual AIDS epidemic, rather than to respond to the existing epidemic among the high risk groups. In the rush to counter public complacency in the face of a small but growing number of cases among heterosexuals, AIDS workers overlooked the facts that the epidemic among gay and bisexual men was actually much larger and was continuing to grow rapidly. As the epidemic expanded, voluntary and statutory sector organisations lost sight of the fact that the heart of the epidemic, where the majority of new infections were continuing to take place, remained squarely among gay and bisexual men. Instead they behaved as though the epidemic had somehow lifted up and moved on, leaving gay men safely behind.

APPLIED EPIDEMIOLOGY

Matters have improved considerably over the last two years. In 1992 a group of gay men set up Gay Men Fighting AIDS (GMFA), the country's first national AIDS organisation devoted specifically to the interests of gay men. With its distinctive propaganda, GMFA has led the campaign to put gay men at the top of the British HIV education agenda, while at the same time launching what is currently the only pan-London gay safer sex project (Stop AIDS London), with an emphasis on peer education, community mobilisation and sex-positivity. The Department of Health has also belatedly issued instructions to the statutory sector stressing the need to target prevention campaigns better and to focus on the high risk groups (Department of Health, 1993). In early 1994 the Health Education Authority commisioned an updated survey of HIV prevention priorities in the UK, which revealed that a dramatic shift had taken place in a period of just two years: no fewer than 86% now reported work targeting gay or bisexual men (Anderson *et al.*, 1994).

These are positive developments, and it is to be hoped that they represent the emergence of a genuinely rational approach to prevention planning, in which prioritisation is based explicitly and concretely on the evidence of epidemiological science.

To some extent, this is how the provision of AIDS treatment and care services is currently planned. Each hospital or clinic which provides care for people with AIDS receives Government funds in proportion to the number of people who are diagnosed with AIDS at that clinic: an attempt, albeit crude, to match resources to need. Moreover, since 1988 the Government has commissioned three major studies estimating current levels of HIV infection and the likely annual number of cases of AIDS in the foreseeable future. The main purpose of these studies is to help NHS staff to plan ahead so that funds and facilities will be available for those who need them in the future (Department of Health and Welsh Office, 1988; Public Health Laboratory Service Working Group, 1990; Public Health Laboratory Service Working Group, 1993).

It is long overdue for this kind of rational approach to service planning to be extended to HIV prevention work. I call this approach 'applied epidemiology' (King, 1993b). The idea of applied epidemiology is that prevention workers should plan campaigns or contract work from other groups strictly on the basis of current need and predictable future need.

This will require workers to base their prioritisation not on their own subjective impressions, but on hard data. Although lip service is now commonly paid to the importance of undertaking a needs assessment before launching a prevention initiative, it is far from clear that work is yet being informed by good assessments, properly planned and implemented and with an emphasis on getting answers that will be of practical value to subsequent campaigns. In addition to surveys of local gay and bisexual men and other forms of behavioural and social research, figures on HIV infection and other sexually transmitted diseases from anonymised seroprevalence surveys as well as the local STD clinic will provide an indication of current patterns of unsafe behaviour and HIV transmission. Trends in the data may provide an indication of future needs and emerging issues, but important as they are it is essential that such trends are not allowed to obscure a proper recognition of current needs. For example, if the proportion of new infections among gay and bisexual men is gradually declining, say from 65% of infections one year to 55% the next, while infections among heterosexuals have increased from 10% to 15%, the scale of the ongoing problem among gay men would mean that it would still be totally irresponsible to deprioritise work with that group.

This approach also raises questions about how useful raw behavioural research data really are. We can investigate ad nauseam who is having unprotected sex, with whom and in what contexts, but that information will not necessarily tell us where our prevention efforts most need to be directed. We will only get a true picture of risk, on the basis of which our prevention campaigns can be prioritised, if we also factor in the likelihood that those people who are having unprotected sex will be exposed to HIV. In other words, unless we take account of where the epidemic of HIV infection is and where it is going, we cannot make proper use of data on potentially risky behaviour.

Obviously there are limitations and these techniques need to be used intelligently, given that we are often working with incomplete data. However, within these restrictions, the principles of applied epidemiology offer an objective means of ensuring that limited funds are put to the best possible use. Rather than being based on inaccurate dogmas such as 'Everyone is equally at risk' or 'AIDS does not discriminate', this approach would at last ensure that our efforts are based upon the HIV epidemic itself, with all its complexities and all its discriminations.

Although the failures I have spoken of so far are most evident in relation to prevention work for gay men, these principles of applied epidemiology should not be misunderstood as 'special pleading' on behalf of gay men. They are a model of good practice that should be applied across the board, with benefits to a range of groups who are currently being inadequately served by HIV prevention. Thus, applied epidemiology is just as important to ensure that prevention campaigns for heterosexuals are properly targeted. In place of the crass generalisations of the mass media with its speculations about whether or not 'heterosexuals' are at risk, most prevention workers have recognised that heterosexual is an unhelpful heterogeneous category. Some heterosexuals are clearly at far greater risk from HIV than others, and it is they who should be prioritised. For example, a proper study of the epidemiology of HIV in London would alert us to the alarming incidence of infection among black women who retain strong links to African countries, and thus to the urgent need for better prevention work for this group.[1]

[1] See Keith Alcorn's analysis of the epidemiology of HIV in the UK in Alcorn, K. (Ed.), *The AIDS Reference Manual*, NAM Publications, London, 1995.

THE NEED FOR TREATMENT INFORMATION

The second area I want to consider is how well AIDS service providers are doing in assisting people with HIV to remain abreast of developments in the field of medical research.

Few can have any doubt of the importance of the provision of accessible, accurate and objective information on treatment choices for people with HIV. Although a proportion of people with HIV prefer to delegate responsibility for medical decisions to their doctors, many more have signalled their desire to be active participants in the decision-making process. What is more, many people with HIV investigate and self-administer so-called 'underground' non-prescription treatments as well as a diverse range of complementary and alternative therapies (Abrams, 1990). For many people with HIV, therefore, access to comprehensive and clear information is the prerequisite to enable them to make their own, properly informed choices about which of the range of treatment options is right for them at any given time.

Although the need for information applies across the range of orthodox and unorthodox treatment options, it can be particularly difficult to get to grips with the constant flow of new information on conventional medical approaches to treating HIV and AIDS. At a time when there are only very limited treatment options available and widely divergent views on the best ways and times to use those treatments, it is potentially a huge task to bridge the gap between this evolving science and the needs of individuals living with HIV who are seeking to be fully informed and able to decide which options they wish to pursue.

Individual physicians clearly have a huge role to play here, and treatment information providers always recommend that decisions should only be made after consultation between the individual and the doctor, as a partnership for health. However, there is now so much information of such complexity that most doctors would probably agree that patients who wish to take an active role in treatment decision-making will usually need to do a fair amount of 'homework' for themselves. Moreover, it is by researching options and identifying questions and uncertainties before clinic visits that the necessarily limited time that a patient has in consultation with his or her doctor can be used to its best.

TREATMENT INFORMATION SERVICES

This is the need that has driven the creation of the range of treatment information services that can be found in the USA and Australia. Initially newsletters such as the San Francisco based *AIDS Treatment News* grew out of underground experimental treatments, reporting on the unproven treatments that people were importing from Mexico or even making for themselves at home, such as AL-721. Others such as *Treatment Issues* published by Gay Men's Health Crisis in New York have focused more on the progress – or lack of progress – in mainstream medical research on AIDS. There are also treatment hotlines, including a federally-funded treatment and trials information line, regular public seminars and updates, activist groups and a carefully constructed system for community consultation on research and drug approval issues that includes representation of people with HIV and their advocates at every level of the treatment development system (Arno & Feiden, 1992).

In countries such as Britain, by contrast, treatment information and advocacy services are relatively under-developed. There are the resources produced by NAM Publications – the *HIV/AIDS Treatments Directory, the Directory of Complementary & Alternative Therapies* and the newsletter *AIDS Treatment Update*, but many of the treatment information services that are provided in other countries – the seminars, public meetings, training events, hotlines and so on – are simply not available in the UK.

All the main AIDS service organisations in the USA recognise that the provision of treatment information is an essential service for people living with HIV, on a par with other client services such as buddying, counselling and welfare rights advice. They have recognised that it is not good enough simply to provide HIV prevention campaigns designed to keep HIV-negative people negative. For people with HIV, treatments information is health education.

While Body Positive has featured treatment information in its newsletter since it started, on the whole self-help groups have not had the resources to prioritise treatment information work. This makes the neglect of this work by the statutory sector and most AIDS organisations all the more regrettable. It is high time that AIDS service providers in Britain and elsewhere in Europe took a hard look at their provision – or lack of it – of treatment information services.

In Britain, there are plenty of warning signs that the neglect of this work is having harmful consequences. For example, a Medical Research Council survey of participants in the Concorde trial of AZT found that a majority of people wanted more information than they had received about the drug. For much of 1993-1994 an ill-informed pair of HIV-positive gay men conducted what amounted to a terrorist campaign against anyone who dared to disagree with their assertion that AZT is a form of deliberate genocide. We should be alarmed that they even attracted equivocal coverage in the gay press from reporters who thought that 'perhaps they had a point'. Perhaps as a consequence of our inadequate ability to counter misinformation, in Britain, the level of withdrawal from the Delta trial of combination antiviral therapy for personal reasons – in other words, not due to disease progression or to side-effects – is substantially higher than in any other participating country.

We also need to examine new ways to encourage intelligent grassroots treatment activism where it has not existed to date. The Medical Research Council already consults patient advocates, but it is unclear who these advocates can in turn consult to ensure that they are adequately representing the interests and concerns of people living with HIV. A more effective mechanism might entail the creation of a pyramid-shaped system, in which those advocates represented the views of a national advisory group itself made up of representatives from specially formed local advisory groups around the UK. Given the evidence that the MRC is committed to community consultation, it seems reasonable to ask for centralised funding for such a scheme to ensure that the MRC's patient representatives can be genuinely in touch with their constituency. As a spin-off benefit, it would hopefully motivate and involve many more people in local and national treatment information and advocacy work. We should also look at ways to bring together existing AIDS service providers to work together on meeting treatment information and advocacy needs, and translating the insights of science into practical services.

CONCLUSION

The points in this paper have focussed predominantly on the situation in the UK – but these problems are reproduced throughout the developed world. Very few AIDS service organisations in Europe can claim to be providing an adequate treatment information service. The harmful consequences of de-gaying can be observed all around the globe, even in cities such as San Francisco where by the early 1990s gay men made up 85% of deaths from AIDS in the state but received only 8% of state funding for prevention (Lee, 1993; Stall, 1994). Closer to home, the epidemic in France continues to devastate that country's gay communities, with a massive 15,000 cases of AIDS already reported – nearly double the number in Germany which has the next highest toll among gay men – yet there still seems to be no sense of the urgency of HIV prevention campaigns for gay men.

I have argued at length for our responses to AIDS to be based firmly in cool scientific objectivity. In advocating this, I would not wish to be seen as dismissing the importance of subjective experience – and especially the significance of the personal motivations that each of us may have. Many of the best responses to AIDS have been born of individuals' own intimate involvement with the epidemic and of the anger and the anguish of living our daily lives in a time of plague. It is by focussing the commitment which springs from these experiences through the lens of rational scientific insight that we will develop the best possible AIDS services.

REFERENCES

Abrams, D. (1990) 'Editorial review: Alternative therapies in HIV infection', *AIDS* 4, 1179-1187.

Alcorn, K. (1995) 'Epidemiology and research' in alcorn, K. (ed.), *The AIDS Reference Manual*, NAM Publications, London.

Anderson, W., Hickson, F., Stevens, C. (1994) *Health Purchasing, HIV Prevention and Gay Men.* Health Education Authority, London.

Arno, P.S. & Feiden, K.L. (1992) *Against the Odds*, HarperCollins, New York.

Department of Health, *Latest AIDS predictions vindicate Government's approach*, press release, London, 14th June 1993.

Department of Health and Welsh Office. (1988) *Short-term Prediction of HIV Infection and AIDS in England and Wales.* HMSO, London.

Gay Men Fighting AIDS, *Unreleased figures highlights AIDS toll among gay men*, press release, London, 3rd June 1994.

King, E., Rooney, M., Scott, P. (1992) *HIV Prevention for Gay Men: A Survey of Initiatives in the UK.* North-West Thames Regional Health Authority, London.

King, E. (1993a) *Safety In Numbers: Safer Sex and Gay Men.* Cassell, London.

King, E. (1993b) 'Fucking by Numbers', *F***Sheet* issue 3, Gay Men Fighting AIDS, London.

King, E. (1994) 'Update on Delta', *AIDS Treatment Update* issue 19, June 1994.

Lee, F. *et al.* (1993) *HIV Provision in California*, Office of AIDS, California Department of Health Services, San Francisco.

Public Health Laboratory Service AIDS Centre – Communicable Disease Surveillance Centre, and Scottish Centre for Infection & Environmental Health, *Unpublished Quarterly Tables* No. 26, December 1994.

Public Health Laboratory Service Working Group, 'Acquired immune deficiency syndrome in England and Wales to end 1993', *Communicable Disease Report*, January 1990.

Public Health Laboratory Service Working Group, 'The incidence and prevelence of AIDS and other severe HIV disease in England and Wales for 1992-1997', *Communicable Disease Report*, 3 (Supplement1), S1-S17, 1993.

Stall, R. (1994) 'How to lose the fight against AIDS among gay men' (editorial), *British Medical Journal*, **357**, 685-686.

15

Nurse-Counsellors' Perceptions Regarding HIV/AIDS Counselling Objectives at Baragwanath Hospital, Soweto

JOANNE STEIN, MALCOLM STEINBERG, CLIFF ALLWOOD, ALAN KARSTAEDT AND PIERRE BROUARD

INTRODUCTION

One of the most critical of the challenges facing health care providers is the need to better define and characterize HIV/AIDS counselling (Bor & Miller, 1988; Balmer, 1992; Schopper & Walley, 1992). In South Africa, feasible and appropriate objectives for counselling services, both within and outside hospital settings, are only beginning to be properly debated and evaluated (Fleming, 1992; Tallis, 1992). For this reason, a study was conducted in which we attempted to gain insight into both the ways in which nurse-counsellors at Baragwanath Hospital in Soweto understand and experience their role as counsellors, and their perceptions of the factors mitigating against achieving their counselling objectives.

This paper, however, will focus only upon research findings relating to nurse-counsellors' perceptions regarding their counselling objectives, and not address the factors they saw as mitigating against achieving these objectives.

THE STUDY SITE

The study was undertaken at Baragwanath hospital, in Soweto, which serves a population of approximately 2.4 million black South Africans in an overcrowded and impoverished urban area of high HIV endemicity (Chimere-Dan, 1993).

Serosurveillance of ante-natal sentinel groups in the area indicate that 8.1% of the sexually active adult population of Soweto were infected at the end of 1993. In the STD sentinel group, 18% of males and 24% of females were infected at this time (National Institute for Virology, 1994). According to demographic modelling of the HIV/AIDS epidemic it is estimated that AIDS will have caused 31,000 to 41,000 deaths in Soweto by the year 2000 (Lee *et al.,* in press). There can be little doubt then that, despite limited resources, Baragwanath hospital will have to cope with increasing numbers of HIV/AIDS patients.

Both the kind and degree of HIV/AIDS counselling training which nurse-counsellors at Baragwanath hospital have received is varied. While some nurse-counsellors have attended five day introductory skills training courses, the majority have attended a series of lectures, but received little in the way of basic practical training. At present, about 20 nurse-counsellors regularly engage in counselling activities. However, 130 nurses have received some degree of informal HIV/AIDS counselling training.

It is also important to point out that counselling services at Baragwanath are generally confined to post-test counselling for HIV-infected patients, and very little pre-test counselling occurs. Doctors are responsible for obtaining informed consent and for informing patients of their HIV positive status and all subsequent post-test counselling is done by nurse-counsellors' (Allwood *et al.*, 1992). As a result, this study is limited to an exploration of nurse-counsellors' perceptions regarding their objectives in post-test counselling alone.

STUDY DESIGN

The study group comprised eight nurse-counsellors from a variety of hospital departments, all of whom had at least one year's counselling experience. All were fully qualified registered nurses, four of whom were in charge of nursing services in their departments. All were black African, second language speakers of English.

The data gathered takes the form of verbatim transcriptions of approximately one-and-a-half hour, semi-structured interviews.[1] The qualitative analysis conducted falls broadly within the parameters of grounded theory methodology and was specifically oriented towards thematic material (Glazer & Strauss, 1967).

RESULTS

The results of the study indicate that the major counselling objectives identified by nurse-counsellors were:

1 The interview schedule can be obtained from the National AIDS Research Programme, Medical Research Council, P.O. Box 1038, Johannesburg, 2000, Republic of South Africa.

* the provision of emotional support
* the provision of information, and
* the provision of guidance in decision-making and problem-solving.

However, in-depth analysis of interview transcripts indicates that these counselling objectives are regularly interpreted as:

(a) the alleviation of distress, and

(b) the facilitation of health promotion goals.

It is the implications of construing their objectives as HIV/AIDS counsellors in these terms, that is the central point for discussion in this paper. Many of these implications will be seen to be negative. It must therefore be pointed out in advance that nurse-counsellors' objectives should be understood in terms of a variety of pragmatic and institutional constraints inherent in their workplace setting.

SUPPORT AS THE ALLEVIATION OF EMOTIONAL DISTRESS

Careful examination of the transcripts makes it clear that nurse-counsellors consistently described their support role in terms which suggest that, for them, support amounts to the alleviation of the patient's immediate distress. Support was thus often described as the provision of "reassurance" and "comfort". What is interesting about this interpretation of support is not merely that it occurs, but the form which it regularly takes.

Firstly, the alleviation of distress was seen to entail an active demonstration of "loving" or "caring", sometimes referred to as "mothering":

"At least to show love and make this person feel she's still wanted in the world." (Interview 5).

Secondly, and for our purposes in this paper, more importantly, strategies for the alleviation of emotional distress were seen to involve the provision of alternative, seemingly preferable ways, for the patient to understand and respond emotionally to his or her situation.

For example, many nurse-counsellors tended to alleviate fear and despair in the face of possible death, by invoking the inevitability of eventual death for all, as well as the uncertainty of its time of arrival:

A: "...and [I] say, 'Look, we are all going to die anyway. Don't you know that?' And then when they say, 'Yes', I say, 'Look now, ... it's only the Lord knows when a person is going to die. I can also die when I go out through the hospital gates and get knocked down by a car." (Interview-6)

Likewise, in order to alleviate guilt, nurse-counsellors considered it necessary to impart the understanding that HIV/AIDS is no different from any other disease, and is, therefore, illegitimately stigmatized:

B: "Like for instance, I might be hypertensive, not because God is punishing me, but because I'm having Hypertension. ... We try to set up simple examples so that to a certain extent she can be able to accept it ... that it's not because of your callousness, it's not a punishment due to your misbehaviours, or what, but it's just an illness. It just happened to you like it could happen to any other person." (Interview 3).

Two points of importance emerge from this data; one directly, and the other by implication. The first concerns the consequences of these interventions for the nurse-counsellor's health promotion and HIV prevention goals. In quotation A, the nurse-counsellor implies that being HIV-positive doesn't put you in a different relation to death from anyone else. The logical extension of this view is that patients need not take any special measures regarding their health, as a result of their HIV status.

In quotation B, the nurse-counsellor's admirable attempt to point out that HIV infection cannot be construed as a "punishment" and that its cause should not be thought of as "misbehaviour" has an equally unfortunate upshot. By comparing HIV infection to hypertension and then stating that, "it could happen to any other person", the nurse-counsellor disguises the important behavioural components implicated in HIV transmission.

Thus, in the interests of alleviating distress what we find is the nurse-counsellors suppressing information regarding both the causes and consequences of HIV infection; information which is essential to behaviour compatible with health promotion goals. Both these examples therefore suggest that interventions geared towards distress alleviation may prove to be at variance with health promotion goals.

The second point of importance here, is that the construal of emotional support as distress alleviation is widely regarded, in contemporary approaches to counselling, as counter-productive. While reassurance and comfort may provide short-term relief, it is now recognised that this is not ultimately conducive to the development of effective coping strategies on the part of the patient (Bor & Miller, 1988). The alleviation of distress *per se* is not only unhelpful to the patient, but may result in repetitive demands for emotional 'first aid' which cannot be sustained by counsellors, especially nurse-counsellors who have heavy work-loads (Bor et al., 1992).

In addition, the comfort offered may be rejected rather than embraced, rendering the counsellor as helpless and ineffective in their supportive function, as some nurse-counsellors themselves attested to:

"Before you say any word of comfort to this person, she knows what you are going to say to her. ... she'll never want to listen to you. So, I have found myself crying with the clients at the clinic when the client was actually telling me about the consequences of the disease, as if I do not know." (Interview 1).

INFORMATION PROVISION AS HEALTH PROMOTION

Nurse-counsellors considered the provision of information regarding HIV/AIDS to be essential to effective health promotion, where health promotion was seen to include both the prevention of further spread of infection, and interventive treatment for those already infected. In some cases, the provision of information was regarded as sufficient for achieving these health promotion goals. As one nurse-counsellor pointed out with regard to the prevention of HIV transmission:

"I feel they must know the cause [of transmission], it's very important ... because once they know the mode [of transmission], I expect them to change their lifestyle." (Interview 2).

For the most part, however, nurse-counsellors felt that the neutral provision of information may often be insufficient to achieve health promotion objectives. As a result, nurse-counsellors felt that they had a further role to play in the process of decision-making and problem-solving which the achievement of these objectives entail. This additional role was commonly described as the provision of 'guidance'.

COUNSELLING AS GUIDANCE

The nurse-counsellors interviewed placed considerable emphasis on the role of guidance in HIV/AIDS counselling. What is of interest here, again, is not only *how* guidance was construed, but the form this construal took.

Nurse-counsellors distinguished between what they call 'guidance' and more authoritarian and didactic methods for achieving health promotion goals, (for example, threatening to break confidentiality and/or contact tracing). While not overtly authoritarian, however, the guidance strategies described do incorporate directive or persuasive health promotion techniques:

> "Its not easy to convince, especially again male people, to use a condom." (Interview 6).
>
> "If you advise them on termination of pregnancy – I've never had anyone give consent to that." (Interview 5).
>
> "When I insist his partner should be tested or use a condom, he says, 'maybe next time', so it's frustrating to keep confidentiality." (Interview 2).

What is noticeable in these examples is not only the use of words like "convince", "advise" and "insist", but the explicitness of the directives given. The result is a situation in which non-compliance, as opposed to compliance, is clearly identifiable:

> "You know, you feel happy that at least I've done something and here's a person who is going to comply." (Interview 7).

> "What is rewarding about it is when I can see I have reached the patient and she agrees also that she is going to abide by the set rules, such as prevention of further spread of disease." (Interview 8).
>
> "My main problem is my patients being non-compliant." (Interview 4).

These quotations demonstrate that nurse-counsellors often referred to their ability to provide effective guidance in terms of the relative achievement of compliance or non-compliance. And certainly, they indicate that nurse-counsellors find counselling interventions in which compliance *is* effected, more rewarding.

This construal of the relation between information provision and guidance, on the one hand, and health promotion goals, on the other, has two important, potentially negative implications.

Firstly, because information provision and guidance are practised in the mode of advice-giving, they are re-incorporated into a compliance model which, if unsuccessful, produces an increased sense of frustration and/or inadequacy on the part of the nurse-counsellor. By contrast, a facilitative approach, which is now widely regarded as definitive of counselling (Nelson-Jones, 1982), does not involve explicit advice-giving and therefore does not have to confront non-compliance in the same way. Because it is not prescriptive, facilitative counselling can, in fact, be successful even in the absence of compliance.

The second consequence of the way in which guidance is construed concerns its implications for the achievement of health promotion. In fact, counselling was introduced into HIV/AIDS care in the light of the now well established failure of traditionally didactic health promotion techniques to achieve health promotion objectives (Rodmell & Watt, 1986; Carballo & Miller, 1989; Taylor, 1990). The re-incorporation of didactic techniques such as instruction and advice-giving into HIV/AIDS counselling, in the interests of health promotion, therefore makes little sense.

GUIDANCE AND SUPPORT: "TRICKY ADVICES"

It is important to point out that the advice nurse-counsellors described does not necessarily take the form of a *standardised* set of instructions. Nurse-counsellors are aware of the very real difficulties faced by those who disclose their HIV status; including the risk of abandonment by partners, loss of employment, and ostracization in general. As a result, nurse-counsellors' advice may often take the form of problem-solving, such that the difficulties of the patient with regard to health promotion are taken into account. What results is a patient-centred form of advice-giving, but advice nonetheless.

The nurse-counsellors' objectives in the provision of this sort of advice are two-fold:

> "We've got to achieve both goals. To prevent *on the one hand*, and, *on the other hand*, we give support at all times." (Interview 1).

What is interesting, once again, is the way in which nurse–counsellors described their attempts to achieve a compromise between these two goals:

A: "Tell him, in a diplomatic manner, that you must use a condom. Not saying that, 'I am HIV positive, please use a condom', or, 'I'm afraid that you're HIV positive.' Just say in general that there is this disease and that we are not sure what's going on, how about doing this and this..." (Interview 5).

B: "I think maybe when the baby's born. Why I at times advise them on that is that if he identifies the baby with him then it motivates him, it makes him feel responsible." (Interview 8).

In quotation A, the counsellor suggests to the patient that the threat of losing her partner may be avoided if she gives excuses for practising safer sex rather than disclosing her HIV status. In quotation B, the nurse-counsellor suggests a strategic delay in disclosure, to avoid the possibility of abandonment.

In both these examples, the nurse-counsellors attempt to reconcile the patient's needs, on the one hand, and the requirements for prevention, on the other. In practice, what is entailed is supporting the patient by giving the kind of advice which takes the potentially negative implications of disclosure into account.

This dual-purpose advice was seen to be appropriately strategic and was vividly described by one nurse-counsellor as "tricky advices". What is important, however, is the fact that what results is a compromise which is less than perfect from the point of view of the provision of either support, or prevention.

CONCLUSION

The findings of this study suggest that where support is read as the alleviation of distress, and health promotion is read as the provision of guidance, the result will be a spontaneous and uneasy form of reassurance and advice-giving which may well be counter-productive. In particular, the research indicates that rather than being properly articulated and inseparable, the two HIV/AIDS counselling goals of support and health promotion are set at variance in unsuspected ways.

It seems unlikely that these difficulties are specific to this particular group of nurse-counsellors alone. To what extent these difficulties are explicable in terms of inadequate training is obviously a key question (Coyle & Soodin, 1992; Burnard, 1992). Clearly, there are numerous other factors in the nurse-counsellors' socio cultural context and workplace setting which may determine the construal of their counselling role. The fact remains that the provision of reassurance and advice would seem to be precisely what any sensitive and intelligent person would do in the absence of counselling training. What differentiates the counsellor from his or her non-professional counterpart is that kind and quality of training which enables the counsellor to perform a different, and potentially more viable function; that of providing the information and conditions in terms of which HIV infected people may best effect a positive relation to their own behavioural resources (Egan, 1990).

The findings of this study therefore indicate that the development of adequate standards for the initial training and ongoing supervision of HIV/AIDS nurse-counsellors in South Africa, as elsewhere, is imperative.

ACKNOWLEDGEMENTS

We wish to thank Dr Robert Bor for commenting upon an earlier draft of this manuscript and Dr Susan van Zyl for her contribution to the final version.

REFERENCES

Allwood, C.W., Friedland, I.R., Karstaedt, A.S., McIntyre, J.A. (1992) AIDS – the Baragwanath experience. Part IV. Counselling and ethical issues, *South African Medical Journal*, **82**, 98-101.

Balmer, D.H. (1992) The aims of HIV/AIDS counselling revisited, *Counselling Psychology Quarterly*, **5**, 203-212.

Bor, R., Miller, R. (1988) Systemic Counselling for Patients with AIDS/HIV Infections, *Family Systems Medicine*, **6**, 21-39.

Bor, R., Miller, R. (1988) Addressing 'Dreaded Issues': a description of a unique counselling intervention with patients with AIDS/HIV, *Counselling Psychology Quarterly*, **1**, 397-406.

Bor, R., Miller, R., Goldman, E. (1992) Theory and Practice of HIV Counselling. *A Systemic Approach*. London: Cassel.

Burnard, P. (1992) AIDS Counselling and Nurse Education, *Nurse Education Today*, **12**, 215–220.

Carballo, M., Miller, D. (1989) HIV Counselling: problems and opportunities in defining a new agenda for the 1990s, *AIDS Care*, **1**, 117–123.

Chimere–Dan, O. (1993) Selected demographic estimates for Soweto 1992. Unpublished data. Department of Sociology, University of the Witwatersrand, Johannesburg.

Coyle, A., Soodin, M. (1992) Training, workload and stress among-HIV counsellors, *AIDS Care*, **4**, 217-221.

Egan, G. (1990) *The Skilled Helper*, Pacific Grove, Ca.: Brooks/Cole.

Fleming, A. (1992) Letter in response to MRC AIDS Bulletin Counselling Guidelines, *AIDS Bulletin*, **1**, 20.

Glazer, B. G., Strauss, A. L. (1967) *The Discovery of Grounded Theory: Strategies for Qualitative Research*, New York: Aldine.

Lee, T., Esterhuyse, M., Steinberg, M., Schneider, H. Demographic Modelling of the HIV/AIDS Epidemic on the Soweto Population, *South African Medical Journal*, in press.

National Institute for Virology (April 1994) Surveillance Records, Johannesburg.

Nelson-Jones, R. (1982) *The Theory and Practice of Counselling Psychology*, London: Cassel.

Rodmell, S., Watt, A. (1986) *The Politics of Health Education - Raising the Issues*, London: Routledge & Kegan Paul.

Schopper, D., Walley, J. (1992) Care for AIDS patients in developing countries: a review, *AIDS Care*, **4**, 89-102.

Tallis, V. (1992) Counselling Guidelines, *MRC AIDS Bulletin*, **1**, 20-21.

Taylor, V. (1990) Health education – a theoretical mapping, *Health Education Journal*, **49**, 13-14.

16

A Family System Approach for Community Health Nursing: Balancing the Complexity of Family HIV/AIDS Care with Human Compassion and Moral Agency

AMANDAH LEA

INTRODUCTION

The World Health Organization estimates heterosexual spread of HIV is increasing among 15 to 24 year olds. More infected young women means inevitably more infants being born at risk for HIV infection, and more families being affected as their loved ones live with the virus or die from AIDS. In turn, this outcome will impact on the provision of health care.

Contrary to popular belief, people living with HIV/AIDS (PLWHIV/AIDS) receive the majority of their care in the community (Adler, 1987). Community health nurses as primary health caregivers in both developing and developed countries are typically the key health care providers. This chapter focuses on the challenge of providing effective nursing care for this growing, diverse client group (Layzell & McCarthy, 1992). A family system approach for community nursing is proposed to enable community health nurses to respond sensitively to different cultures and to balance the complexity of HIV/AIDS care for families with human compassion and moral agency.

IMPACT OF HIV/AIDS ON FAMILIES

Research on the impact of HIV/AIDS on families of homosexuals and intravenous users as well as families from sub-Saharan Africa (Bor, 1993), reveals the diversity of family structure. In this chapter, the term 'family' is defined broadly to encompass the varying arrangements in which individuals form interpersonal, supportive bonds. Essentially, "family is what the patient says it is" (Wright & Leahey, 1988:11).

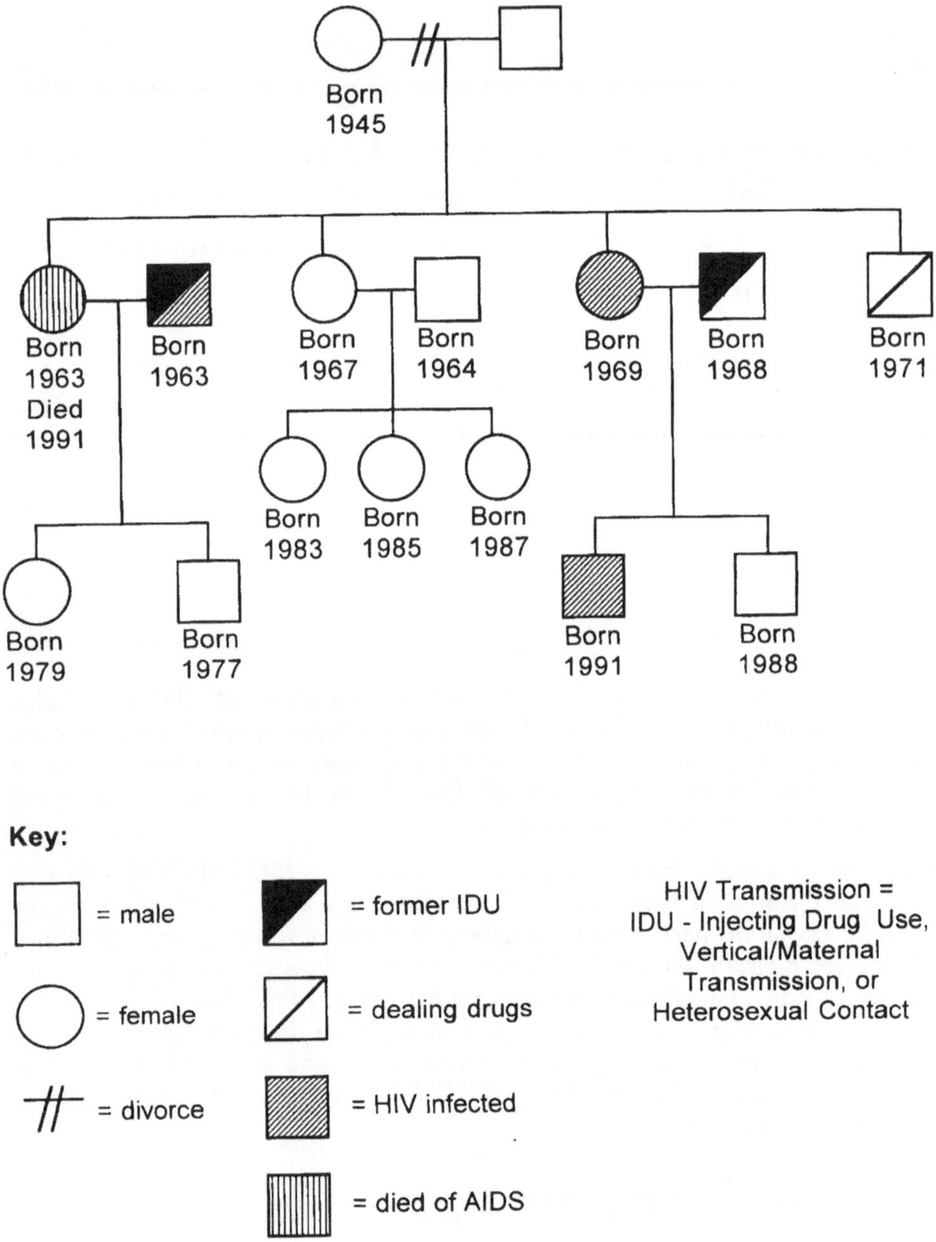

Fig. 16.1 A family affected by HIV/AIDS in Edinburgh (1992)

Families affected by HIV infection may encounter financial hardship, housing problems, or ostracism from 'AIDS phobia' (Brown & Powell-Cope, 1991). The challenges of this life-threatening illness may further confront the ill persons and their families about the meaning of life and death (Jones, 1989). Such existential concerns may contribute to personal anxiety and depression (Flaskerud, 1989; Govoni, 1988). Consequently, people living with individuals infected by the virus often need to respond to PLWHIV/AIDS' emotional reactions as well as cope with the burden of the illness.

Disclosure about HIV/AIDS diagnosis is a prominent issue for both PLWHIV/AIDS and their families due to fear of stigma and perhaps resultant loss of economic and social support (Bor, 1991,1993; Chekryn, 1989; Lippmann, James, & Frierson, 1993; Salisbury, 1986). Research about the effects of disclosure or non-disclosure on interactions between family members, family groups or their communities has been limited (Bor, 1993) or isolated to particular groups such as homosexuals (Govoni, 1988) or intravenous drug users (Morrison, 1991). However, when one or both parents are infected, studies have shown that this predicament negatively affects children's health (Bor, 1993). With the relationship between health problems and family functioning well-documented (Catford, 1994; Feetham *et al.*, 1993) and the social stigma of AIDS negatively impacting on PLWHIV/AIDS and their families, it is inevitable that community health nurses are required to provide care that meets the needs of both the individual family members and the family unit.

FAMILY SYSTEM APPROACH FOR COMMUNITY NURSING CARE

Community health nurses consider the family to be the major source of stress and social support for an individual's growth and development or illness recovery (Friedemann, 1989). Family nursing is based on the scientific model of linear causality and on the belief that health is self-contained in the individual or family (Robinson, 1994). The aim of nursing is to provide a cure or solve the family health problem, and to sustain family norms. However, this implicit nursing strategy of gaining family conformity is criticised for being 'paternalistic' (MacPherson, 1991) and may contribute to the burden of family care.

Two assumptions of traditional family nursing models are: family responses may 'cause' ill member's responses (Robinson, 1994); and equality is a norm that exists in the family (MacPherson, 1991). As a result, the individual's needs may be ignored, as nurses focus on family care rather than enabling the ill member as an autonomous individual within the family. Further, 'family compliance', the hallmark of success for family nursing care, may be problematic for both families and nurses. For example, nurses may interpret 'family deviance' as nurses' failure to meet the needs of PLWHIV/AIDS and their families. In reality, non-compliance by these families may relate to the previously discussed issues about fear of stigma and disclosure of HIV status.

In family system nursing, the family is viewed as functioning as a 'mutually connected whole' (Friedemann, 1989; Leahey & Wright, 1987; Robinson, 1994). A pattern of circular causality is observed with change in a family member, the family or environment affecting the entire family system's interactional processes. Hence, the multiplicity of messages and actions inherent in nurse-family reactions rather than predictable, family behaviour are emphasised (Watson, 1992; Knafl *et al.*, 1993).

In using family system nursing, the nurse gains insights about the dynamics of family processes as well as the way a particular family interfaces with the environment in order to understand a family's responses to a particular acute or chronic condition such as HIV/AIDS. The nurse may intervene at the individual level to promote personal well-being and physical health, at the interpersonal level to improve decision-making or clarify family roles, or at the family system level to reinforce postive interaction patterns with the environment. In turn, the level for intervention is based on the greatest system change for enhancing family functioning (Friedemann, 1989). The nurse's role thus shifts from being the 'expert' to being the 'change facilitator'. The nurse is neutral rather than prescriptive and focuses on what the family does rather than their verbal explanations about why they do it. The nurse can then reinforce behaviour, (for example, the family's positive interaction patterns for utilising health services;) or help families discover their own solutions for coping with the impact of illnesses, such as HIV/AIDS.

ISSUES RELATED TO FAMILY SYSTEM NURSING

The organisation of health care reflects the western socio-economic system with its stratified workforce, its division of labour and specialisation (MacPherson, 1991) and its cultural bias of self-contained individualism. Western health care is also underpinned by the biomedical model which emphasises the doctor's role as a scientist who diagnoses the problem (diseases) and prescribes a solution (medical treatments). Consequently, when phenomena such as community health nursing care are viewed within a systems framework, conflict may occur. This arises from the problem-solving, 'cure' or outcome orientation of Western medicine ignoring the interactional processes involved in the provision of health care.

Material and power relations, such as the self-interests of professional groups, or competition for political power between interest groups and primary health care members, including community health nurses, may further hinder a system approach. In other words, the overall modus operandi is supported by explicit roles and responsibilities of the health care employees as well as the implicit ways in which the professional carers relate, communicate and function with each other. From a system perspective, any change in community health nursing would thus impact on the overall provision of health care in the community.

Community health nurses have currently busy workloads (Wolf, 1989). Further, HIV/AIDS is a chronic, fatal condition which demands long term care provided mainly in the home. As a result, nurses require an approach that optimises rather than exploits care provided by family members or significant others. Nurses also need to be able to respond flexibly to the increasingly diverse client group's health and nursing needs which may extend anywhere from a few months to several years (Adler, 1987).

When using a family system nursing approach, nurses could enhance quality of life for individuals affected or living with the virus. By considering the social context of family health and illness, this approach for nursing care can overcome the lack of continuity and integration of care characteristic of western health care systems. Anticipation of necessary assistance and support based upon knowledge about the entire family system's capabilities would also promote social well-being and could perhaps prevent costly hospitalisation for either PLWHIV/AIDS or their caregivers.

Despite these advantages, community health nurses may perceive the shift from linear to circular causality required in using family system nursing complicates rather than simplifies problem-solving; and the shift from caring for individuals within a family context to both individuals and their families creates more work for their busy caseload. In addition, issues such as confidentiality, ethics and the natural course of AIDS in the context of family system nursing add further complexity and challenge nurses' competency to provide professional care. These issues will now be discussed in order to explore ways to resolve them.

Health professionals promise implicitly that they are competent, their competency is in the patient's interest, and that they will not abuse the vulnerable, ill or disabled person who is in their care (Pellegrino, 1985). However, if none, or only a few, selected members know about a member's HIV status, the nurse encounters the problem of confidentiality while working with the whole family system. Alternatively, respite care requested by the primary caregiver may not be supported by the rest of the family. As the nurse faces what ought to be done, additional confusion may also arise from the perception of conflicting responsibilities and competing rights within a family unit.

Nurses may refer to the major bioethical principles of autonomy, justice, beneficence or non-maleficence and ethical norms such as the right to privacy, confidentiality and fidelity to resolve ethical dilemmas (Beauchamp & Childress, 1989). However, any decision based on a bioethical principle or ethical norm is likely to be inadequate because the nurse-patient relationship encompasses the whole family. For example, respite care is arranged for the primary caregiver to enhance quality of life and family functioning. However, other family members may resent this assistance and their response is to increase their demands of the primary caregiver rather than to allow this individual respite.

The practical realities of ethical decision-making thus relate to the nature of the relationship between the nurse and the whole family system. Given the previously discussed vulnerability of PLWHIV/AIDS from fear of stigma, multiple losses, increasing physical and emotional dependency, a covenantal relationship model is proposed. A covenant is interpreted as a binding agreement between a community health nurse and a PLWHIV/AIDS and their family that involves reciprocity (Fry, 1989; Tunna & Conner, 1989). In this regard, community health nurses are committed, competent and bound implicitly not to abandon PLWHIV/AIDS and their familes who share intimate aspects of their lives. As a result of this experience, both covenantal partners mutually benefit. Community health nurses are able to develop a sense of moral agency from their professional obligations and from a commitment to their own moral well-being while PLWHIV/AIDS and their families receive safe and supportive care.

Underpinning this covenantal agreement is an 'ethic of care' that influences a community health nurse's receptivity to a patient's situational context (Condon, 1992; Cooper, 1990). Nurses' actions are based on providing individualised care guided by 'virtue ethics', including moral integrity, good character and the private norms of friendship, love and care (Cooper, 1991). However, the policies and structures of the work environment may constrain nurses' ability to meet the commitment of a covenantal agreement (MacPherson, 1991).

The covenantal relationship model provides a foundation for family system nursing care. By appreciating a family's predicament and being effective communicators, nurses enable families to share narratives about their lives. Together, they imagine possibilities for coping with the impact of HIV/AIDS (Walker, 1989). In turn, the partners of the covenantal relationship gain mutual understanding and adaptation as positive, family system change occurs and the nurse acquires insights about being an active moral agent.

To explore how a family system approach for community nursing could balance the complexity of HIV/AIDS care with moral agency and human compassion, two cases studies are presented. To provide the context for each case study, the AIDS epidemic for the respective communities will be compared. Each case study will then be presented to illustrate how a family system perspective is applied in community nursing.

THE AIDS EPIDEMIC IN RURAL BRITISH COLUMBIA AND EDINBURGH, SCOTLAND

Canada's population, an estimated 27 million, (1991 Census) is less than half of UK's population, an estimated 57 million, (1991 Census; Whitaker, 1994). However, Canada has an estimated 13,282 more HIV cases and an estimated 842 more AIDS cases than the UK (Bhatia, 1994; The Scottish Centre for Infection and Environmental Health (SCIEH), 1994). Overall, 0.129% of Canada's population is estimated to be living with HIV and 0.035% are living with AIDS (Bhatia, 1994) compared to UK's population with 0.037% estimated living with HIV and 0.015% estimated living with AIDS (SCIEH,1994).

In rural British Columbia (BC) in Canada, some aboriginal (First Nation) and non-aboriginal communities are in close proximity. These communities may support each other economically and share diverse yet common social networks. In this regard, the extent of HIV infection among aboriginal peoples in Canada is noted. An estimated 3.7% of Canada's population represent aboriginal peoples (Bhatia, 1994). One percent of the total known AIDS cases in Canada is among aboriginal peoples (Bhatia, 1994) and 40% of these cases live in BC (Rekart, 1994). However, the actual number of cases is considered to be greater than the number reported because ethnicity has not been reported before 1988 (AIDS Education and

Prevention Unit (AEPU), 1994). The number of aboriginal peoples living with the virus are unknown (Bhatia, 1994). Nevertheless, aboriginal peoples are considered at risk for becoming infected with HIV (AEPU, 1994).

In BC, the majority of aboriginal peoples live in isolated First Nation communities (Seaton *et al.*, 1991). Their life expectancy, which is 10 years less than the general population, results from being a marginalised group and socio-economically deprived (Seaton *et al.*, 1991). Further, the average rate of sexually transmitted diseases is three times greater for aboriginal peoples than mainstream Canadians (Health and Welfare Canada, 1987). High rates of sexually transmitted diseases, teen pregnancy and abuse of alcohol and other drugs may also occur in both aboriginal and non-aboriginal communities, for example, in northwest BC (Skeena Health Unit, 1989). Despite race and cultural boundaries, the aforementioned high risk behaviours indicate HIV transmission by sexual contact is a threat in rural communities.

With limited resources to service communities that are located in remote areas of BC, community health programmes are often collaborative projects. Health education initiatives may be sporadic, and may ignore specific cultural needs (Seaton *et al.*, 1991). With only a few known PLWHIV/AIDS for each public health unit area beyond the urban areas of southern BC (Wong *et al.*, 1995), HIV/AIDS care is generally integrated within local health services. It is noted that fear of stigma and 'AIDS phobia' prevails partly due to ignorance and partly due to entrenched bias that result from lack of contact with homosexuals, intravenous drug users, or prostitutes in rural communities. There is the assumption that only those kinds of individuals get HIV infection. Given the lack of HIV/AIDS awareness and lack of specific HIV/AIDS health and support services, it is inevitable that people with or affected by HIV/AIDS experience loneliness and isolation in BC's rural communities.

In contrast, Lothian region which includes Edinburgh has Scotland's highest prevalence of HIV infection and AIDS cases (Lothian Health Board, 1992). This region has only 15 percent of the Scottish population. The high prevalence of HIV infection is associated with drug misuse in Edinburgh and has resulted in a medical response for a social problem, including methadone maintenance, extensive research to monitor transmission and the natural course of AIDS among drug users (Huby *et al.*, 1994). Health and support services for individualised care of the HIV infected person are understandably a priority. However, poor communication and poor co-ordination among service providers contributes to inconsistent, fragmented care (Morrision, 1991). PLWHIV/AIDS and their families are often from marginal and socio-economically deprived areas which may reinforce common notions that they are 'problems' rather than people who have resources for coping with the impact of AIDS. Little is known about the majority of PLWHIV/AIDS who do not access services, nor about their families who care for them (Huby *et al.*, 1994).

In the next section, the 'family genogram' is introduced as a means for assessing family functioning. Community health nurses, PLWHIV/AIDS and their families are also able to identify resources and limitations within the family system in terms of mobilising more effective care for PLWHIV/AIDS, individual family members, and the family unit.

THE FAMILY GENOGRAM

The family genogram reveals the intergenerational family system, family health history and identifies family resources (Thomas, Barnard, & Sumner, 1993).This description of family structure or family relationships provides the context for assessing a family's responses to a family member's chronic, deteriorating condition such as AIDS. Communication, cohesion and adaptability within the family system may also be examined to describe family processes (Frude, 1991). For example, communication may range from being supportive and clear to being critical and vague among family members. Cohesion entails both emotional bonding between family members and their individual autonomy while adaptability refers to family roles and rules which change in response to situational and developmental events. The nurse considers these dimensions of family functioning by referring to family genograms and asking "circular and sometimes hypothetical questions" (Goldman, Miller, & Lee, 1993: 80) or questions about family decision-making. In turn, the nurse may facilitate communication among family members or identify who could provide care directly or indirectly as the HIV infected member's health deteriorates.

To explore a family system approach for community nursing, two case studies are presented. No names are used, nor the specific location of the rural community in British Columbia identified to protect rights of privacy and confidentiality. The Edinburgh case study describes issues pertaining to Edinburgh's high prevalence of HIV infection associated with drug misuse (Lothian Health Board, 1992). The case study from rural British Columbia depicts the isolation experienced by people with or affected by HIV/AIDS resulting from cultural and social stigma. Together, these case studies exemplify the nurse's neutral rather than prescriptive response to what families do and to what families are capable of doing given the context of their situations.

CASE STUDY FROM EDINBURGH

In 1992, a young woman from Edinburgh, age 23, shared her experience of being an HIV infected mother with a visiting, community health nurse. To facilitate discussion and to explore family resources with this woman, the nurse prepared a family genogram (Figure 16.1). During this process, it was discovered that the young woman felt 'guilty' for her sister's drug use and HIV status, refused to talk about her sister's death and cared for her sister's children. Her mother's acute grief and the chaotic lives of her siblings also meant family members were unreliable sources of support.

Fear of stigma and potential rejection from her partner and her siblings prevented this woman from making major changes in her life or accessing community services.

The local health visitor was her main source of support, albeit tenuous, given appointments were missed frequently. The health visitor's role entailed listening compassionately to the woman's fears and validating her efforts in parenting as she struggled from one crisis to another.

The nurse did not interact with the partner or family of the woman, nor observe their communication patterns. However, a family system approach, facilitated by the use of a family genogram, took into consideration the drug subculture and her family's health beliefs. Through this process, the nurse also learned that this woman felt powerless about escaping from the drug culture milieu and believed HIV infection was her lot in life. Her fatalistic outlook may have related to living in a marginalised and socio-economically deprived area of Edinburgh. Further, the woman remarked that this nurse's approach for discussing her situation helped her see things differently and helped her identify personal, inner strengths and resources in the community that she could draw upon in the future.

CASE STUDY FROM RURAL BRITISH COLUMBIA

Diverse First Nation communities are located in rural British Columbia. When a community health nurse works in these communities, the aboriginal peoples' beliefs and cultural practices that influence family functioning need to be considered. For example, a matrilineal system identifies the hereditary leaders, who are responsible for maintaining traditional laws of governance. Familiarity of the major 'clans' which are divided into 'family houses' enables the nurse to support family members with their familial duties, or to understand how families respond collectively to an individual member's illness. The nurse may also depend on the indigenous, community health representative (CHR) to inform the nurse about cultural beliefs and practices. However, manipulation of information or opinions may occur during the process of translating beliefs, interactions or conversations from families by the CHR for the nurse (Browning & Woods, 1993).

Direct inquiries about a particular family's heritage by the nurse may result in reticent responses due to generations of cultural invasion (Freire, 1985), for example, by Catholic priests. Nevertheless, by attending community events and responding respectfully and confidentially to family problems, the nurse may become accepted as a trustworthy health professional. In other words, by modelling the behaviours of these people (Browning & Woods, 1993), the nurse empathises to learn the ways of these people.

In the early 1990s, a community health nurse was approached by an aboriginal family who suspected a family member was infected with HIV. However, this individual refused to be tested for HIV because confidentiality about an individual's health status is sometimes impossible in a rural community. Initially, circular or hypothetical questions were asked to enable family members to voice their concerns and to improve communication within the family. Information about the etiology of HIV was given to dispel misconceptions and to support this family member to act on the best choice for this complex situation. Arrangements were also made to ensure that the HIV test would only involve the local physician. However, the positive HIV test result paradoxically ended frustration of the unknown only to establish the uncertainty inherent with the illness trajectory of HIV infection.

To cope with this disease and its related social stigma, the family chose to remain isolated with minimal involvement with the nurse. To mitigate the perceived fears of this family and to promote family system change, the nurse focused on the community. Since the elders are considered the community gatekeepers, the nurse met with them and explained the nature of HIV infection and its potential threat to the area. In response, the elders recalled vividly the sickness and family suffering of past generations that resulted from tuberculosis and syphilis. In their minds, the potential harm of HIV in their community was no different from these diseases. Hence, they urged the nurse and CHR to initiate a comprehensive health education about HIV/AIDS.

Despite increased community awareness about the virus, the family kept the HIV status of their family member a secret. Decisions were made about which clan members were privy to this information. Medical care was sought from the regional rather than the local hospital which was located several hundred kilometers away from home; an intervention perhaps to maintain family privacy. Alternatively, it may have arisen from the belief that a wider range of technological equipment, health and social services meant better care. However, during hospitalisation, the family member developed an AIDS-related condition and died with significant family members at the bedside.

Research suggests that patients often react to their family's responses to their illness rather than their actual condition (Wright & Leahey, 1990). In this situation, the grief and feelings of shame and guilt shaped by cultural and social stigma may have influenced the response of the family member living with HIV. Further, the family's resilience may have been eroded by its inability to control the uncertainty inherent in the virus (Reiss, Gonzalez, & Kramer, 1986).

CONCLUSION

From the descriptions of the two case studies, each family's unique way of relating, communicating and meeting its needs influenced the quality of life of the family member living with HIV/AIDS. Problems with relationships and communication among family systems also transcended cultural differences (Goldman *et al.*, 1993). This suggests the potential attached to recognising patterns of family response to chronic and acute conditions through research.

These case study descriptions may not be generalisable to other people living or affected by HIV/AIDS. Nevertheless, they demonstrate how a family system approach widens the lens for recognising the complex and multiple ways HIV/AIDS may affect families, and in turn, offers greater possibility for community health nurses to enable families as they cope with the losses, stress and social stigma associated with the virus. Further, these narratives expose family 'distress' from the impact of HIV/AIDS which is neither relieved nor resolved through time, but may be comforted by nurses' human compassion and moral agency.

ACKNOWLEDGEMENTS

This research was supported in part by a grant from the British Columbia Health Research Foundation. The author gratefully acknowledges the support of Dr. Joan Bottorff. She also thanks Alistair Cant for his assistance in preparing the illustration and the families from Edinburgh and rural British Columbia for contributing to the case studies.

REFERENCES

Adler, M.W. (1987) Care for patients with HIV infection and AIDS, *British Medical Journal*, **295**, 27-30.

AIDS Education & Prevention Unit (AEPU) (1994) *Information about AIDS and Aboriginal Peoples*, Ottawa: National AIDS Clearinghouse.

Beauchamp, T.L. & Childress, J.F. (1989) *Principles of Biomedical Ethics, 3rd Edn.*, New York: University Press.

Bhatia, R. (1994) *Personal Communication from HIV/AIDS Program Specialist*, Ottawa: Epidemiology & Community Health Specialities, Indian and Northern Health Services, Medical Services Branch.

Bor, R. (1991) Amsterdam Summaries: The impact of HIV/AIDS on the family, *AIDS Care*, **4**, 453-456.

Bor, R. (1993) Berlin Summaries: HIV/AIDS and the family, *AIDS Care*, **5**, 482-484.

Brown, M.A. & Powell-Cope, G.M. (1991) AIDS family caregiving: Transitions through uncertainty, *Nursing Research*, **40**, 338-345.

Browning, M.A. & Woods, J.H. (1993) Cross-Cultural Family-Nurse Partnerships, in: Feetham, S.L., Meister, S.B., Bell, J.M., & Gillis, C.L. (Eds) *The Nursing of Families*, London: SAGE Publications.

Catford, J. (1994) Promoting emotional health and family relationships- an even greater challenge for the 1990s, *Health Promotion International*, **9**, 1-3.

Chekryn, J. (1989) Families of people with AIDS, *The Canadian Nurse*, **9**, 30-32.

Condon, E.H. (1992) Nursing and the caring metaphor: gender and political influences on an ethics of care, *Nursing Outlook*, **40**, 14-19.

Cooper, M.C. (1990) Reconceptualizing Nursing Ethics. *Scholarly Inquiry for Nursing Practice*, **4**, 209-218.

Cooper, M.C. (1991) Principle-oriented ethics and the ethic of care: A creative tension, *Advances in Nursing Science*, **14**, 22-31.

Flaskerud, J.H. (Ed.) (1989) *AIDS/HIV Infection, A Reference Guide for Nursing Professionals*, Philadelphia: W.B. Saunders Co.

Feetham, S.L., Meister, S.B., Bell, J.M., & Gilliss, C.L., (1993) (Eds) *The Nursing of Families*, London: SAGE Publications.

Friedemann, ML. (1989) The concept of family nursing, *Journal of Advanced Nursing*, **14**, 211-216.

Friere, P. (1985) *The Politics of Education*, Handsmill: Macmillan Pub. Ltd.

Frude, N. (1991) *Understanding Family Problems, A Psychological Approach*, Chichester: Wiley & Son.

Fry, S.T. (1989) Toward a theory of nursing ethics, *Advances in Nursing Science*, **11**, 9-22.

Goldman, E., Miller, R., & Lee, C.A. (1993) A family with HIV and haemophilia, *AIDS Care*, **5**, 79-85.

Govoni, L.A. (1988) Psychosocial issues of AIDS in the nursing care of homosexual men and their significant others, *Nursing Clinics of North America*, **23**, 749-765.

Health and Welfare Canada. (1987) *Health Status of Canadian Indians and Inuit*, Update: Ottawa.

Huby, G., van Teijlingen, E., Porter, M., & Bury, J. (1994) *Community-Based Services For People Living With HIV Infection In Lothian*, Edinburgh: University of Edinburgh, Dept. of General Practice.

Jones, A. (1989) AIDS and death: some important considerations, *Senior Nurse*, **9**, 14-17.

Knafl, K.A., Gallo, A.M., Zoeller, L.H., Breitmayer, B.J., & Ayres, L. (1993) One Approach to Conceptualizing Family Response to Illness: in Feetham, S.L., Meister, S.B., Bell, J.M., & Gilliss, C.L. (Eds.) *The Nursing of Families*, London: SAGE Publications.

Layzell, S. & McCarthy, M. (1992) Community-based health services for people with HIV/AIDS: a review from a health service perspective, *AIDS Care*, **4**, 203-215.

Leahey, M. & Wright, L.M. (1987) Families and chronic illness: Assumptions, assessment and intervention: in Wright, L.M. & Leahey, M. (Eds.) Families & Chronic Illness, Springhouse: Springhouse Corporation.

Lippmann, S.B., James, W.A. & R.L. Frierson. (1993) AIDS and the family: Implications for counselling, *AIDS Care*, **3**, 71-78.

Lothian Health Board (1992) *An HIV/AIDS Strategy For Lothian* (Edinburgh).

MacPherson, K. (1991) Looking at caring and nsg through a feminist lens, in: Neil, R.M. & Watts, R (Eds) *Caring & Nsg: Explorations In Feminist Perspectives*, New York: National League for Nursing Press.

Morrison, V. (1991) The impact of HIV upon injecting drug users: a longitudinal study, *AIDS Care*, **3**, 193-201.

Pelligrino, E.D. (1985) The caring ethic: The relation of physician to patient, in: Bishop, A.H. & Scudder, J.R. (Eds) *Caring, Curing, Coping: Nurse, Physician, Patient Relationships*, Alabama: University of Alabama Press.

Reiss, D., Gonzalez, S., & Kramer, N. (1986) Family process, chronic illness, and death: On the weakness of Strong Bonds, *Archives of General Psychiatry*, **43**, 795-804.

Rekart, M.L. (1994) *Personal Communication from Director, Division of STD/AIDS Control*, Vancouver: The B.C. Centre for Disease Control.

Robinson, C.A. (1994) Nursing interventions with families: a demand or an invitation to change? *Journal of Advanced Nursing*, **19**, 897-904.

Salisbury, D.M. (1986) AIDS: Psychosocial implications, *Journal of Psychosocial Nursing*, **24**, 13-16.

Seaton, Justice P.D., Evans, R.G., Ford, M.G., Fyke, K.J., Sinclair, D.R. & Webber, W.A. (1991). *Closer To Home: The Report of the British Columbia Royal Commission on Health Care and Costs*, Victoria: Crown Publications Inc.

Skeena Health Unit. (1989) *A Health Profile for Hazelton Area*, Terrace: BC.

The Scottish Centre for Infection and Environmental Health. (1994) *Personal Communication*, Glasgow: Ruchill Hospital.

Thomas, R.B., Barnard, K.E., & Sumner, G.A. (1993) Family nursing diagnosis as a framework for family assessment, in: Feetham, S.L., Meister, S.B., Bell, J.M., & Gilliss, C.L. (Eds.) *The Nursing of Families,* London: SAGE Publications.

Tunna, K. & Conner, M. (1989) You are your ethics, *Canadian Nurse,* **89**, 25-26.

Walker, M.U. (1989) Moral Understandings: Alternative 'epistemology' for a feminist ethics. *Hypatia,* **4**, 15-28.

Watson, W.L. (1992) Family Therapy, in: Bulechek, G.M. & McCloskey, J.C. (Eds.) *Nursing Interventions: Essential Nursing Treatments, 2nd Edn.*, Philadelphia: W.B. Saunders.

Whitaker & Sons, Ltd. (1994) *Whitaker's Almanack,* London: Whitaker & Sons Ltd.

Wolf, Z.R. (1989) Uncovering the hidden work of nursing, *Nursing Health Care,* **10**, 463-467

Wong, E., MacDougall, R.G., Patrick, D.M., & Rekart, M.L. (1995) *AIDS UPDATE. Quarterly Report, Second Quarter 1995,* Vancouver: British Columbia Centre for Disease Control Division of STD/AIDS Control.

Wright, L.M. & Leahey, M. (1988) *Nurses and Families: A Guide to Family Assessment and Intervention,* Philadelphia: F.A. Davis Co.

Wright, L.M. & Leahey, M. (1990) Trends in nursing of families, *Journal of Advanced Nursing,* **15**, 148-154.

17

Human Immunodeficiency Virus (HIV) Infection in the Brain: Pathological and Clinical Features

IAN P. EVERALL

INTRODUCTION

The importance of the brain as a target of infection by HIV can easily be forgotten. Understandably drug and vaccine development are seen as crucial, and brain disorders may be perceived as only affecting a small number of people. However, in reality the thought of developing dementia often causes alarm to those with HIV disease or acquired immune deficiency syndrome (AIDS). The burden of care is often left to partners, friends and family who may feel isolated and be unaware of the few resources available.

In the second decade of the epidemic, our understanding of the cause of HIV associated dementia is still limited, there are no effective therapies for either treatment or prevention, and the survival time of those with dementia, unlike many other illnesses that occur in AIDS, has not improved. This latter point ironically, can appear to minimise the problem. Fortunately, the survival time for those with AIDS has lengthened, and consequently the population has increased. As those with dementia still die rapidly, the percentage of the AIDS population with dementia has apparently fallen (McArthur & Harrison, 1994) whereas the real picture is more likely to be of a rapidly changing demented population which is increasing in size. This chapter will highlight the progress made so far in clarifying the pathological features of HIV associated brain disorders and the clinical manifestations.

PATHOLOGICAL CHARACTERISTICS OF HIV

HIV infects nervous tissue and cells of the immune system, resulting in symptomatic disease after a latent period of months to years. The virus has a number of regulatory genes, tat, rev, nef, vif, vpr and vpu. It also has three structural genes: gag which codes for core viral proteins; pol encoding for the reverse transcriptase; and env for the envelope glycoproteins. The external membrane glycoprotein gp120 recognises and binds to host cell receptors, principally the CD4+ receptor on T-helper immune system cells. Following target cell binding the RNA genome enters the cell and viral reverse transcriptase synthesises a double stranded DNA copy which is integrated into the host DNA to form a provirus (for review Atwood *et al.*, 1993). Subsequent activation of T cells facilitates expression of HIV and virus production, allowing more cells to be infected and increasing the viral load. It was assumed that the virus entered the brain within a few weeks after infection as viral antigen could be detected at this time in the cerebrospinal fluid (CSF) (Ho *et al.*, 1985). It is still not clear whether this may be the consequence of a limited meningeal involvement (Achim *et al.*, 1991), or infection of the brain. Provirus has been identified occasionally from the brain of asymptomatic individuals (Sinclair *et al.*, 1991), but viral load in the brain usually remains undetectable until symptomatic disease (Donaldson *et al.*, 1994), and virus recovered early replicates slowly and at low levels (Asjo *et al.*, 1986). This low level may explain the lack of neutralising antibodies in the CSF at early stages of infection (Ljunggren *et al.*, 1989). With progression to HIV disease the virus changes to rapid replication, high titres (Chiodi *et al.*, 1991) and develops increased virulence, including proliferation in monocytes and macrophages (Cheng-Mayer *et al.*, 1988). It is these cells, together with microglia and multinucleated giant cells, which harbour the virus in the brain.

NEUROPATHOLOGY

Central nervous system (CNS) disorders are diagnostic of AIDS (CDC, 1987). They include a wide range of opportunistic infections, the commonest being toxoplasma gondii, cryptococcus, cytomegalovirus, and JC virus, as well as a high occurance of primary CNS B-cell lymphoma. These secondary disorders, as opposed to the primary effects of HIV on the CNS, are reviewed by Everall and Lantos (1991) and Gray (1992).

Non-specific changes are found in asymptomatic individuals, which can include myelin pallor, reactive astrocytosis, and mineralisation of vessel walls (Gray *et al.*, 1992). However, it is not until the late symptomatic stage of the disease that a range of HIV specific disorders may develop (Budka *et al.*, 1991). These pathological disorders are:

1) ***HIV encephalitis*** – which consists of inflammatory cell infiltrates, including macrophages, microglia and multinucleated giant cells. The latter are the hallmark of this disorder, but in their absence demonstration of HIV antigen or nucleic acids, by immunocytochemistry or in situ hybridisation, are also confirmatory.

2) ***HIV leukoencephalopathy*** – the dominant feature is diffuse white matter damage, primarily resulting in myelin loss, accompanied by similar inflammatory changes as described above. While categorised as a distinct entity the encephalitis and leukoencephalopathy probably represent two ends of a spectrum of inflammatory pathology. A rare variant of the leukoencephalopathy has been noted with numerous vacuolar myelin swellings and macrophages. This is called vacuolar leukoencephalopathy.
3) ***Diffuse poliodystrophy*** – this refers to cortical damage with accompanying reactive astrocytosis, gliosis, and microglial activation. Neuronal loss was included, as it was assumed to occur, this has subsequently been confirmed.
4) ***Lymphocytic meningitis*** – the leptomeninges, including the perivascular space are infiltrated with lymphocytes. No opportunistic pathogens are ever identified, and clinically this is presumed to be associated with the aseptic meningitis that can occur during seroconversion.
5) ***Cerebral vasculitis including granulomatous angiitis*** – blood vessel walls are infiltrated with multinucleated giant cells and lymphocytes. There may be accompanying necrosis, and so clinically, this may produce focal neurological deficits.
6) ***Vacuolar myelopathy*** – this disorder occurs in the spinal cord, predominantly in the dorsolateral spinal tracts. There are multiple areas of numerous vacuolar swellings with macrophages. A number of the macrophages can reside inside the vacuoles.

It has been assumed that these HIV specific disorders, especially HIV encephalitis, underlie the clinical dementia. However, less than 50% of those individuals with dementia have autopsy proven HIV encephalitis (Glass *et al.*, 1992). Therefore, other factors may also be important, such as HIV associated neuronal damage and loss.

HIV ASSOCIATED NEURONAL LOSS

Quantitative studies of neurons have been undertaken to clarify whether, as in other neurodegenerative diseases, neurons are damaged by HIV. An initial morphometric study of the fronto-orbital region of the brain in individuals who had died of AIDS (Ketzler *et al.*, 1990), revealed an 18% loss of neurons. However, whether this was the cause of dementia remained speculative as the brains were affected by a wide range of opportunistic infections, lymphomas as well as HIV encephalitis. Thus, they could not exclude the possibility that the multitude of pathologies in these brains was the cause of the cortical changes.

This was clarified by stereological studies, which are more sensitive than traditional quantitative morphometric techniques in estimating neuronal number. In the frontal cortex a 38% reduction in the neuronal density in the HIV infected group was observed, and this occurred regardless of the presence of HIV encephalitis (Everall *et al.*, 1991). Importantly, none of the cases studied had evidence of CNS opportunistic infections or neoplasms. In addition, there were varying degrees of loss in other neocortical areas (Everall *et al.*, 1993): 30% loss in the primary visual area of the occipital lobe and 18% decrease in the superior parietal lobule, but no change in the inferior temporal gyrus. Similar degrees of loss have been observed in studies of brains investigating the effect of HIV encephalitis (Wiley *et al.*, 1991). This loss appears to occur during the symptomatic stage of the disease. Examination of the frontal region of the brain in a series of symptom free HIV infected drug users, none of which had neuropathological evidence of HIV induced disorders (Gray *et al.*, 1992), revealed no evidence of loss (Everall *et al.*, 1992). This was the same area which in those who died of AIDS had demonstrated 38% neuronal loss (Everall *et al.*, 1991).

There are several other indices of cortical and neuronal damage, including reduced neocortical grey matter width (Wiley *et al.*, 1991) and an increase in the mean neuronal volume in areas with cortical neuronal loss in the brain of patients who died of AIDS (Everall *et al.*, 1993). This volume shift may be due to neuronal damage, possibly prior to loss, as there is also a 40-60% decrease in dendritic spine density in the frontal cortex (Masliah *et al.*, 1992a). It has been suggested that the level of HIV in the cortex, as demonstrated by HIV gp41 envelope protein, rather than the presence of multinuleated giant cells, may be responsible, either directly or indirectly, for the neuronal damage and loss (Masliah *et al.*, 1992b). Immunocytochemistry for parvalbumin and neurofilament proteins has revealed selective vulnerability of neurons (Masliah *et al.*, 1992c). The activity of astrocytes and microglial cells has been found to be increased in the frontal lobe in all, including asymptomatic, HIV-infected cases. The degree of these glial changes could be correlated with the severity of lesions in the white matter (Ciardi *et al.*, 1990). Interestingly, neuronal loss has also been observed in areas outside the cerebral cortex, including the substantia nigra (Reyes *et al.*, 1991) and possibly the cerebellum (Grauss *et al.*, 1990).

MECHANISMS OF HIV ASSOCIATED NEUROTOXICITY

The establishment, within the brain, of virulent viral strains during the development of HIV disease provides the pathological substrate for neurological and psychiatric disorders. It is proposed that neurotoxicity may be either due to direct neural injury by the virus, or indirect injury mediated by the production of factors from either macrophages, microglial cells and possibly astrocytes (Lipton, 1991a). In vitro studies have revealed that the envelope glycoprotein gp120 is neurotoxic (Brenneman *et al.*, 1988) possibly via calcium channels (Dreyer *et al.*, 1990), especially those activated by glutamate through the N-methyl-D-aspartate (NMDA) receptor (Lipton, 1991b). The calcium entry can be blocked by calcium channel antagonists (Dreyer *et al.*, 1990). In the CSF of patients with HIV associated cognitive impairments, elevated levels of quinolinic acid, a glutamate agonist, have been found (Heyes *et al.*, 1991), thus implying that an endogenous NMDA excitotoxin is involved in neuronal damage and death. Furthermore, administration of purified gp120 to rats caused dystrophic dendritic changes of pyramidal neurons in all cortical areas and the development of behavioural retardation (Hill *et al.*, 1993).

Indirect neurotoxicity involves macrophages, microglia and astrocytes, which following infection by HIV, secrete immune mediators such as cytokines, oxidative radicals, and proteases, all of which are capable of neuronal damage (Grimaldi *et al.*, 1991; Lipton, 1991b; Saito *et al.*, 1994). However, the involvement of cytokines in producing neuronal damage and cognitive deficits has yet to be substantiated. Whilst they have been found to be increased in patients who died of AIDS there was no correlation with those who had dementia (Tyor *et al.*, 1992). As with neuronal damage the load of the virus in the brain may influence the clinical state. Pang *et al.* (1990) have proposed that there is direct relationship between the load of viral DNA in the brain and the severity of the clinical dementia, but this hypothesis has yet to be substantiated.

HIV AND DEMENTIA

The ultimate aim of understanding the development and cause of the brain damage is to clarify the aetiology of the progressive dementing illness associated with HIV infection. Abnormalities affect cognitive, behavioural and motor domains, causing memory loss with impaired information manipulation and retrieval, and general slowing of thought processes. Behaviourally there may be apathy and social withdrawal, while motor abnormalities can affect hand writing, balance and result in a tendency to trip or be clumsy. Neurological examination is usually normal in the early stages, but with increasingly severe dementia there is increased tone, especially in the lower limbs, tremor, clonus and frontal release signs.

Attempts at clinico-pathological correlations have been frustrated by the differing diagnostic classification systems that exist. Firstly, there is AIDS dementia complex (ADC), this is divided into four stages (Price and Brew, 1988) which are wide, may be difficult to define, and dependent on subjective assessment. Furthermore, an equal importance is placed on both cognitive and motor disorders, and so a diagnosis of severe dementia could be made solely on the presence of marked motor problems without cognitive impairments. Secondly, the World Health Organisation (1990) have defined HIV-1 associated dementia, derived from the ICD-10 diagnosis of dementia with a number of modifications. Finally, the American Academy of Neurology AIDS Taskforce (1991) published a specific operational definition for dementia in HIV disease, called HIV-1 associated cognitive-motor complex. It has a main category of HIV-1 associated dementia complex, for individuals with predominantly cognitive abnormalities, while the subcategory HIV-1 associated myelopathy is retained for those with mainly motor problems. HIV-1 associated dementia complex is divided into a number of stages and includes probable and possible categories. The possible category is applied when other causes such as opportunistic infections and neoplasms cannot be excluded. Understandably, the definitive diagnosis is made at autopsy. These classification systems are reviewed elsewhere (Catalan, 1991; Everall, 1995).

EPIDEMIOLOGY AND COURSE OF HIV ASSOCIATED DEMENTIA

Initially, there was an over-estimate that up to 60% of patients with AIDS would suffer dementia (Price & Brew, 1988). Currently, it has been shown to be in the region of four to 15 percent (Catalan *et al.*, 1993; McArthur *et al.*, 1993). Dementia is a late manifestation of HIV disease, occurring earlier in those with the shortest survival time (McArthur *et al.*, 1993), and even those with mild cognitive impairments may have a worse prognosis (Mayeux *et al.*, 1993). The prognosis of dementia remains poor, with death on average occurring within three to six months. In the majority, there is a relentless progression from mild to severe cognitive impairments, but a few develop a stable mild dementia until death (McArthur & Harrison, 1994). There is no association between dementia and either a specific AIDS defining illness, such as Kaposi's sarcoma or pneumocystis pneumonia, or with multiple AIDS related illnesses, CD4+ cell count, or with markers of immune activation (serum β2-microglobulin or neopterin levels). There is an association with an older age, lower body mass index, anaemia and constitutional symptoms prior to the diagnosis of AIDS (McArthur *et al.*, 1993).

INVESTIGATIONS

In the CSF a mononuclear pleocytosis occurs in about 20% of individuals, and increased protein is found in two-thirds. More importantly, β2-microglobulin elevated over 3.8mg/L, in the absence of opportunistic infections, is probably the most reliable predictive marker for the onset of dementia (McArthur & Harrison, 1994).

On magnetic resonance imaging major findings are atrophy, often ventricular as well as sulcal, and white matter abnormalities. These may progress in parallel with the clinical course. The white matter lesions may indicate blood-brain barrier alterations (McArthur & Harrison, 1994). While more brain lesions occur during AIDS, white matter abnormalities are found in both asymptomatic and seronegative homosexual individuals (Manji *et al.*, 1994). Thus, care must be taken in interpreting lesions in asymptomatic individuals as they may not be indicative of HIV brain involvement (McArthur *et al.*, 1989). Magnetic resonance spectroscopy (MRS) has shown a reduced ratio of adenosine triphosphate to inorganic phosphate (Deicken *et al.*, 1991), and decreased levels of N-acetyl aspartate, a putative neuronal marker (Menon *et al.*, 1990), which were more marked in the presence of cognitive impairments. Similarly, single photon emission computed tomography (SPECT) reveals hypoperfusion in the cerebellum and cortex which may correlate with the severity of the cognitive impairments (Maini *et al.*, 1990). While MRS and SPECT reveal functional changes there is still no characteristic or consistent imaging abnormality that is pathognomonic of HIV dementia.

The neuropsychological tests which often detect abnormalities in HIV associated dementia include fine motor control (Grooved Pegboard and Finger Tapping tests), rapid sequential problem solving (Trail Making and Digit-Symbol tests), spontaneity (verbal fluency), visuospatial problem solving (Block Design test), and visual memory (visual perception). While two studies had previously found cognitive impairments in asymptomatic HIV infected individuals (Grant *et al.*, 1987; Saykin *et al.*, 1988), these have not been supported by large scale cohort studies (McArthur *et al.*, 1989; Janssen *et al.*, 1989). Finally, EEG findings have been found to be rather non-specific (for review Baldeweg & Lovett, 1991), and the majority of abnormalities occur in the later stages of HIV disease. They consist of slowing of the posterior background activity, increase in delta and theta slow wave activity, and sometimes hemispheric asymmetry. Those with dementia can also display non-specific changes including generalised or predominantly anterior symmetrical slow wave activity, and abnormal evoked potentials.

DIFFERENTIAL DIAGNOSIS AND TREATMENT

A diagnosis of HIV associated dementia can only be applied following exclusion of the multiple infections and disorders to which individuals with AIDS are susceptible. A CNS opportunistic infection is suggested by a more acute presentation over a few weeks with features such as headache and drowsiness. Examination of the CSF is helpful in excluding meningitis, other opportunistic infections, such as CMV, JC virus (which causes progressive multifocal leukoencephalopathy), and neurosyphilis. Cryptococcal antigen can be identified from either CSF or serum. In conjunction, neuroimaging is useful in excluding focal lesions such as progressive multifocal leukoencephalopathy, lymphomas and toxoplasma abscesses.

It must be remembered that endocrine and metabolic disorders, medication side effects, substance misuse, and depression can result in apparent dementia. Nevertheless, a first episode of hypomania, in an individual without a personal or family history of mania, may not be a separate illness but an initial presention of dementia (Lyketsos *et al.*, 1993).

Antiretroviral agents, AZT, didanosine and dideoxycytidine, have been advocated for the treatment of HIV associated dementia. However, their benefits are still being assessed. While AZT may have reduced the frequency of HIV encephalitis (Gray *et al.*, 1994) it has not been shown to protect neuronal density (Everall *et al.*, 1994). Clinically, administration of AZT, may improve the cognitive state, especially when given in high doses (Sidtis *et al.*, 1993). However, clear evidence that AZT is effective in consistently producing a definite or sustained improvement in activities of daily living is still lacking. Therapeutic trials for the treatment of dementia are still in their infancy, but with greater understanding of the pathogensis of dementia, and the numerous drugs now entering clinical evaluation the prognosis of those with dementia will hopefully improve.

REFERENCES

Achim, C.L., Schrier, R.D., Wiley, C.A. (1991) Immunopathogenesis of HIV encephalitis. BrainPathol., **1**, 177-184.

American Academy of Neurology AIDS Taskforce (1991) Nomenclature and research case definitions for neurologic manifestations of human immunodeficiency virus-type 1 (HIV-1) infection. *Neurology,* **41**, 778-785.

Asjo, B., Morfeldt-Manson, L., Albert, J., Biberfeld, G., Karlsson, A., Lidman, K., *et al.* (1986) Replicative capacity of human immunodeficiency virus from patients with varying severity of HIV infection. *Lancet,* **ii**, 660-662.

Atwood, W.J., Berger, J.R., Kaderman, R., Tornatore, C.S., Major, E.O. (1993) Human immunodeficiency virus type 1 infection of the brain. *Clinical Microbiology Reviews,* **6**, 339-366.

Baldeweg, T., Lovett, E. (1991) Psychophysiology and neurophysiology of HIV infection. *Int Rev Psychiatry,* **3**, 331-342.

Brenneman, D.E., Westbrook, G.L., Fitzgerald, S.P., Ennist, D.L., Elkins, K.L., Ruff, M.R., *et al.* (1988) Neuronal cell killing by the envelope protein and its prevention by vasoactive peptide. *Nature,* **335**, 639-642.

Budka, H., Wiley, C.A., Kleihues, P., Artigas, J., Asbury, A.K., *et al.* (1991) HIV associated disease of the nervous system and proposal for neuropathology based terminology. *Brain Pathol.,* **1**, 143-152.

Catalan, J. (1991) HIV-associated dementia: review of some conceptual and terminological problems. *Int Rev Psychiat.,* **3**, 321-330.

Catalan, J., Meadows, J., Singh, A., Burgess, A. (1993) Prevalence of HIV associated dementia in a central London health district in 1991. *Clin Neuropath.,* **12**, S27.

Centers for Disease Control. Revision of the CDC surveillance case definition for acquired immunodeficiency syndrome. *Morbidity Mortality Weekly Report,* **36**, 3-15.

ChengMayer, C., Levy, J.A. (1988) Distinct biological and serological properties of human immunodeficiency viruses from the brain. *Ann Neurol.,* **23**, S58-S61.

Chiodi, F., Fenyo, E.M. (1991) Neurotropism of human immunodeficiency virus. Brain Pathol, **1**, 185-191.

Ciardi, A., Sinclair, E., Scaravilli, F., Harcourt-Webster, N.J., Lucas, S. (1990) The involvement of the cerebral cortex in human immunodeficiency virus encephalopathy: a morphological and immunohistochemical study. *Acta Neuropathol,* **81**, 51-59.

Deicken, R.F., Hubesch, B., Jensen, P.C., Sappey-Marinier, D., *et al.* (1991) Alterations in brain phosphate metabolite concentrations in patients with human immunodeficiency virus infection. *Arch Neurol,* **48**, 203-209.

Donaldson, Y.K., Bell, J.E., Ironside, J.W., Brettle, R.P., *et al.* (1994) Redistribution of HIV outside the lymphoid system with onset of AIDS. *Lancet,* **343**, 382-385.

Dreyer, E.B., Kaiser, P.K., Offermann, J.T., Lipton, S.A. (1990) HIV-1 coat protein neurotoxicity prevented by calcium channel antagonists. *Science,* **248**, 364-367.

Everall, I.P. Neuropsychiatric aspects of HIV infection. *J Neurol Neurosurg Psychiat,* 399-402.

Everall, I.P., Lantos, P.L.L. (1991) The neuropathology of HIV: a review of the first 10 years. *Int Rev Psychiat.,* **3**, 307-319.

Everall, I.P., Luthert, P.J., Lantos, P.L. (1991) Neuronal loss in the frontal cortex in HIV infection. *Lancet,* **337**, 1119-1121.

Everall, I.P., Gray, F., Barnes, H., Durigon, M., Luthert, P., Lantos, P. (1992) Neuronal loss in symptom-free HIV infection. Lancet, **340**, 1413.

Everall, I.P., Luthert, P.J., Lantos, P.L. (1993) Neuronal number and volume alterations in the neocortex of HIV infected individuals. J Neurol Neurosurg Psychiatry, **56**, 481-486.

Everall, I.P., Glass, J.D., McArthur, J., Spargo, E., Lantos, P. (1994) Neuronal density in the superior frontal and temporal gyrii does not correlate with the degree of human immunodeficiency virus-associated dementia. Acta Neuropathol., **88**, 538-544.

Glass, J.D., Wesselingh, S.L., Selnes, O.A., McArthur, J.C. (1993) Clinical-neuropathological correlation in HIV-associated dementia. Neurology, **43**, 2230-2237.

Grant, I., Atkinson, J.H., Hesselink, J.R., Kennedy, C.J., *et al.* (1987) Evidence for early central nervous system involvement in the acquired immunodeficiency syndrome (AIDS) and other human immunodeficiency virus (HIV) infections. Studies with neuropsychologic testing and magnetic resonance imaging. *Ann Intern Med.,* **107**, 828-836.

Graus, F., Ribalta, T., Abos, J., Alom, J., *et al.* (1990) Subacute cerebellar syndrome as the first manifestation of AIDS dementia complex. *Acta Neurol Scand.,* **81**, 118-120.

Gray, F. (1993) Atlas of the Neuropathology of HIV Infection. Oxfird University Press,

Gray, F., Lescs, M.C., Keohane, C., Paraire, F., *et al.* (1992) Early brain changes in HIV infection: neuropathological study of 11 HIV - seropositive non AIDS cases. *J Neuropathol Exp Neurol.,* **51**, 177-185.

Gray, F., Belec, L., Keohane, C., de Truchis, P., *et al.* (1994) Zidovudine therapy and HIV encephalitis a 10 year neuropathological survey. *AIDS,* **8**, 489-493.

Grimaldi, L.M.E., Martino, G.V., Franciotta, D.M., Brustia, R., *et al.* (1991) Elevated alpha-tumor necrosis factor levels in spinal fluid from HIV-1 infected patients with central nervous system involvement. Ann Neurol., **29**, 21-25.

Heyes, M.P., Brew, B.J., Martin, A., Price, R.W., *et al.* (1991) Quinolinic acid in cerebrospinal fluid and serum in HIV-1 infection: Relationship to clinical and neurological status. Ann Neurol., **29**, 202-209.

Hill, J.M., Mervis, R.F., Avidor, R., Moody, T.W., Brenneman, D.E. (1993) HIV envelope protein-induced neuronal damage and retardation of behavioural development in rat neonates. Brain Res., **603**, 222-233.

Ho, D.D., Rota, T.R., Schooley, R.T., Kaplan, J.C., *et al.* (1985) Isolation of HTLV-III from cerebrospinal fluid and neural tissues of patients with neurologic syndromes related to the acquired immunodeficiency syndrome. New Engl J Med, **313**, 1493-1497.

Janssen, R.S., Saykin, A.J., Cannon, L., Campbell, J., *et al.* (1989) Neurological and neuropsychological manifestations of HIV-1 infection: associations with AIDS-related complex but not asymptomatic HIV-1 infection. *Ann Neurol.,* **26**, 592-600.

Ketzler, S., Weis, S., Haug, H., Budka, H. (1990) Loss of neurons in the frontal cortex in AIDS brains. Acta Neuropathol., **80**, 92-94.

Lipton, S.A. (1991a) HIV-related neurotoxicity. Brain Pathol., **1**, 193-199.

Lipton, S.A. (1991b) Calcium channel antagonists and human immunodeficiency virus coat protein-mediated neuronal injury. Ann Neurol., **30**, 111-113.

Ljunggren, K., Chiodi, F., Broliden, P.A., Albert, J., *et al.* (1989) Presence of antibodies mediating cellular cytotoxicity and neutralisation in cerebrospinal fluid in HIV infection. AIDS Res Human Retroviruses, **5**, 629-638.

Lyketsos, C.G., Hanson, A.L., Fishman, M., Rosenblatt, A., *et al.* (1993) Manic syndrome early and late in the course of HIV. Am J Psychiat, **150**, 326-327.

McArthur, J., Harrison, M.J.G. (1994) HIV associated dementia. Current Neurology, **14**, 275-320.

McArthur, J.C., Cohe, B.A., Selnes, O.A., Kumar, A.J., *et al.* (1989) Low prevalence of neurological and neuropsychological abnormalities in otherwise healthy HIV-1 infected individuals: results from the multicenter AIDS cohort study. Ann Neurol., **26**, 601-611.

McArthur, J.C., Hoover, D.R., Bacellar, H., Miller, E.N., *et al.* (1993) Dementia in AIDS patients. Neurology, **43**, 2245-2252.

Maini, C.L., Pigorini, F., Pau, F.M., Volpini, V., *et al.* (1990) Cortical cerebral blood flow in HIV-1 related dementia complex. Nuclear Medicine Communications, **11**, 639-648.

Manji, H., Connolly, S., McAllister, R., Valentine, A.R., *et al.* (1994) Serial MRI of the brain in asymptomatic patients infected with HIV: results from the UCMSM/Medical Research Council neurology cohort. J Neurol Neurosurg Psychiatry, **57**, 144-149.

Masliah, E., Ge, N., Morey, M., DeTeresa, R., Terry, R.D., Wiley, C.A. (1992a) Cortical dendritic pathology in human immunodeficiency virus encephalitis. *Lab Invest.,* **66**, 285-291.

Masliah, E., Achim, C.L., Ge, N., DeTeresa, R., Terry, R.D., Wiley, C.A. (1992b) Spectrum of human immunodeficiency virus-associated neocortical damage. *Ann Neurol.,* **32**, 321-329.

Masliah, E., Ge, N., Achim, C.L., Hansen, L.A., Wiley, C.A. (1992) Selective neuronal vulnerability in HIV encephalitis. *J Neuropathol Exp Neurol.,* **51**, 585-593.

Mayeux, R., Stern, Y., Tang, N-X., Todak, G., Marder, K., *et al.* (1993) Mortality risks in gay men with human immunodeficiency virus infection and cognitive impairment. *Neurology,* **43**, 176-182.

Menon, D.K., Baudouin, D., Tomlinson, D., Hoyle, C. (1990) Proton MR spectroscopy and imaging of the brain in AIDS: evidence of neuronal loss in regions that appear normal with imaging. *J Comp Assist Tomography,* **14**, 882-885.

Pang, S., Koyanagi, Y., Miles, S., Wiley, C., Vinters, H., Chen, I.S.Y. (1990) High levels of unintegrated HIV-1 DNA in brain tissue of AIDS dementia patients. *Nature,* **343**, 85-89.

Price, R.W., Brew, B.J. (1988) The AIDS dementia complex. *J Infect Dis.,* **158**, 1079-1083.

Reyes, M.G., Faraldi, F., Senseng, C.S., Flowers, C., Fariello, R. (1991) Nigral degeneration in acquired immune deficiency syndrome (AIDS). *Acta Neuropathol.,* **82**, 39-44.

Saito, Y., Sharer, L.R., Epstein, L.G., Michaels, J., Mintz, M., *et al.* (1994) Overexpression of nef as a marker for restricted HIV-1 infection of astrocytes in postmortem pediatric central nervous tissues. *Neurology,* **44**, 474-481.

Saykin, A.J, Janssen, R.S., Sprehn, G.C., Gwen, C., Kaplan, J.E. (1988) Neuropsychological dysfunction in HIV infection: characterization in a lymphadenopathy cohort. *Int J Clin Neuropsychol.,* **10**, 81-95.

Sidtis, J.J., Gatsonis, C., Price, R.W., Singer, E.J., Collier, A.C., *et al.* (1993) Zidovudine treatment of the AIDS dementia complex: results of a placebo controlled trial. *Ann Neurol.,* **33**, 343-349.

Sinclair, E., Scaravilli, F. (1992) Detection of HIV proviral DNA in cortex and white matter of AIDS brains by non-isotopic polymerase chain reaction: correlation with diffuse poliodystrophy. *AIDS,* **6**, 925-932.

Tyor, W.R., Glass, J.D., Griffin, J.W., Becker, S.P., McArthur, J.C., *et al.* (1992) Cytokine expression in the brain during the acquired immunodeficiency syndrome. *Ann Neurol.,* **31**, 349-360.

Wiley, C.A., Masliah, E., Morey, M., Lemere, C., DeTeresa, R., *et al.* (1991) Neocortical damage during HIV infection. *Ann Neurol.,* **29**, 651-657.

World Health Organisation. (1990) Report of the Second Consultation on the Neuropsychiatric Aspects of HIV-1 infection, Geneva, 11-13 January 1990: WHO.

18

Ethical Dilemmas for Psychiatrists: Assisted Suicide in AIDS

ALEXANDRA BECKETT

INTRODUCTION

In the United States over the last two years, tremendous changes have taken place in the public debate over assisted suicide and euthanasia. We have seen the so-called "suicide doctor" Jack Kevorkian – the Michigan pathologist who since 1990 has participated in 20 suicides of chronically, though not necessarily terminally ill persons – tried in a court of law, and acquitted of the charge of assisted suicide (New York Times 1992). Perhaps more importantly, we have seen him tried in the court of public opinion which has expressed massive support for the principle of helping fatally ill persons to die.

Although assisted suicide and euthanasia in the United States are virtually underground activities, it is estimated that 3% to 37% of American doctors help their patients commit suicide (New York Times 1992) despite the legal ramifications in some states. Twenty-three percent of a sample of San Francisco physicians indicated that they would grant an AIDS patient's request for assisted suicide (Slome *et al.,* 1992), and public attitude surveys demonstrate that 65% of Americans support voluntary active euthanasia (Painton *et al.,* 1990). In the Netherlands, where euthanasia can be administered without legal consequences provided certain conditions are met (de Wachter, 1989), at least 3% of those granted euthanasia suffer from AIDS (Van de Wal *et al.,* 1991) and 20% to 25% persons with AIDS die by euthanasia (Van Ham, 1994). While it is clear that a majority of Americans believe in the "right to die" for persons with incurable illness, and that a sizeable number endorse the principle of physician assistance in expediting death under such circumstances, we are still a great distance from a consensus over whether, when, and how physician-assisted suicide and euthanasia might be administered.

Meanwhile, researchers have found that suicide rates among persons with HIV and AIDS have reached significant levels – and, it is widely believed among clinicians working with the HIV/AIDS population, that many of these suicides are assisted, whether by a physician, nurse, other health care provider, lover, family member, or friend - or more commonly, by a group of such individuals. So while we await the legal solutions to the questions of where, when, and how to help those with terminal illness to die, the practice is surreptitiously taking place.

Two recent articles in the New York Times have underlined the potential horrors attendant to assisting AIDS suicides. Social worker Russel Ogden (Farnsworth, 1994) discovered that half of 34 assisted suicides among men with AIDS in Vancouver were botched, with resultant increased suffering for both patient and those who tried to assist. He attributed the suicide failures to insufficient medical knowledge and unavailability of appropriate drugs, and likened these failed attempts at euthanasia to back-street abortions. In a second New York Times article (Kolata 1994), reporter Gina Kolata describes the terror of friends and family instructed by the intended victim to cover his head with a dry cleaning bag if he failed to die within six hours of his overdose. While in that case the suffocation was unnecessary, I know of several instances where well-intentioned friends or family felt compelled to smother their loved one when the appearance of an agonal breathing pattern caused them to think that the drugs were starting to "wear off". These individuals suffer Post Traumatic Stress symptomatology, with intrusive thoughts, flash backs, and nightmares.

It is a rare AIDS care provider who has not been approached by a patient with an inquiry about suicide techniques or a request for help in committing suicide. It is a troubling moment for most of us; even participating in such conversations can feel like an act of conspiracy. These discussions by necessity involve legal, ethical, clinical and psychological difficulties. Although there are no data regarding doctor-patient conversations about assisted suicide, it is my experience that such discussions occur with greater frequency in AIDS than in other medical illnesses.

What are the clinician's responsibilities in the face of the AIDS patient who wishes to die? In particular, what is the role of the mental health clinician confronted with such an individual? Traditionally, psychiatry has viewed suicide as a psychopathological act. Moves to confine the suicidal individual have seldom met with public or legal opposition, because it is assumed that such individuals require our intervention and will benefit as a result. But in AIDS work, mental health professionals encounter patients for whom all treatments, medical and psychiatric, have been exhausted and who wish most of all for death. Is there a limit to what we can or should do to prevent suicide? Is there such a thing as a rational suicide? What is to be our role in resolving these dilemmas, both individually and as a profession?

Whether we wish it or not, mental health providers occupy a central position in the controversy over assisted suicide. It is inevitable that our patients will confide in us when questions of suicide arise. It is likely that some will ask for our support, whether by word or deed. Just as importantly, our medical colleagues expect something of us – we are, in their eyes, suicide experts. They need us to evaluate patients who contemplate suicide; perhaps to sanction a decision to write the requested barbiturate prescription; sometimes to discuss a patient whom they have helped to die. In his moving 1991 New England Journal article (Quill 1990, Altman, 1991) Dr. Timothy Quill described his decision to prescribe a lethal dose of barbiturates at the request of his terminally ill patient, Diane. He had known her long before she developed a particularly aggressive leukemia for which she chose not to undergo chemotherapy. Whereas many instances of reported physician-assisted suicide have met with harsh criticism from the medical community (Jama, 1988), Dr. Quill's revelations were met with much greater acceptance, in part because he and his patient consulted a psychologist before he honoured her request.

Our attempts to navigate these turbulent waters are best undertaken with an understanding of the clinical phenomenon of assisted suicide and a knowledge of the relevant legal and ethical principles. I will attempt to place assisted suicide in the greater context of suicide in AIDS. I will briefly ask you to consider a case in which some difficult issues were raised. Finally, I will address some of the legal, ethical, and clinical considerations involved in such cases.

THE WISH TO DIE IN TERMINAL ILLNESS

There are, to date, no systematic studies of the wish to die and its relation to psychopathology among individuals in the terminal stages of AIDS. The "pathologic" versus "rational" nature of the wish to die and suicidality among the medically ill remains controversial. In one study of 44 terminally ill cancer patients, 11 had wished for death to come early – and all 11 were found to suffer from clinically significant depressive illness (Brown *et al.,* 1986). In other studies, investigators concluded that only a small minority of cancer patients who commit suicide do so in the absence of diagnosable psychopathology (Hietanen *et al.,* 1991). In Marzuk's data on 12 AIDS suicides in New York City in 1985 (Marzuk *et al.,* 1988) more than half of the cohort was profoundly depressed during the month before committing suicide, and fully half had seen a psychiatrist within 4 days of death.

SUICIDE IN AIDS

If we hope to distinguish a rational wish to die from an impulsive or pathological one, it is important to be familiar with the constellation of suicidal behaviours associated with HIV infection and AIDS. What are the reasons for the elevated suicide rates in AIDS? For the most part, suicide in HIV/AIDS is associated with the same risk factors that have been known to elevate suicide risk since before the advent of this particular illness. These include demographic, psychosocial, psychopathological, and medical factors. It is further likely that certain AIDS specific factors convey an additional probability of suicide. As one enumerates these factors, it becomes increasingly apparent why persons with AIDS are often multiply at risk for suicide.

SUICIDE RATES IN AIDS AND OTHER ILLNESS

The association between medical illness and suicide is well-known, and it is thought that the reported rates of suicide in the medically ill are lower than actual rates – deaths of persons with fatal illness are often attributed to natural causes and are therefore unlikely to be ascertained as suicide, particularly if the death results from a non-traumatic cause such as medication overdose. In AIDS, medication overdose increasingly is the mode of suicide, accounting for 16% of AIDS related suicides in New York City in 1985 but for over half in 1987 (Marzuk 1991). Likewise, among known substance abusers, suicide by drug overdose is likely to be erroneously classified as accidental death.

Estimated suicide rates in AIDS range from seven and a half times that of the general population, reported by Cote and colleagues (Cote *et al.*, 1992), to 17 times that of a control group, reported by the California Department of Health Services (Kizer *et al.*, 1988), to an astounding 36 times that of age-matched controls and 66 times that of the general population found by Marzuk's group (Marzuk 1988).

Elevated suicide rates have, of course, been demonstrated in a variety of medical illnesses. In cancer, for example, the suicide rate is up to 4 times (Fox *et al* 1982, Marshall *et al.*, 1983) higher, while in Huntington's Disease, rates have been estimated up to 23 times higher than those of the general population (Schoenfeld *et al.,* 1984). The parallels between Huntington's and AIDS should not escape our notice: the occurrence of both can be predicted before their onset by a laboratory test. In addition, both disorders are slow in onset and affect the central nervous system, with consequent deterioration in motor control and cognitive ability. Finally, both Huntington's and AIDS patients are likely to have witnessed the death of at least one friend or relative with the disease.

DEMOGRAPHIC FACTORS

The demographic factors associated with suicide include male gender, Caucasian race, and homosexuality. While Blacks and Hispanics constitute a disproportionately large segment of those with HIV/AIDS, in the United States and Europe the disease still overwhelmingly strikes gay white men, the demographic group at highest risk for suicide.

PSYCHOPATHOLOGY

With regard to psychopathological factors, studies have consistently found that the vast majority of persons who commit suicide do so while mentally ill (Black *et al.*, 1990) and that these individuals are observably disturbed prior to their suicide (Barraclough *et al.,* 1974). Depressive illness is identified in almost half, alcoholism in about 20%, and schizophrenia in 10% of completed suicides (Clark *et al.*, 1992).

Hopelessness has an even higher predictive value for eventual suicide than does depression (Maltsberger *et al.*, 1986; Beck *et al.*, 1985; Beck & Steer, 1989; Kovacs *et al.*, 1975; Brown *et al.*, 1992; Belkin *et al.*, 1992). While hopelessness is often a feature of depression, it may exist in the absence of diagnosable psychopathology. For example, an individual with an incurable illness may feel hopeless about the possibilities for recovery, or may realistically anticipate inexorable physical deterioration, without having other symptoms of psychiatric illness.

Several researchers have found that persons with HIV/AIDS are prone to depression. Brown's cohort of largely asymptomatic HIV-infected United States Air Force personnel (Belkin *et al.*, 1992) were found to have elevated rates of mood disorders both antedating and subsequent to seroconversion in comparison population base rates. The lifetime prevalence of major depression among the Air Force cohort was almost double that of the general population, while a current diagnosis of major depression diagnosis was made three times as often in the Air Force group.

Belkin and colleagues interviewed 831 HIV-infected individuals, most of whom had AIDS (Belkin *et al.*, 1992) and found that 42% were depressed. The likelihood of depression increased with the number of self-reported AIDS-related physical symptoms including weakness or numbness, fever, chills, night sweats, shortness of breath, diarrhoea, weight loss, and difficulty with cognition.

ALCOHOL ABUSE AND DEPENDENCE

The evidence linking alcohol and suicide is extremely strong (Carrera 1992, Kessel, 1961), and the coexistence of alcoholism and depression elevates suicide risk beyond that of either disorder alone (Fowler *et al.*, 1980). Alcohol use, with or without alcoholism, occurs in up to 30% of all suicides (Clark *et al.*, 1985). Alcohol is also significant in attempted suicide; studies have found that up to 64% of those attempting suicide consume alcohol before the attempt (Roizen *et al.*, 1982).

In Brown's HIV-seropositive United States Air Force cohort (Brown *et al.* 1992), the lifetime rate of alcohol abuse was 29%, nearly double the population base rate. It is important to note that a study of randomly selected Air Force personnel (Pace *et al.*, 1990) found a significant increase in new onset alcohol abuse disorders after a diagnosis of HIV seropositivity.

INTRAVENOUS DRUG USE

An increased suicide attempt rate has also been found among intravenous drug users. The use of intravenous drugs is associated with an eight-fold increase in suicide attempts compared to no drug use, controlling for the presence of comorbid disorders (Dinwiddie *et al.*, 1992). As with alcoholism, comorbidity with psychiatric disorders is common.

ASSISTED SUICIDE

What is to be our stance when confronted with a request for assisted suicide? After a careful assessment for treatable suicide risk factors has been completed, can or should those trained in mental health abandon the assumption that the wish to die is prima facie evidence of psychopathology? Let's consider the following case with these questions in mind.

VIGNETTE

A medical resident in her last year of training approached me to discuss a case. She proceeded to tell me about John a much beloved patient with AIDS who had died the month before.

John was assigned to Dr. D. during her internship year in family medicine. A proud, independent, and somewhat eccentric man, he lived in the woods in a trailer, without running water, his only companion a pet wolf. He had been diagnosed with AIDS during the previous month. Though he had never undergone serologic testing, John was not at all surprised that he had AIDS, given a high risk sexual history; nor was he surprised that his CD4 count was 7, suggesting that he had been HIV-seropositive for many years. His only longterm partner had died 4 years previously of AIDS, and in the last year of his life, already blind from retinitis, had suffered tremendously with nausea, abdominal pain, and headaches.

John told Dr. D. that he was looking for a physician who would support his freedom of choice, which might include a decision to discontinue treatment or even to end his life were it not to seem worth living. Having grown up on a farm in rural New England, he wondered why sick human beings were not accorded the kindness extended to ailing and aged animals through euthanasia.

He asked Dr. D. whether she could work with him under the condition that she would never interfere with his freedom to choose death by suicide and that she promise not to document or speak with any other health care providers about this contract without his permission.

Though uneasy at being sworn to secrecy, Dr. D. admired John's quest for autonomy and control, and believed in the right of terminally ill patients to die. She agreed to become John's physician.

Over the next two years, John contracted both usual and unusual opportunistic illnesses. He had further bouts of pneumonia, and developed severe drug allergies. He had recurring, painful rectal herpes. A pustular skin rash was diagnosed as disseminated Histoplasmosis, and treatment entailed daily calls from a visiting nurse. However, one day she was attacked by the patient's wolf, and all home-based care was withdrawn.

Though Dr. D. begged him move from his trailer to an apartment with running water, John refused. While he tolerated the ongoing discomforts related to his condition for a period of several months, with the onset of severe, chronic diarrhoea, John told his doctor that his life was becoming progressively less tolerable. He decided to commit suicide within the next month unless his condition improved, and asked Dr. D. whether she would be willing to prescribe barbiturates for him.

She asked John to meet with a psychiatrist to determine whether his decision was influenced by depression or another treatable psychiatric condition, but he declined. He told her that he was certain about his decision. He assured her that he was not depressed, and understood her reticence to help. He had a gun, and though prepared to use it was worried about the aftermath – he didn't want to expose emergency personnel to his HIV-infected blood.

Dr. D. decided that she could not prescribe the barbiturates. A week later, she received word that he had been found dead of a shot gun wound.

DISCUSSION

What are the ethical, legal, and clinical issues in this case? How might a mental health professional have dealt with John and Dr. D.?

Clinical Considerations: the Role of the Mental Health Professional

Most HIV-infected individuals consider suicide. In this sense, suicidal thoughts can sometimes be considered a normal aspect of coping with the diagnosis – reserving the "right" to commit suicide, and, for some individuals, acquiring the means to do so, often provides comfort without increasing the risk of actual self-destruction. John's initial conversation with his doctor is clearly to be understood in this light.

Was there a potentially treatable psychiatric illness that contributed to this patient's wish to die? A detailed psychiatric history and mental status examination is vital, and while Dr. D. was competent to evaluate her patient from a medical perspective, she would have been well-served to have the consultation of a psychiatric colleague. Though she attempted to get psychiatric input later on, she was hampered by her promise to keep John's confidence regardless of the circumstances. As honorable as her intentions may have been, no clinician should allow herself to be isolated from her peers.

Suicidal ideation in AIDS increases in bereavement and in proportion to the number of friends with the disease; and as friends and loved ones die, the patient's support system may disintegrate. Whom does the patient turn to for support? In John's case, his enduring and apparently unconflicted choice was for a life with few significant others, and though Dr. D. may have wished him more company he was unlikely to choose it for himself.

What are the current treatments, medications, and side effects? Has the treatment become a source of suffering? How much physical pain does the patient experience and what attempts have been made to remedy it? For John, daily life had become uncomfortable in the extreme, and short of hospice care, which he consistently refused, Dr. D. had maximized palliative measures.

How does the patient make sense of the current medical situation; how bad does he think it is? How long does he think he has to live? What does he think lies ahead? What does he fear? John's appraisal of his condition and prognosis were realistic, and his concerns about the future were valid.

Should Dr. D. have written a prescription and assisted John in a peaceful death?

Ethical Considerations

There is considerable divergence of opinion in the medical community regarding assisted suicide. A commonly held view is that the wish for assisted suicide or euthanasia is a result of inadequate palliative care provided to dying patients. From this perspective, the proper response to a patient who wishes for death is psychosocial support, palliative medicine, and hospice service (Milne, 1993; Callahan, 1989; Illich, 1976). On the other side, there are those like physician ethicist Christine Cassel who believe that the debate over assisted suicide and euthanasia must focus on the needs and values of patients, recognizing the limits of modern medicine and the inevitability of death. She writes, "For many people, the transcendent or spiritual meaning of life (and afterlife) creates a context in which death is not the enemy, and is in fact sometimes to be welcomed as an appropriate and timely end, either to a life fully lived or to a life cut short by the ravages of incurable disease. The refusal of physicians to deal with their patients at the level of the personal meaning of life and death is a reflection of how sterile and technological our profession has become." (Cassel & Meier, 1990).

Legal Considerations

Laws prohibiting physician-assisted suicide exist in at least 26 of the United States, though the sale of "how-to" books such as Final Exit is unrestricted. Attempts to enact voluntary euthanasia legislation at the state level have thus far been unsuccessful, despite public opinion polls which would seem to indicate sufficient support for such measures.

Those who favor the legalization of euthanasia often point to the Netherlands as an example where euthanasia has been successfully legitimized. One should be clear that euthanasia remains illegal in Holland, but a mechanism has been evolved whereby it can be administered without legal consequences provided certain conditions are met. There must be physical or mental suffering which the patient finds unbearable; he must clearly understand his condition and treatment options, and he must find no other solution acceptable. A repeated, sustained, uncoerced wish to die must be documented in writing, and the physician involved must consult another doctor with whom he has no professional or social relationship. Finally, only a doctor may prescribe or administer the drugs, and the time and manner of the death must not cause avoidable misery to the patient's family, who must be kept informed (de Wachter, 1989).

CONCLUSION

Is there a limit to what we can or should do to prevent suicide? Is there such a thing as a rational suicide? This question confronts psychiatry at the very limits of its therapeutic tradition. Sullivan and Younger recently wrote, "For the intractably suffering terminally ill patient, activities providing pleasure may no longer be available. One may be unable to help oneself or others in any meaningful way. Intolerable symptoms may in fact persist for the short remainder of one's life. One may have no real future." (Sullivan & Younger 1994).

When psychopathology is not present, the psychiatrist can be put in the uncomfortable position of validating a patient's request to die. But how are we to do this? How far should such validation extend? Do we advise about suicide techniques, caution against engaging loved ones in activities, such as suffocation, which might traumatize? Do we write a prescription, or bid others to do so?

Unless or until we have mutually agreed upon guidelines, we are left to our own devices. In the era of AIDS, it is important to remember that these problems are too complex for clinicians to bear alone. They are also too common to be ignored. How psychiatry will continue to formulate its response to these challenges constitutes a central risk for the profession in the coming years.

REFERENCES

Altman, L.K. (1991) A doctor agonized, but provided drugs to help end a life. New York Times, March 7, 1991.

Barraclough, B., Bunch, J., Nelson, B., Sainsbury P. (1974) A hundred cases of suicide: clinical aspects, *Br J Psychiatry*, **125**, 355-373.

Beck, A.T., Steer, R.A., Kovacs, M., Garrison B. (1985) Hopelessness and eventual suicide: a 10-year study of patients hospitalized with suicidal ideation. *Am J Psychiatry*, **142**, 559-563.

Beck, A.T., Steer, R.A. (1989) Clinical predictors of eventual suicide: a 5- to 10-year prospective study of suicide attempters. *J Affective Disord*, **17**, 203-209.

Belkin, G.S., Fleishman, J.A., Stein, M.D., Piette, J., Mor, V. (1992) Physical symptoms and depressive symptoms among individuals with HIV infection. *Psychosomatics*, **33**, 416-427.

Black, D.W., Winokur, G. (1990) Suicide and psychiatric diagnosis. In: Blumenthal S.J., Kupfer D.F., eds. Suicide Over the Life Cycle: Risk Factors, Assessment, and Treatment of Suicidal Patients. Washington, DC: American Psychiatric Press, Inc, 135-153.

Brown, G.R., Rundell, J.R., McManis, S.E., Kendal, S.N. *et al.* (1992) Prevalence of psychiatric disorders in early stage of HIV infection. *Psychosomatic Med.*, **54**, 588-601.

Brown, J.H., Helteleff, P., Barakat, S., Rowe, C.J. (1986) Is it normal for terminally ill patients to desire death? *Am J Psychiatry*, **143**, 208-211.

Callahan, D. (1989) Can we return death to disease? *Hastings Center Report Jan/Feb special supplement*: **4-6**.

Carrera, R.N. (1992) Prediction of suicide in military medical facilities. *Mil Med.*, **157**, 139-141.

Cassel, C.K., Meier, D.E. (1990) Sounding Board: Morals and moralism in the debate over euthanasia and assisted suicide. *NEJM*: 750-752.

Clark, D.C., Fawcett, J. (1992) An empirically based model of suicide risk assessment for patients with affective disorder. In Jacobs D., ed. *Suicide and Clinical Practice*. Washington, D.C.: American Psychiatric Press.

Clark, M.A., Campagnari, K.D., Jones L.M. (1985) The major causative role of ethanol and the minor of other drugs in the deaths of military personnel in San Diego County, California. *Mil Med.*, **150**, 487-491.

Cote, T.R., Biggar, R.J., Dannenberg, A.L. (1992) Risk of suicide among persons with AIDS: a national assessment. *Journal of the American Medical Association*, **268**, 2066-2068.

de Wachter, M.A., (1989) Active euthanasia in the Netherlands, *Journal of the American Medical Association*, **262**, 3316-3319

Dinwiddie, S.H., Reich, T., Cloninger, C.R., (1992) Psychiatric comorbidity and suicidality among intraenous drug user. *J. Clin Psychiatry*, **53**, 364-369.

Farnsworth, C.H. (1994) Vancouver AIDS suicides botched. *New York Times*, June 14, 1994, C12.

Fowler, R.C., Liskow, B.I., Tanna, V.L., (1980) Alcoholism, depression, and life events. *J Affective Disord*, **2**, 127-135.

Fox, B.H., Stanek III, E.J., Boyd, S.C., Flannery, J.T. (1982) Suicide rates among cancer patients in Connecticut. *J Chron Dis.*, **35**, 89-100.

Hietanen, P., Lonnqvist, J. (1991) Cancer and suicide. *Ann Oncol.*, **2**, 19-23.

Illich, I. (1976) Limits to Medicine – Medical Nemesis: the Expropriation of Health, London: Penguin Books, 111.

It's over Debbie, A Piece of My Mind. *Journal of the American Medical Association*, **1988**, 259-172.

Kessel, N., Grossman, G. (1961) Suicide in alcoholics. *British Medical Journal*, 1671-1672.

Kizer, K.W., Green, M., Perkins, C.I., Doebbert, G., Hughes, M.J., (1988) AIDS and suicide in California (letter). *Journal of the American Medical Association*, **260**, 1881.

Kolata, G. (1994) AIDS patients seek solace in suicide but many find pain and uncertainty. *New York Times*, June 14, 1994, P. C1

Kovacs, M., Beck, A.T., Weissman, A. (1975) Hopelessness: an indicator of suicidal risk. *Suicide*, **5**, 98-103.

Maltsberger, J.T., (1986) Suicide Risk: the Formulation of Clinical Judgment. New York: New York University Press.

Marshall, J.R., Burnett, W., Brasure, J. (1983) On precipitating factors: cancer as a cause of suicide. *Suicide Life Threat Behav.*, **13**, 15-27.

Marzuk, P.M., Tierney, H., Tardiff, K., Gross E.M. *et al.* (1988) Increased risk of suicide in persons with AIDS. *Journal of the American Medical Association*, **259**, 1333-1337.

Marzuk, P.M. (1991) suicidal behavior and HIV illnesses. *International Review of Psychiatry*, **3**, 365-371.

Milne, D., (1993) Better care would reduce requests for assisted suicide. *Psychiatric News, December 17, 4.*

Pace, J., Brown, G.R., Rundell, J.R., Paolucci, S. *et al.*, (1990) Prevalence of psychiatric disorders in a mandatory screening program for infection with human immunodeficiency virus: a pilot study. *Mil Med.*, **155**, 76-80.

Painton, P., Taylor, E., (1990) "Live or Let Die." *Time*, March 19, 1990.

Personal communication, Dr. P. van Ham, Netherlands, July, 1994,

Quill, T.C. (1990) Death and dignity. *NEJM.*, **322**, 1881-1883.

Roizen, R. (1982) Estimating alcohol consumption in serious events. In: *Alcohol Consumption and Related Problems, Alcohol and Health Monograph*, National Institute on Alcohol Abuse and Alcoholism. Washington, D.C.: U.S. Government Printing Office.

Ruling favours doctors who aided in suicides. New York Times, February 18, 1992: A21.

Schoenfeld, M., Myers, R.H., Cupples, L.A., Berkman, B. *et al.* (1984), Increased rate of suicide among patients with Huntington's disease. *J Neurol Neurosurg Psychiatry*, **47**, 1283-1287.

Slome, L., Moulton, J., Huffine, C., Gorter, R., Abrams, D. (1992) Physicians' attitudes toward assisted sucide in AIDS. *J of Acquired Immune Deficiency Syndromes*, **5**, 712-718.

Suicide device inventor faces murder charges. New York Times, February 2, 1992: A21.

Sullivan, M.D., Younger, S.J. (1994) Depression and the right to refuse treatment. *Am J Psychaitry*, **151**, 971-978.

Van der Wal, G., van Eijk, J.T., Leenen, H.J., Spreeuwenberg C. (1991) Euthanasia and assisted suicide by physicians in the home situation. I. diagnoses, age and sex of patients. *Netherlands J Med.*, **135**, 1593-1598.

19

HIV Infection in Psychiatric Inpatients

JOSE L. AYUSO-MATEOS, ISMAEL LASTRA MARTÍNEZ, FRANCISCO MONTAÑES RADA AND JUAN J. PICAZO DE LA GARZA

Although the classification of Human Immunodeficiency Virus cases in relation to the so-called "risk groups" can be useful for epidemiological studies, excessive emphasis on them can lead researchers to overlook the existence of other populations which have not been included in the traditional risk group categories, but whose conduct makes their infection with HIV highly possible..

Among these populations, patients suffering from psychiatric disorders must be included. These patients are vulnerable to HIV infection for several reasons; prominent among these is their frequent substance abuse, since intravenously administered drugs are often used by psychiatric patients, and the close association between shared needles and HIV is notorious. As to the relationship between HIV infection and high-risk sexual contacts, this is also relevant to mental patients, because their psychiatric symptoms can affect their ability to perceive that their behaviour puts them at risk for contracting the AIDS virus.

In this paper, we will refer to risk behaviour that could be related to the spread of the epidemic in this population group. We will also present data provided recently by various task forces, ours among them, which show the high rate of HIV infection found in samples of mental patients. We will review strategies for preventing and controlling the epidemic in this group of patients, and finally we will discuss the ethical problems derived from the presence of this infection in a psychiatric patient.

HIGH-RISK BEHAVIOUR IN PSYCHIATRIC PATIENTS

Patients suffering from serious mental disorders are at higher risk for HIV infection due to a number of reasons, two of them indicated above. For example, a psychiatric

Table 19.1
Studies on risk factors in mental patients for HIV infection

	Kelly *et al.*, 1992	Kalichman *et al.*, 1994	Cournos *et al.*, 1991	Di Clemente and Ponton, 1993
Sample procedence	outpatient	outpatient	outpatient	Hospitalized
Time of study	1 year	1 year	6 months	Lifetime
% non-affective psychosis	70%	82%	100% Schizophrenia	—
% male	53%	52.6%	74%	—
Mean age	35.8	39.3	18-39=63% 40-59=67%	adolescents
Number of patients	60	95	95	76
Sexually active during last year	62%	54%	44%	52.6%
Intravenous drug users	5%	4%	Substance abuse = 67%	9.2%
Never use condoms	82-88%	29%	19%	45%
Had sex in exchange for money, drugs or a place to stay	13%	18% received 27% given	22%	4%
Was pressured into unwanted sex	15%	43%		
Had sex after using alcohol or drugs	20%	36%	45%	—
Anal sex*	3%	1.3%	—	—
Male homosexuality	6.25%	22%	10%	10.5%
Risk partner: HIV positive, IDU, Sexually transmitted disease (STD)	7% (IDU only)	6% HIV positive, 8% IDU, 7% STD	12.6% (no STD)	10.5% (only IDU)
Has sexually transmitted disease	33%	27-32%	—	7%
Multiple partners in a year**	42% male 19% female	27-32.6% (two or more)	62%	62.5% (3 or more in lifetime)

* For male and female ** no definition in Kelly *et al.* and Cournos *et al.* articles.

diagnosis is often linked to substance abuse, with a two-way cause-and-effect relationship: chronic substance abuse can aggravate and even trigger psychotic episodes, while some authors support the hypothesis of self-medication in mentally ill drug-users. The use of intravenously-injected opiate derivatives is frequently seen in psychiatric patients. In this context, it is interesting to note that the estimated rate for HIV infection among intravenously-injected drug users (IVDU) in the Madrid region is 60%.

Seriously ill mental patients' sexual conduct also puts them at risk for contracting HIV. Recent clinical and descriptive studies have associated schizophrenia, bipolar and major personality disorders with impulsive and indiscriminate sexual activity. Chronic psychiatric patients who do not exhibit inappropriate sexual conduct may present personality deficiences which increase their vulnerability to being victims of sexual abuse or engaging into casual or coercive relationships.

In addition to these factors, chronic psychiatric patients tend to live in districts with a very low socioeconomic level. In Spain these districts are associated with high rates of substance abuse, alcoholism, and sexually-transmitted diseases.

Yet another factor for a poor prognosis in the management and evolution of a psychiatric patient's illness is the lack of awareness of these issues on the part of the medical personnel responsible for their care, as shown in several studies carried out in the USA (Kelly *et al.*, 1992).

Table 19.1 shows major studies on risk factors in psychiatric patients that have been carried out till the present day, and which have proven the high rate of risk behaviours associated with contracting HIV. In a recent study on the risk of HIV infection among adults suffering from psychiatric illnesses in the USA, Kalichman *et al.* (1994) found that 27% of all patients had had two or more sex partners in the previous year and 18% had received money or drugs for sex. High rates of illicit drug use were also found, with frequent use of drugs or alcohol in association with sexual activity, so that the risk of HIV among psychiatric patients appears to be mediated by illicit substance abuse. They stress the fact that these patterns of HIV risk are alarming because they occur in the context of high rates of HIV seroprevalence among psychiatric patients and in the inner city areas were many patients live.

These authors (Kelly *et al.*, 1992; Kalichman *et al.*, 1994) have also pointed out that in this population risk behaviour occurred in a context of misinformation about HIV transmission and perceptions of personal invulnerability of becoming HIV-infected. Mass media campaigns designed to produce a reduction in risk behaviours in the general population appear to have had little effect on the psychiatric population.

PREVALENCE OF HIV INFECTION IN PSYCHIATRIC PATIENTS

The significant increase in the number of HIVpositive patients who are admitted to the psychiatric units of general hospitals over the last few years has led numerous task forces to carry out anonymous seroprevalence studies or chart reviews in order to examine the true prevalence of this pathology. In addition to the known cases, in some studies there has been a number of HIV infected patients who have gone undetected.

Table 19.2 shows the detected HIV infection prevalence in various work centres, inducting our own, with rates that oscillate between 5% and 7% in acute psychiatric units. The rate is higher if the seroprevalence study is carried out among homeless pychiatric patients, or in an alcohol rehabilitation unit. It should be noted that all of the anonymous seroprevalence studies conducted to date in acute psychiatric units show a very low percentage of HIV infected patients who are not detected during their hospitalization.

Table 19.2
Seroprevalence studies in psychiatric inpatients

Authors	Patients	Method	Seroprevalence%
Ayuso, 1993	Acute psychiatric unit	chart review	23/652 = 3.5%
Ayuso, 1994	Acute psychiatric unit	anonymous seroprevalence.	13/286 = 4.5%
		chart review	13/286 = 4.5%
Cournos, 1991	Acute and chronic psychiatric unit	anonymous seroprevalence.	25/350 = 5.5%
		chart review	7/350 = 1.5%
Empfield, 1993	Homeless.	anonymous seroprevalence.	13/203 = 6.4%
Mahler, 1994	Alcohol rehabilitation unit.	anonymous seroprevalence.	31/300 = 10.3%
		chart review	7/300 = 2.3%
Sacks, 1992	Acute psychiatric unit	anonymous seroprevalence.	25/350 = 7%
		chart review	17/350 = 4.8%
Schleifer, 1990	Unit for alcohol treatment but not with simultaneous use of other drugs	anonymous seroprevalence.	3/68 = 4.5%
	Unit for alcohol treatment with intravenous drug use currently or in the past.	anonymous seroprevalence.	13/27 = 48.1%

PREVENTION AND INTERVENTION

In general, and above all in Spain, epidemiological data show that the HIV epidemic continues to spread among IVDUs and their heterosexual partners. This growth in new cases over the last decade, in spite of the many preventive programmes established, indicates clearly the difficulty of introducing changes in the behaviours that put people at risk. In addition, many HIV carriers and others at risk of becoming infected are unaware of this situation – something which is particularly striking in the case of HIV infected psychiatric patients.

Therapeutic studies carried out to date have shown that early treatment with anti-retroviral agents and prophylactic medication against the most frequent opportunistic infections improve both patients' quality of life and life expectancy, while delaying the disease's advance. Therefore, it is obvious that psychiatric patients who are HIV positive carriers would benefit from an early diagnosis of the infection. Psychiatric care services, whether outpatient clinics or hospitals, are the centres best able to identify psychiatric patients with high-risk behaviour and to initiate early preventive measures, by providing advice and treatment.

In light of the information available regarding the frequency of high-risk behaviour and the prevalence of HIV infection among mental patients, the necessity of establishing preventive programmes aimed at this population becomes clear. These programmes should centre on providing adequate information aimed at raising the level of HIV awareness of the population in contact with psychiatric services regarding the problems deriving from HIV infection, and at trying to produce a reduction in the risk behaviours identified in these patients. In addition to these general information measures mental health personnel should incorporate personalised evaluation of patients' possible risk behaviours into their clinical activity in order to develop specific training techniques to reduce these behaviours.

ETHICAL ASPECTS

Measures have been proposed which are aimed at integrating preventive programmes and health care for HIV infected patients at all levels, inducting mental health centres. It is clear that general hospital psychiatric departments are the ideal centres for identifying psychiatric patients who run a high risk of contracting the infection, and initiating preventive measures, evaluation and treatment, as necessary (Ostrow, 1992). However, even though the need for these activities has been recognised, the debate has shifted to whether or not diagnostic tests for HIV antibodies should be carried out on all patients admitted in order to control the spread of the epidemic associated with these patients. Protective measures should be increased during their hospitalisation, and early therapeutic intervention initiated, given the the high rate of risk behaviour in the psychiatric inpatient population. This has been associated with their lack of knowledge regarding AIDS and the situations which put them at risk of becoming infected (Sacks *et al.*, 1992).

The recomendations which various institutions (American Psychiatric Association, Royal College of Psychiatrists) have made until now emphasise the need for evaluating the presence of risk factors and obtaining the patient's informed consent in order to carry out a test if it is considered necessary. They also emphasise the need to respect confidentiality at all times.

Some authors have suggested that obligatory HIV detection tests should be administered to all psychiatric patients upon admission (Strain *et al.*, 1991), saying that it is not necessary to obtain informed consent from these patients, above all from those presenting aggressive behaviour, delirium, or organic cerebral syndromes compatible with HIV related damage to the central nervous system, or those who continue their high-risk behaviour while in hospital. Other authors are opposed to the generalisation of routine serological tests for psychiatric patients, due to the following arguments:

1) Discrimination against HIV infected mental patients, by their families and health personnel, increases the social stigma which they already carry due to their psychiatric illness.
2) Difficulty in maintaining confidentiality in this group of patients.
3) Distortion of the relationship between the patients and the psychiatrist if such an compulsory measure should be instituted.
4) False positives.
5) Difficulty in providing the mental patient with adequate care once HIV infection has been diagnosed. This argument, despite its relevance to the situation in the USA is less important in Spain, where the public health system provides universal coverage and where antiretroviral medication for asymptomatic carriers is free of charge.

Although there are no regulations in Spain regarding this matter, our own view – derived both from the literature and our experience treating HIV infected psychiatric patients and considering the ethical norms involved in treating HIV positive individuals generally – is that the most appropriate practice is to evaluate the presence of risk behaviours in every psychiatric patient admitted, on a case-by-case basis, and ask for a verbal authorisation from the patient to carry out a test if the presence of such risk behaviours are detected. If the patient has an organic cerebral syndrome which could be due to an AIDS related affectation of the CNS, the test should be carried out even if the patient is not able to give his or her consent, since the results could have a major impact on the diagnosis and decisions regarding specific treatment.

Another question which has arisen due to the existence of a growing group of HIV-infected psychiatric patients is: Under what conditions should norms of confidentiality be infringed when dealing with these patients? Strict respect for confidentiality is based on the assumption that more people would seek out evaluation and treatment if confidentiality has guaranteed. If not, potentially infected individuals might avoid evaluation, diagnostic and treatment services for fear of stigmatisation and discrimination.

However, recent legal precedents in the USA and several infrequent situations which arise when treating this type of patient have led to the development of a series of norms regulating the conditions under which confidentiality may be compromised. These norms attempt to find a balance between society's interest in controlling the spread of HIV, and the need to encourage individuals who may have been exposed to the virus to seek evaluation and treatment. The recommendations of the American Psychiatric Association 1992 on this matter state that:

"In situations where a psychiatrist has received convincing clinical information that the patient is infected with HIV, the psychiatrist should advise and work with the patient either to obtain agreement to cease behavior that places others at risk of infection or to notify individuals who may be at continuing risk of exposure. If a patient refuses to agree to change behavior or to notify the person(s) at ongoing risk or if the psychiatrist has good reasons to believe that the patient has failed to or is unable to comply whith this agreement, it is ethically permissible for the psychiatrist to notify identificable persons who the psychiatrist believes to be in danger of contracting the virus, or to arrange for the public health authorities to do so".

Similar criteria were previously defended by the Center for Disease Control (1987) and the American Medical Association (1987), and later adopted by other entities such as the Canadian Medical Association (1989). In any case, these guidelines will surely prove inadequate for resolving the multitude of ethical and legal problems derived from the treatment of these patients (Weinstock *et al.*, 1990).

On the other hand, the AMA (1987), following several studies (such as Perry *et al.*, 1988), concluded that physicians cannot trust seropositive patients to inform their sexual partners or to change their high-risk behaviour, in spite of the fact that they say they will do so. This has led the AMA, along with other authors (Kermani *et al.*, 1989) to advocate the creation of a public health agency in charge of collecting reports on such cases and subsequently taking the necessary measures when other parties are at risk. Still, the APA (1990) categorically rejects a regulation which would make it obligatory to report HIV positive patients to the authorities in any other case.

More recently, Botello *et al.*, (1990) have proposed the following criteria for identifying situations in which confidentiality could be compromised:

1) A patient knows that he or she is tested for HIV and has been informed about medical recommendations concerning AIDS-related safety precautions (for example, "safer sex", no needle-sharing).
2) The HIV positive patient has a psychiatric disorder.
3) There are reasonable grounds to believe that the psychiatric disorder has significantly impaired or may significantly impair the patient´s ability to behave along the lines of the AIDS related medical safety recommendations. Under these circumstances, there is a significant likelihood for potential danger to others.

In the previous cirumstances, there is a high probability that the patient could infect other people, and the clinician could infringe confidentiality in order to protect identifiable persons who could be endangered in the future. .

An even more difficult situation is presented by cases in which the patient does not know his or her serological condition, and in the course of a psychotherapeutic relationship, exhibits the coexistence of risk behaviour that could affect other people as well as a refusal to be tested for HIV. In this case, some authors (such as Kleinman, 1991), recommend the psychotherapist, inform and advise the patient in the course of treatment. If this is not possible due to the to the nondirective nature of the psychotherapy (e.g. psychoanalysis), then the patient must be sent to another health care professional who could do this.

The complications derived from the spread of HIV infection among psychiatric patients, which have become increasingly problematic over the last year years, signify yet another challenge in psychiatry. This challenge can only be approached correctly from a perspective which integrates the information supplied regarding the most appropriate prevention strategies and treatment of the epidemic in the general population with consideration of the special circumstances of the mentally ill, and in the organisation of psychiatric care under the aegis of strict respect for the patient's right to confidentiality.

ACKNOWLEDGEMENT

Research supported by Grant 93/0116 from the Fondo de Investigacion Sanitaria, Spanish Department of Health.

REFERENCES

American Medical Association (1987) Report of the board of trustees. Report YY, (A-87).

American Psychiatric Association (1988) Committee on AIDS Policy: Confidenciality and disclosure. *Am J Psychiatry*, **145**, 541.

American Psychiatric Association (1990) APA opposes reporting names in cases of HIV. *Hospital and Community Psychiatry*, **41**, 209.

American Psychiatric Association (1992) AIDS Policy: Guidelines for inpatient psychiatric units. *Am J Psychiatry*, **149**, 722.

Ayuso-Mateos, J.L., Lastra, I., Montanes, F. (1993) HIV infection in the psychiatric inpatient . *Clinical Neuropathology*, **12**, S 26.

Ayuso-Mateos, J.L., Montanes, F., Lastra, I. (1994) HIV seroprevalence in an acute psychiatric unit. 2nd International Conference on Biopsychosocial Aspects of HIV Infection, S5.5 (Abstr.)

Botello, T., Weinberger, L., Gross, B. (1990) A proposed exception to the AIDS confidentiality laws for psychiatric patients. *Journal of Forensic Sciences*, **35**, 653-660.

Canadian Medical Association (1989) Acquired immunodeficiency syndrome. *Canadian Medical Association Journal*, **140**, 64A-64B.

Center for Disease Control (1987) Guidelines for counseling and antibody testing to prevent HIV infection AIDS, *MMWR*, **36**, 509-515.

Cournos, F., Empfiels, M., Horwath, E., Mckinnon, K. *et al.* (1991) HIV seroprevalence among patients admitted to two Psychiatric Hospitals. *Am J Psychiatry*, **148**, 1225-1230.

Di Clemente, R. & Ponton, L. (1993) HIV-related risk behaviours among psychiatrically hospitalised and school-based adolescents. *Am J Psychiatry*, **150**, 324-325.

Empfield, M., Cournos, F., Meyer, I., Phil, M., Mckinnon, K. *et al.* (1993) HIV seroprevalence among patients admitted to a psychiatric inpatient unit. *Am J Psychiatry*, **150**, 47-52.

Kalichman, S.C., Kelly, J.A., Johnson, J.R. *et al.* (1994) Factors associated with risk for HIV infection among chronically mentally ill adults. *Am J Psychiatry*, **151**, 221-227.

Kelly, J.A., Murphy, D.A., Bahr, G.R., Brasfield, T.L., *et al.* (1992) AIDS/HIV risk behaviour among the chronic mentally ill. *Am J Psychiatry*, **149**, 886-890.

Kermani, E.J., Weiss, B.A. (1989) AIDS and confidentiality: legal concept and its application in psychotherapy. *Am J Psychotherapy*, **43**, 25-31.

Kleinman, I. (1991) HIV transmission: Ethical and legal considerations in psychotherapy. *Can J Psychiatry*, **36**, 121-123.

Mahler, J., Yi, D., Sacks, M., Dermatis, H., Stebinger, A., Card, C., Perry, S. (1994) Undetected HIV infection among patients admitted to an alcohol rehabilitation unit. *Am J Psychiatry*, **151**, 439-440.

Ostrow, D.G. (1992) HIV counselling and testing of psychiatric patients: time to reexamine policy and practices. *General Hospital Psychiatry*, **14**, 1-2.

Perry, S.W., Markowitz, J.C. *et al.* (1988) Counselling for HIV testing. *Hospital and Community Psychiatry*, **39**, 731-739.

Recommendations for HIV testing services for inpatients and outpatients in acute-care hospitals settings; and technical guidance on HIV counselling.(1993) *MMWR Morb Mortal Wkly Rep.*, **42** (RR-2), 1-17.

Sacks, M., Dermatis, H., Looser-Ott, S., Burton, W., Perry, S. (1992) Undetected HIV infection among acutelly ill psychiatric inpatients. *Am J Psychiatry*, **149**, 544-545.

Schleifer, S., Keller, S., Franklin, J.E., LaFarge, S., Miller, S.I. (1990). HIV seropositivity in inner-city alcoholics. *Hosp. Community Psychiatry*, **41**, 248-249.

Strain, J., Forstein, M. (1991) Yes and No. Viewpoints-Crossfire: It's time to require HIV mandatory testing of all hospitalized inpatients. *Psychiatric News*, March 15, pp. 9-30.

Weinstock, R., Leong, G.B. & Silva, J.A. (1990) Psychiatric patients and AIDS: the forensic clinician perspective. *Journal of Forensic Sciences*, **35**, 644-652.

Zamperetti, M. (1990) Attemped suicide and HIV infection: Epidemiological aspects in a psychiatric ward, in Abstracts VI International Conference on AIDS. Los Angeles.

Index